The Health Care Professional
as Friend and Healer

Building on the Work of
Edmund D. Pellegrino

T0199934

The Health Care Professional as Friend and Healer

Building on the Work of Edmund D. Pellegrino

DAVID C. THOMASMA
JUDITH LEE KISSELL

Editors

GEORGETOWN UNIVERSITY PRESS/WASHINGTON, D.C.

Georgetown University Press, Washington, D.C.
© 2000 by Georgetown University Press. All rights reserved.
Printed in the United States of America

10 9 8 7 6 5 4 3 2 1   2000

This volume is printed on acid-free offset book paper.

Library of Congress Cataloging-in-Publication Data

The health care professional as friend and healer : building on the work of
    Edmund D. Pellegrino / edited by David Thomasma, Judith Lee Kissell.
        p. cm.
    Includes index.
    ISBN 0-87840-809-6 (cloth : acid-free paper)—
    ISBN 0-87840-810-X (paper : acid-free paper)
    1. Medical ethics.   2. Physicians—Attitudes.   3. Humanism.
  4. Medical education.   I. Pellegrino, Edmund D., 1920-   II. Thomasma,
  David C., 1939-   III. Kissell, Judith Lee.
  R724 .H3476 2000
  174'.2dc21   00-026362

*This book is dedicated to
Edmund D. Pellegrino, M.D.
—physician, friend, and healer.*

Acknowledgments

We wish to thank John Monagle, Ph.D., for helping to conceptualize this book. Marti Patchell, of the Center for Clinical Ethics at Georgetown University, was very helpful in suggesting possible authors for the book and obtaining contact information. Her enthusiasm and support were constant. We wish to thank David Miller of Georgetown University as well. Robbin Hiller, research assistant, and Doris Thomasma, managing secretary of the Medical Humanities Program at Loyola University of Chicago Stritch School of Medicine, were essential in fostering and completing the book. Robbin, in particular, helped shepherd the manuscript's day-to-day progress; she was the contact person for all of the authors, as well as an unflagging source of cheerful support. Many of our colleagues were especially cooperative in reading the manuscript and suggesting revisions; we thank them as well. We also are grateful to the director of Georgetown University Press, John Samples, Ph.D., for his support and encouragement in adding our work to a growing and distinguished series on ethics and health care.

Contents

PART III: CURRENT CHALLENGES

PART IV: MEDICAL EDUCATION

Contributors

William S. Andereck, M.D.
Chairman, Institutional Ethics Committee
California Pacific Medical Center
San Francisco, California

Lazare Benaroyo, M.D.
Senior Lecturer on Medical Ethics
School of Medicine
University of Lausanne
Lausanne, Switzerland

Patricia Benner, R.N., Ph.D.
Professor, School of Nursing
Department of Physiological Nursing
University of California
San Francisco, California

Jeffrey Blustein, Ph.D.
Associate Professor of Bioethics
Albert Einstein College of Medicine
Adjunct Associate Professor of Philosophy
Barnard College
Columbia University
New York, New York

Chester R. Burns, M.D., Ph.D.
James Wade Rockwell Professor of Medical
    History
Institute for the Medical Humanities
University of Texas Medical Branch
Galveston, Texas

Courtney S. Campbell, Ph.D.
Associate Professor
Department of Philosophy
Oregon State University
Corvallis, Oregon

F. Daniel Davis, Ph.D.
Associate Dean, Education Planning
Director, Continuing Professional
    Education
Office of the Dean of Academic Affairs
School of Medicine
Georgetown University Medical Center
Washington, D.C.

G. Kevin Donovan, M.D., M.L.A.
Director
Oklahoma Bioethics Center
Professor and Vice-Chair
Pediatric Department
The University of Oklahoma
Tulsa, Oklahoma

Glenn C. Graber, Ph.D.
Professor of Philosophy
University of Tennessee
Professor of Medicine
University of Tennessee Medical Center
Knoxville, Tennessee

John Collins Harvey, M.D., Ph.D.
Professor of Medicine, Emeritus,
    Georgetown University
Senior Research Scholar, Kennedy
    Institute of Ethics
Physician, Emeritus, Georgetown
    University Hospital
Senior Research Scholar, Center for
    Clinical Bioethics
Georgetown University Medical Center
Washington, D.C.

Rodger L. Jackson, Ph.D.
Assistant Professor of Philosophy
Richard Stockton College of New Jersey
Pomona, New Jersey

George Khushf, Ph.D.
Humanities Director
Center for Bioethics
Assistant Professor of Philosophy
University of South Carolina
Columbia, South Carolina

Judith Lee Kissell, Ph.D.
Assistant Professor of Philosophy
Georgia College and State University
Milledgeville, Georgia

Erich H. Loewy, Ph.D.
Professor and Endowed Alumni
    Association Chair of Bioethics
Associate, Department of Philosophy
University of California
Davis, California

Richard A. McCormick, S.J.
John A. O'Brien Professor of Christian
    Ethics
University of Notre Dame
Notre Dame, Indiana

Thomas K. McElhinney, Ph.D.
Consultant
Philadelphia, Pennsylvania

Leo J. O'Donovan, S.J.
President
Georgetown University
Washington, D.C.

Ruth B. Purtillo, Ph.D.
Director and C. C. and Mabel L. Criss
    Professor
Center for Health Policy and Ethics
Creighton University
Omaha, Nebraska

Marian Gray Secundy, Ph.D.
Professor and Director
Program in Clinical Ethics
Howard University College of Medicine
Washington, D.C.

Bradford R. Smith, Ph.D.
Chaplain Resident, Clinical Pastoral
    Education Program
Department of Pastoral Care
University of Tennessee Medical Center
Knoxville, Tennessee

Daniel P. Sulmasy, O.F.M., M.D., Ph.D.
Sisters of Charity Chair in Ethics at Saint
    Vincents
Professor of Medicine and Director
Bioethics Institute of New York Medical
    College
New York, New York

David C. Thomasma, Ph.D.
The Fr. Michael I. English, S.J., Professor
    of Medical Ethics
Director, Medical Humanities Program
Stritch School of Medicine
Loyola University Chicago
Maywood, Illinois

Robert M. Veatch, Ph.D.
Senior Research Scholar
Professor of Medical Ethics and
    Philosophy
Joseph and Rose Kennedy Institute of
    Ethics
Georgetown University
Washington, D.C.

Jos V. M. Welie, J.D., Ph.D.
Associate Professor
Center for Health Policy and Ethics
Department of Community and
    Preventive Dentistry
Creighton University
Omaha, Nebraska

Preface

This book originally was conceived by John F. Monagle, Ph.D., who was one of the first clinical ethicists in the field of bioethics. During years of working closely with health care professionals, hospitals, and (later) hospital associations and corporations, Monagle clung to the notion that there was something very special about the relationship between healer and patient. For Monagle, that special character lay in the idea of friendship. This insight is controversial. Many critics would argue that friendship could get in the way of the objectivity that is required in health care. Yet Monagle articulated a conception of medical ethics that included friendship at its core within an Aristotelian ethic of a role model.

Inspired by Monagle's ideas, we decided to develop this book on the grounds of friendship and role modeling. Our friend and model is Edmund D. Pellegrino, M.D., to whom the book is dedicated.

We asked many persons who have been touched by Dr. Pellegrino's leadership, friendship, and support to write on topics that have interested Dr. Pellegrino over the years in his capacity as physician, educator, president of a university, ethicist, and philosopher of medicine. Yet this volume is not a *Festschrift;* we did not request contributions about Dr. Pellegrino's thinking per se. Instead, we offered to potential contributors a slate of Dr. Pellegrino's interests—from bioethics to education—and asked them to write from their own perspectives, perhaps as influenced by his leadership in the area. Because one of Dr. Pellegrino's primary interests was helping to formulate the role of the humanities in medical education, some of the contributions fall into this general category.

We approached many of Dr. Pellegrino's friends and colleagues about contributing to this volume. Those who, for one reason or another, could not meet our deadlines still wished to underline their deepest respect for Dr. Pellegrino. This regard is universal. In 1998, Dr. Pellegrino received the first Lifetime Achievement Award from the newly constituted American Society of Bioethics and Humanities at its annual meeting in Houston, Texas.

In effect, this book recognizes Dr. Pellegrino's prominence as a role model by developing ideas about the health care professional as role model, friend, and healer in the new century.

David C. Thomasma, Ph.D.   Judith Lee Kissell, Ph.D.
Chicago, Illinois   Milledgeville, Georgia

A Profession of Trust: Reflections on a Fundamental Virtue

Leo J. O'Donovan, S.J.

There is a profound similarity between physicians and educators: The coin of both our realms is trust. Trust is at the heart of being a good doctor; it also is at the heart of being a good educator. In this essay, I reflect on the importance and value of trust in our lives and in our work.

Depending on one's perspective, of course, trust can be defined in different ways. According to political theorist Mark Warren, trust means accepting "vulnerability to the potential ill will of others by granting them discretionary power over some good."[1] According to another writer, in almost all cases trust involves a "confidence or reliance upon someone or something" without full investigation or evidence.[2] In religious terms, trust can be defined as "the reliance upon the integrity, compassion, ability, or strength of another person"—and ultimately, of course, upon God.[3] Such reliance, which allows us to care for each other—indeed, to minister to each other—is at once a necessity and a virtue.

In each case, we notice, trust implies being vulnerable and taking a risk, a leap of confidence—sometimes without any evidence that you will land on your feet. Where does the capacity for this leap of trust come from? According to Erik Erikson, we learn it from our mothers at the earliest stage of our development. We build our self-confidence on this basic trust; it is the foundation for successful communication throughout our lives. This same basic trust, adapted in sophisticated and complex ways, is an essential and positive element in every civil society.

Thus far I have defined trust as a proper noun; in fact, however, it is a very active verb. Every day, to form social relationships and interact, to communicate effectively, to care for ourselves, to conduct business, to get along in a civil society, we trust—we must trust—each other, institutions, and, most important, ourselves.

Consider the small child learning how to swim who jumps into his mother's arms in water that is well over his head . . . the parents dropping off a beloved daughter on the first day of college in an unfamiliar city, among people they have never met before . . . the

Conley Lecture, American Academy of Otolaryngology Head and Neck Surgery, September 7, 1997. Reproduced from *Otolaryngology Head Neck Surgery* 118 (1998): 565–70, with permission from Mosby, Inc. Previously published in *Vital Speeches of the Day* 64, no. 6 (1998): 178–82.

patient suffering from throat cancer who agrees to be anesthetized for more than four hours while an otolaryngologist works to save his voice box . . . the negotiator of a peace agreement who is asked to agree to a demobilization of arms and a cease fire. In each of these instances—some ordinary, some not so ordinary—trust is working hard.

We depend on trust every day, sometimes in ways we barely realize. One need only drive on a freeway or an interstate to see trust in action. Vast numbers of drivers obey the same laws—some quite intricate—because they trust that these laws ensure their safety and may even save their lives. We trust the necessity of such laws, but we also trust many things that are beyond our immediate understanding. We trust that the digital clock will accurately tell us the time in the morning so that we can arrive on time for work each day. We trust the uses to which scientific advances are put, even though we know that science has regularly revised itself from Galileo to Newton to Einstein to Hawking. Even as we become increasingly aware of the relativity of scientific knowledge, we still board the latest Boeing aircraft—and our astronauts still launch into space.

We trust medical research in a similar way. We trust that scientists and researchers will give us the right information as we care for our aging bodies. We don't question how exactly the Tylenol or the Inderol we take works, we just trust that it will; we trust the science behind it.

Trust allows us to function socially as individuals in a complex society. There is also an important moral dimension to trust that should not be overlooked, however. How we trust and whether we are trustworthy depend on something deeper than need. Philosopher Michael Polanyi rightly emphasizes that women and "men are valued . . . according to their moral force"[4] and that moral rules affect our whole selves, not just the exercise of our faculties. "To comply with a code of morality," Polanyi tells us, "is to live by it in a far more comprehensive sense" than is involved in stopping at a red light, say, or adhering to the speed limit.[5]

Our success as a society depends on the extent to which our lives are ordered not just by laws and customs but by a shared moral code of thought and behavior that requires a deeper trust. As the distinguished medical ethicist Edmund Pellegrino reminds us, every genuine moral community is built on the trust that its members will look beyond personal interests and individual concerns toward a truly common good.[6]

We can be morally responsible people only to the extent that we reflect on our obligations and then conscientiously fulfill them. This process involves trusting oneself in a radical sense: feeling comfortable—and confident—that one will reflect and respond accordingly, that one will follow sound judgments with responsible decisions. It also involves trusting and relying on others, however. If we do not enter social interaction with a sense that people will follow a common moral code, we will be fundamentally mistrustful—and fragmented.

Thus, trust is similar in structure to the religious notion of faith. We trust in, believe in, commit ourselves to God—if we do—because God has entrusted divine life to us, and boundlessly. Scripture presents a God who is passionately involved in our lives and history, who invites us to absolute trust. The early Church and the Biblical nation of Israel, in particular, are frequently called upon to make that trust a way of being, especially in the face of peril and need. A passage from the prophet Isaiah (43:1–2) illustrates the depth of this trust:

But now thus says the Lord,
He who created you, O Jacob,
He who formed you, O Israel:
Do not fear, for I have redeemed you;
I have called you by name, you are mine.
When you pass through the waters, I will be with you;
And through the rivers, they shall not overwhelm you;
When you walk through fire you shall not be burned,
And the flame shall not consume you.

Of course, faith can be—and has been—interpreted in many ways, and the way of our faith will affect not just our thought but our conduct. In a similar way, trust is a fundamental attitude that affects how we think, how we relate to other persons, and how we develop a community. In both cases—faithful conduct and trusting action—there is an ongoing interaction of practice, reflection, and fundamental attitude.

Like faith, trust is untrue to itself when it is blind. A blind faith that every scientific discovery, every medical innovation will be beneficial would surely be dangerous and almost certainly lead to our neglect of the ethics involved in every trust relationship. Whether in our cars or our classrooms, our laboratories or our liturgies, trust involves a moral concern that transcends the interests of the self and embraces the interests of the community.

People in the medical profession know this. Medical professionals, especially physicians, live it. They participate every day in trust relationships that call on them routinely to transcend personal concerns and answer to a higher standard. They understand that the patient's concerns come first—before the physician's own concerns, before those of the hospital, and, yes, even before the interests of managed care organizations. Medical professionals understand that the patient who comes to them with acute otitis or head and neck cancer is extremely vulnerable; to help that patient, the physician must first protect that vulnerability.

Physicians widely understand that their highest priority is to apply their medical knowledge and skill for the patient's benefit—a benefit that can never be measured adequately on an economic scale. They understand that to make informed decisions about what is medically good for a patient, they need to consider the whole person. Quality-of-life issues and personal values that are important to a patient routinely help physicians determine individualized care and treatment.

Medical professionals understand that the research they do and the medicine they practice require not just scientific knowledge but also an ethical consideration of its application and use. The mere availability of a new radiation therapy does not require one to use it in every case. The morbidity associated with radiating the larynx, for instance, may not be worth it for a patient who is an operatic tenor or an accomplished trial attorney. People in the medical profession understand that "doctors do not treat diseases, they treat patients."[7] From consultation to recovery and beyond, they understand the unique ethical responsibility of their role as trusted physician.

The centerpiece of the medical profession, therefore—and the heart of the doctor's relationship with the patient—is trust. Yet all physicians practice in a society in which the corrosive signs of mistrust are ever present and ever powerful.

MISTRUST

In reflecting on the mistrust we all regularly encounter, I seek what the theologian Edward Schillebeeckx called "understanding by contrast." To begin, I note that the challenge we Americans face in thinking beyond individual concerns is not new. It dates to the time of our earliest colonial settlements. Shortly after the Plymouth Colony was founded in 1620, its members sought to dissolve their cherished communal life and opt for the parceling of land. William Bradford lamented in his journal, *Of Plymouth Plantation,* that members of the colony who once were bound together by a "sacred bond and covenant of the Lord"[8] no longer trusted the value of caring for others and were weakened by individual interests. Bradford wrote in an aged hand in his journal, "O sacred bond, whilst inviolably preserved! How sweet and precious were the fruits that flowed from the same! But when this fidelity decayed, then their ruin approached."[9]

Bradford's lament has been echoed through the centuries. Today, it seems, more and more people admit that they do not trust those around them. This lack of trust is evident in headline after headline, news story after news story. We've seen mistrust of law enforcement and the criminal justice system during and after the O.J. Simpson case. We've seen mistrust of politics in campaign finance coverage. We've seen mistrust among nations and peoples obstructing peace processes in Bosnia, Kosovo, Rwanda, Northern Ireland, and, certainly, the Mideast.

Reasons for mistrust abound. Some people say that specific events, especially crimes and scandals, have fueled our mistrust. We've seen mistrust of government escalate after events such as Watergate or the admission of former Secretary of Defense Robert Mac-Namara that military data were intentionally and unethically manipulated during the Vietnam War. We've seen mistrust of medical research intensify after the 1972 disclosure of the federal government's Tuskegee experiments on patients with syphilis and later revelations about government radiation studies.

Other commentators find that today's lessening of our social connectedness has a correlation with declining social trust.[10] In his tour of the United States more than a century ago, Alexis de Tocqueville observed and admired the willingness of Americans to volunteer and come together as citizens.[11] We live in a vastly changed world today, however, and our impulse to unite and help one another has gradually eroded under the considerable strains of modern society. We live busier, more complex lives; many families are fractured; parents are working longer and commuting longer hours; there are fewer hours to be with children, enjoy family dinners, volunteer for civic activities, care for neighbors. Neighborhoods are no longer as cohesive as they once were; our citizens live in isolation and view each other as competitors for limited resources. This loss of connectedness makes it harder for us to trust each other and the institutions that guide civic life.

More and more often we face situations in which mistrust is apparent. Just as health care has experienced dynamic changes in the past decade that have upset traditional notions about medicine and those who practice it, education likewise faces new challenges that sometimes threaten the trust we have in our educational institutions. The distribution of finite resources to cover the cost of educating an increasing number of students is strikingly similar to the challenge people in medicine face to make health care available to more and more citizens with funds that are limited and highly regulated. With the incredible growth in both fields, patients and students alike have come to ask—understandably—whether their individual interests are lost in an institutional groundswell of bureaucratic regulations.

As in medicine, greater technological advances in higher education have meant bigger bills for those we serve. Bigger bills, of course, mean many more questions about trust: Am I getting my money's worth? Do our colleges and universities focus on knowledge that matters, or have they been hijacked by faculty members that simply conform to political correctness and the latest pedagogical fads? Are institutions of higher education too focused on athletics? Do our educational institutions have a higher purpose beyond preparing students for productive economic lives? Are colleges just glorified job training centers, or do they inspire the growth of other values as well?

These questions are real—and serious. Some arise out of deep mistrust of "the system," others out of understandable doubts and fear and lack of information. During the ten years I have served as Georgetown University's president, one lesson I have certainly learned is that we must not ignore such questions. To renew trust in higher education, we must confront head-on the real issues, the real fears, the real anger that people have. By *confront* I mean candid communication, regular dialogue, willingness to remain open to change.

Consider, for example, the question of why tuition costs have been rising faster than the rate of inflation. Some educators blame this thorny issue on the media and wish it would just go away. I disagree. The question arises out of parents' legitimate concerns that they will not get what they paid for—or, worse, that they will not be able to provide for one of the most important stages of their child's development.

Although we may be uncomfortable doing so, we in higher education need to take the time to explain to the public exactly why college costs what it does. We need to talk to people about the new regulatory environment that reduces the flow of federal support for universities. We need to show them graphs that illustrate the large reduction of revenue for teaching hospitals associated with managed care. We need to lay out pie charts that show the overall cost of educating a student to be much greater than the price of tuition and fees. We need to remind them that aging buildings and outdated technology cannot be neglected. We need to explain dollar costs and the invaluable benefits of financial aid.

We need to remind people about the extraordinary range of essential new services that have indeed driven up the cost of education: new advanced computer technology, new library services, new laboratories, new research centers, new career counseling services, new campus ministry programs, new residence halls, new campus security measures, new academic programs in every field under the sun. All of these advances costs money—but it's worthwhile because these investments have improved the quality of American higher education and help young people realize their God-given potential.

Truly confronting the tuition issue means not only speaking forthrightly but listening carefully to our constituents as well as doing everything we can to keep higher education—particularly medical education—affordable. As we pursue better communication and fiscal responsibility, we must do something else to renew trust: We must engage our community in the fundamental process of discerning, articulating, and strengthening our core mission and aspirations.

For Georgetown University, our mission is the soul of our community. More than 200 years ago, when John Carroll (America's first Catholic bishop) founded his "Academy at George-Town," he was animated by a remarkable vision that education mattered profoundly to our destiny as a nation. Archbishop Carroll sought to create an academic community that would emphasize intellectual development and what he called the "cultivation of virtue." He sought to create an academic community that was truly diverse—a community that would be open to "every class of citizens" and "students of every religious profession." He also wanted that community to serve the Church *and* society—because it would invest in the minds and hearts of talented young people and help them develop their full potential as students and as citizens.

The Jesuit maxim *ad majorem Dei gloriam inque hominum salutem* lies at the heart of Georgetown's mission—challenging us to live and learn "for the greater glory of God and the well-being of humankind." At Georgetown we seek to renew this vision of education in fresh and creative ways. Our greatest task is to communicate its importance and enduring value to the students who come to us, to their parents, and to the community beyond our campus gates. We must be involved together in the university's mission. And so too with other institutions, if we are to restore the trust in higher education that is eroding around us.

Similarly challenging questions face people in the medical profession. Patients increasingly wonder: Why does my treatment cost so much? Is my family's health care in jeopardy because of runaway costs in the health care system? Can I trust the business practices of HMOs, insurance companies, lawyers, hospitals, and the government? Whom can I really trust, when all I read is bad news: doctors accused of malpractice, HMOs accused of fraud, therapies that fail, studies that contradict each other, services that cost more than I have? Do doctors still care about my individual needs, or has the sacred doctor-patient relationship been destroyed?

Here again, communication that is direct, candid, and to the point is at least part of the answer. Many people do not realize the radical improvements we have made in health care in just one generation. Before World War II, there were no intensive care units or coronary care units in our nation's hospitals. There were no MRIs, no sonograms, no routine mammograms. The unraveling of the molecular structure of DNA was only in its infancy. In medical schools, fields such as molecular biology, cell biology, molecular genetics, and biophysics were just being created. Bioethics was still in the future. To explain current changes in health care costs, one must understand these tremendous advances in medical knowledge and technology. Medical care today is costly in part because we are so much better at treating disease; we have more accurate and sophisticated diagnostic tests, and we can offer more and better treatment to patients. All of this is morally good.

A wider understanding of these improvements—and the cost that comes with them—would help clarify the state of health care today and renew patients' trust in the work of medical professionals and in our health care system. When I reflect on how many physicians have helped me care for my body over the years, I am reminded of what has always been important to me: not just the fact that my physicians have those impressive diplomas hanging on the wall or that they work at Georgetown University Medical Center but that they take the time to listen to me, to answer my questions, to instruct me, and finally to reassure me. The result is not merely that I leave their office well-informed and better able to look after myself, but that I appreciate the care I have received. The trust I have in my physician is reinforced and in a sense renewed through our connection—a connection forged by mutual respect, openness, and honesty.

The problem is that this special communication we all enjoy and value between ourselves and our doctors is increasingly threatened. It is a difficult time for doctors to give individualized care. The new pressures on the medical profession are well known: from the threat of malpractice to the scrutiny physicians face simply to submit a bill. It must be terrible to have to refrain from offering hope in uncertain circumstances because malpractice has taught us, "better safe than sorry." It is understandable that many doctors have developed a reticence that jeopardizes the human bond they need with their patients. Nonetheless, it is saddening that some doctors today are less likely to reassure patients, to offer encouragement, and to bolster courage—all essentials when one is half naked on an examining table, possibly in pain, struggling to regain health.

None of us would want to return to the time when we did not have a polio vaccine or accurate tuberculosis tests—or, for that matter, when we could not effectively treat sinus ailments and trachea problems. We all can benefit, however, from protecting the special communication that builds trust and has always been an essential feature of the physician-doctor relationship.

People miss the old-time physician who made house calls not because (as one physician recently put it) they long for "a wise old man with a little black bag and a few harmless (and useless) nostrums" but because they yearn for a time when physicians could communicate freely in a common language.[12]

Our position in education and medicine is paradoxical, in a sense. We have the world's best systems of higher education and health care, yet the widespread perception is otherwise. Changing that perception is among our greatest challenges. To do so, we must remember our great strength: There is no better place to be than the United States if you have a history of throat cancer in your family, or are at risk of a heart attack, or have been injured in a car crash. If you're going to break your neck, for that matter, there's no better place to do it than in America!

For the past five years there has been a great debate about health care—about Medicare and Medicaid, about managed care, about the cost of prescription drugs, about the direction of biomedical research, about whether patients should have the right to choose their doctors, about how we pay for health care in what gerontologists call our aging society. This debate is important and necessary, but I know a place where we definitely have steered off course. For the past five years, it has been clear that most elected officials have not grasped one central fact: The fact that the primary motivation of America's physicians and surgeons is moral, not economic—that the well-being of patients is at the top, not the bottom, of the list of reasons that physicians enter the profession.

Public officials of all political persuasions do not understand how physicians cherish the moral foundation of their work: the sacred relationship of doctor and patient—a relationship built on trust. The moral foundation of our doctors' vocations ultimately is the real strength of our still-great health care system—not simply our scientific and technical knowledge—and all of us in public life need to do a better job communicating that aspect of our professional commitment. By emphasizing the roots and the core of our career choices, we can begin to break down some of the mistrust that impedes our work and colors our national debates about health care and education. Only when we have personally reflected on and renewed our moral commitment to our vocations, however, can we restore what Sir William Osler called the physician's "well-deserved title of the Friend of Man."[13]

CONCLUSION

Some concluding reflections may be useful as educators and physicians seek to minister to those in need—physically, spiritually, and intellectually—and as we seek to renew trust in our lives and in our professions. First, we would all benefit by taking time each day for personal reflection—time to renew the vows we took when we entered our professions and dedicated ourselves to the service of others. I know a medical student who centers herself in the middle of a taxing day by going to an afternoon Mass at our chapel. Another friend I know simply listens to Bach's *Goldberg Variations*—a total of 38 minutes—any time she's in need of rejuvenation. For my own part, each morning I say in Latin the vows I took more than thirty-five years ago. Sometimes I need to hear the words so I can translate their meaning in new ways; at other times I am simply invigorated by knowing that they have become a part of me.

Second, those of us in medicine and education are called, are we not, to inspire the next generation. We must seed the future. As role models for future otolaryngologists, future teachers, and future theologians, we need to show younger people trust in action. We cannot alleviate the mistrust around us and inspire the caring and trusting leaders of the future if we wilt beneath current challenges. Albert Schweitzer got it right when he said, "Example is not the main thing in influencing others. It is the only thing."[14]

Third, we must learn to act in trusting concert, as a community. Although individually we may all at times feel undervalued and dispirited, helpless to change the things that threaten our vocations, nevertheless we have together great collaborative strength. Our collective voice and determination, our collective commitment to our patients and students, will—and must—be heard.

Fourth, let us be willing to risk truly for what is truly most important: our desire to make a difference in the lives of those we help. The sacred relationships between doctor and patient, between teacher and student, between friend and friend, must be cherished, protected, and strengthened at any cost. We need to know that some of the people who come to us may experience what Tennyson aptly called "pains that conquer trust,"[15] and we need to take the risks necessary to comfort and reassure them.

Last, we need to trust *trust*. We all learn trust by trusting. And so we need to trust even more in ourselves and our families, our profession and our colleagues, our fellow human beings—and whoever it is we call our God.

Since we first fell into the arms of our mothers and fathers—thanks to a caring attending physician or nurse—we have been meant to, and needed to, trust. Today and forever, lovers fall into each other's arms because of trust. Patients visit their physicians because of trust. Every believing human being, encouraged by some community of faith, can face suffering and death with courage because we trust that we shall finally fall not into a dark emptiness but into the creative and redemptive hands of God. So let us trust, and keep learning to trust—for the love of God and all our fellow human beings.

NOTES

1. Mark E. Warren, "Introduction," in *Democracy and Trust,* ed. Mark E. Warren (Cambridge: Cambridge University Press, 1999).

2. Larry R. Churchill, in *The Illusion of Trust: Toward a Medical Technological Ethics in the Post-Modern Age,* ed. E. R. DuBose (Dordrecht, The Netherlands: Kluwer Academic Publications, 1995), 3.

3. C. W. Brister, "Trust in Pastoral Relationships," in *Dictionary of Pastoral Care and Counseling,* ed. Rodney J. Hunter (Nashville, Tenn.: Abingdon Press, 1990), 1288.

4. Michael Polanyi, *Personal Knowledge: Towards a Post-critical Philosophy* (Chicago: University of Chicago Press, 1958), 215.

5. Ibid.

6. Edmund D. Pellegrino, "Being a Physician: Does it Make a Moral Difference?" *Advances in Otolaryngology—Head and Neck Surgery* 6 (1992): 1–10.

7. Eric J. Cassell, *The Nature of Suffering and the Goals of Medicine* (New York: Oxford University Press, 1991), 20.

8. William Bradford, *Of Plymouth Plantation: 1620–1647* (New York: Random House, 1981), 34.

9. Ibid.

10. Robert D. Putnam, "Bowling Alone: America's Declining Social Capital," *Journal of Democracy* 6 (1995).

11. See Joshua Mitchell, *The Fragility of Freedom: Tocqueville on Religion, Democracy, and the American Future* (Chicago: University of Chicago Press, 1995).

12. Jerome Lowenstein, *The Midnight Meal and Other Essays about Doctors, Patients, and Medicine* (New Haven, Conn.: Yale University Press, 1997), 22.

13. William Osler, "Teacher and Student," in *Aequanimitas* (Philadelphia: Blakiston Company, 1943), 41.

14. Albert Schweitzer, *Out of My Life and Thought: An Autobiography* (New York: Henry Holt, 1949).

15. Alfred Lord Tennyson, "In Memoriam," in *The Works of Alfred Lord Tennyson, Vol. III* (New York: MacMillan, 1899), 343.

PART I

The Nature of the Health Care Professional

The Physician-Patient Relationship

G. Kevin Donovan

The relationship between a physician and his or her patient is the heart and the soul of medicine. This relationship is the mundane stuff of daily practice as well as the transcendent spirit of the medical profession. It is rightly the object of insight and analysis, for by seeing this relationship in its best light, we see medicine at its best. Conversely, if we believe medicine is somehow going awry, we should not blame scientific or societal influences but look at their influence on the ideal healing interaction that occurs in the coming together of a virtuous healer and an individual in need of healing—the physician and the patient.

THE PHYSICIAN

Good definitions are a prerequisite for a good discussion, so we should begin by defining what we mean when we say *physician* or *doctor.* Similarly, we will need to define what we mean by *patient.*

Physician, which is derived from the Latin *physic,* indicates a person who is skilled in the art of healing. The Latin word *docere*—the root for the English word *doctor*—means to teach or to appear right, fitting, or decent.[1] The ideals suggested by these terms are integral components of what it means to be a medical professional.

The term *professional* historically was reserved for practitioners of medicine, law, divinity, and (eventually) teaching. Professionals did not produce goods for sale or artistic pleasure; instead, they were guides and healers to individuals, particularly in times of personal crisis. The traditional professions were characterized by the acquisition of systematic and valuable knowledge (knowing), the practice or application of this knowledge through technical skill and training (doing), and the value placed on putting this knowledge and skill to work in the service of others (helping).[2] A profession's high degree of internal control of its members' behavior was integral to this concept; typically, each profession developed its own code of ethics to govern practice, and limited entry into the profession—even expelling members who did not meet the required ideals of the profession. Consequently, professionals have a great deal of autonomy in judgment and authority. We must examine how the term finds application today; in particular, when we examine the relationship between physicians and patients, we must decide if using alternative terms such as "health care provider" support or detract from the attributes we wish to find in our physicians.

We can easily find some consensus about characteristics that are desirable in one's physician. Qualities such as competency, compassion, confidentiality, and caring have long been considered essential. In the words of Francis Peabody, "The essential quality of the clinician is interest in humanity, for the secret of caring for the patient is in caring about the patient."[3] Yet medicine is attractive not only to dewy-eyed humanistic scientists; it clearly has its own rewards. Some of these rewards are monetary, to be sure (if slightly less so in the present era), but the honorary rewards are as important. The physician occupies a privileged place in society, with access to a patient's most private thoughts and body parts and the right and privilege of even entering that body in a fashion that would be considered an assault in any other context. If a knife-wielding stranger were to accept money from the layperson, it would be a matter for the police; in the context of medicine, we call it surgery.

In our scientific and technological age, we sometimes lose sight of the similarity between the role of the priest and physician in ancient times. Nevertheless, we maintain sacerdotal symbols such as the stethoscope (often carried unused by senior staff during rounds) and especially the robe of office: the white coat. Donning the physician's white coat signals acceptance of the respect traditionally accorded to the profession and often serves as a sign of reciprocal respect for the patient—surely a more likely symbol than a doctor examining the patient while wearing a T-shirt and running shoes. Such putative respect for the patient is instantly negated, however, if it is not consistent with other courtesies such as introducing oneself, shaking hands, and using an adult's first name only when invited to do so (or only when the physician expects to be addressed in similar fashion).

The privileges of the profession are not unbounded, however. Boundaries have been set by the profession itself, often with input from the public at large. Some boundaries—such as the terms by which we address patients—may seem trivial, whereas others have greater significance. Physicians in training, for instance, sometimes violate these limits by using demeaning terms such as "crock" and "gomer" for undesirable patients; the most serious and extreme form of boundary violation involves unwarranted sexual contact. Many other behaviors exploit the dependency of the patient on the physician and the inherent power differential. These behaviors range from the apparently trivial, such as lack of timeliness for appointments, to the more serious—such as excessive involvement with patients, inappropriate gift-giving or self-disclosure on the part of the physician, and lack of care for the patient's privacy during the physical exam. Other inappropriate situations may entail dual relationships in the physician-patient relationship (such as treating one's own family members), dating patients, and especially conflicts of interest in relation to payors.[4]

We must recognize that as physicians, we are moral agents who are responsible for our own actions and our own values; we are humans acting in a human context. We require humility in our actions, knowing that God or nature is primarily responsible for our successes and acknowledging that our knowledge is always incomplete. Such humility serves as a healthy balance to the natural arrogance to which we are tempted when arrogating to ourselves the right to treat patients according to our judgment. The evolution of evidence-based medicine may help to provide scientific balance to our individual judgment.

Coupled with this humility—and acting as a frequent stimulus to it—is the knowledge of our own fallibility and mistakes. Mistakes in medical practice not only happen; they happen with what may appear to be alarming frequency.[5] Nevertheless, the medical culture still has difficulty dealing with them. Part of the problem is endemic in medical culture itself. The profession and the public regard medicine with the expectation of perfection in practice. Yet we are all bound to make errors in our careers, despite our best intentions. To teach that perfection is the norm is unrealistic; such expectations interfere with honesty with patients as well as with improvements in practice, and they lead to physician stress and burnout.

Too little attention has been given to the role of the physician as nonprofessional—that is, someone with a life and interests outside the professional practice. Unlike some priesthoods, the physician's role does not require or encourage celibacy. In fact, physicians should lead a balanced life and develop other interests. Efforts to foster self-awareness, strengthen the ability to share feelings as well as responsibilities, learn to take care of oneself, nurture one's personal values, and place limits on professional and external demands contribute to the physician's mental and physical health.[6]

Other significant pressures exist for the deprofessionalization of medicine. One of the foremost of these pressures is the devaluation of the concept of the professions themselves. In the industrial and technological age, the term *professional* is not limited to the learned professions of the Middle Ages. Today, anyone who can be paid for his or her work is considered a professional: This language extends not only to professional plumbers and professional athletes but even to the "world's oldest profession"! Obviously, this usage confuses the concept greatly; today's physician would hardly want to be regarded as one who might prostitute himself or herself for profit or a third-party payor.

More important, the crucial link between medicine's professionalism and its autonomy is being eroded, for economic and technological reasons. Physicians increasingly find themselves part of a large medical organization—either a corporation or a hospital system—that delivers care. Their role is frequently relegated to that of valued employee, and their function is considered interchangeable with any other similar physician, without regard to any personal relationship with the patient. Compounding this trend is increased outside regulation of medical practice, the incursion of other health care professionals competing in areas of physician practice, and the inclination of many patients to seek medical information independently (e.g., through the Internet) and to diagnose and treat themselves. Such trends do not bode well for society. If physicians are not ultimately responsible for health care, who will be responsible—the government or the insurance payors? If so, can this situation be regarded as any improvement for the patients?[7]

Last, but not least, the act of profession itself defines the role of the physician. That is, a professional can be rightly described as one who professes. When young medical graduates are awarded their degrees, they make a public avowal by taking an oath such as the Hippocratic Oath; they then officially become members of the profession. In ancient times, this oath-taking was a public declaration of belief in and intent to practice certain ideals, as well as a public declaration that one possessed the skills required and would place them in the service of others. In taking such an oath, medical students avow competence to heal, binding themselves publicly to competence as a moral obligation and placing the well-being of those they would help above their own personal gain.

This concept of the medical professional defines the nature of the physician-patient relationship. Moreover, the actual or perceived failure to act in accordance with the full meaning of the word *profession* leads to concerns about malpractice, governmental regulation, and consumerism and underlies much of the public disquietude with medicine today.[8]

THE PATIENT

The physician must be defined in terms of his or her relationship to patients. Simply put, physicians would have no practice, and no purpose, without patients. The word *patient* comes from the Middle English *paycent,* which is derived from the Latin. This word indicates not only "a suffering or sick person under medical treatment" but also "one who bears trials steadfastly or calmly."[9]

Health care workers and most of our society seem to admire the "cheerful stoic" who is afflicted with illness or injury. There is a discrepancy, however, between what people say and what they do with regard to pain. According to a study reported in *Pain in America: A Survey of American Attitudes toward Pain* (1998), 62 percent of people said they would rather bear pain than take action to relieve it.[10] Yet although 80 percent of the respondents said they tried to avoid taking medication, the same number had at least one over-the-counter pain medication on hand, and one-third said they had a prescription specifically for pain relief. Moreover, most people believe they are more courageous than everyone else. The survey showed that 33 percent of respondents believed that they could withstand a lot more pain than most people, and 27 percent believed they could stand a little more pain than most people. Yet whenever an individual's pain exceeds the point of tolerance, that individual becomes a patient and seeks out another person who has professed to help. The patient is defined in some way by the fact of illness, as well as by being "one who awaits or receives medical treatment."

This existential condition of the patient demands primacy, and the fact of illness demands some response from the physician. This interaction between the physician and the patient defines the right and good relationship between the two. We have seen what the physician wants: to practice the art and science of medicine, to put his or her skills at the service of others, to reap the rewards—intellectual, fiscal and prestigious—that accrue to this role. What does the patient want? The patient wants healing—but healing means more than a physical cure. The state of illness also inflicts psychological, social, and even spiritual challenges to the ill individual. To heal is to become whole again and to return as far as possible to what one considers a normal life. Ideally, healing involves a cure, but when a cure is not possible, it still involves restoring function, maintaining function, or, at the very least, regaining the sense of balance and the integration of meaning and living. Therefore, the therapeutic activity of medicine need not cease even in a patient who is terminally ill.[11]

Illness can be acute or chronic and obviously will affect different patients in different ways. The effects of illness include anxiety, discomfort, pain, and threats to one's lifestyle, independence, and income. The individual becomes dependent—primarily on the physician, but perhaps also on others around him or her. The patient comes to the doctor as a supplicant, sits patiently in an aptly named waiting room, then typically is placed half-dressed in an examining room where uncomfortable and embarrassing things are done to his or her body. This process does *not* entail a relationship of equality. The inequality of power places an inequality of obligation on the participants, with the greater obligation placed on the physician. Nevertheless, patients also have obligations to the physician and responsibilities to the relationship. In American culture, a good patient is defined as one who communicates honestly and fully with the physician, cooperates with the treatment plan, and takes personal responsibility for helping himself or herself and paying the bills.[12] Clearly, the dependent nature of this role places a significant moral duty on those who profess the knowledge and willingness to help.

Finally, no discussion on the role of the patient would be complete without asking ourselves, "Who is the patient?" As anyone who cares for children knows, patients come in different sizes and degrees of competency. Some patients, such as children and the retarded, have never been competent or able to formulate their own values. Some become incompetent and unable to participate in medical decision making or to enforce their pre-determined values. Those of us who deal with such situations on a daily basis can readily understand that the patient is often a single part of a more complex relationship. We accord family members the right to make decisions on their behalf, in part because we assume they will always place the best interests of the patient foremost. We are less ready to acknowledge that their ability to participate also depends on the effect of the illness on themselves and the rest of the family. Too often, we fail to acknowledge socioeconomic, ethnic, cultural, and gender differences among our patients, their reactions to illness, and their ways of coping with it.

When we understand that the doctor-patient relationship involves more than a single individual as the patient, the relationship becomes not only more complex but more open to including others in the decision-making process. In fact, given certain ethnic and cultural preferences, the delivery of bad news and decision making may come to and from the patient via other family members, even when the patient is a competent adult. In such situations, we must remember that the focus of decision making must always be on the patient's benefit. Only this approach lends weight to the family's participation in the decision-making process. Alternately, differences in attitudes toward autonomy, illness, and the value of independence may prevent some patients, particularly males, from even seeking care at all.

THE RELATIONSHIP

The physician-patient relationship is the heart of medicine and the healing process. Healing takes place in this interactive relationship more than in the unilateral or parallel actions of a competent physician or needful patient. A proper healing relationship is a critical factor in restoring a patient to health. This fact seemed clear to ancient practitioners of the art, but it must be rediscovered in the present age. Perhaps the development of more effective drugs and surgery have made the physician's role seem less personal. Certainly the intrusion of insurance companies and government payors—which make treatment affordable—has also diminished the immediacy of the relationship between what had previously been only two parties. Little wonder that contemporary observers have sought to reinterpret or redefine the physician-patient relationship in view of these developments. Let us review some of these proposed new models before examining the model that I would argue best meets the needs of the physician, the patient, and the community.

As summarized by Edmund Pellegrino and David Thomasma in their landmark work *For the Patient's Good: The Restoration of Beneficence in Health Care* (1988), different models of health care condition the practitioner's view of his or her roles and principles, as well as the virtues we might expect the good doctor or the good patient to exhibit.[13] We must first acknowledge that the normal relationship is not balanced, and it is this inherent imbalance that places additional obligations on the physician, legally and morally. It is fair to ask why medicine and the health professions should be called to a higher standard of moral behavior than the society around them. Pellegrino and Thomasma reply that effacement of self-interest is central to the medical profession, epitomizing the central distinguishing moral feature of medical activity—the healing relationship between the one who is ill and the one who professes to help and heal.[14] This healing relationship must balance self-interest against self-effacement, and the balance must tilt in favor of the patient. Pellegrino and Thomasma cite five features characterizing this relationship and providing medicine with its moral imperatives: the inequality of the medical relationship, the fiduciary nature of the relationship, the moral nature of medical decisions, the nature of medical knowledge, and the moral complicity of the physician in whatever happens to a patient.

The existential fact of illness creates vulnerability in the sick person and a consequent inequality in the medical relationship. Patients experience dis-ease, loss of freedom, and dependency on the physician for access to specialized knowledge and skill. This vulnerability imposes moral obligations on the physician. Unlike the world of business, medicine requires its practitioners to offer protection, not exploitation, when they encounter weakness.

Because patients are vulnerable, they are forced to trust physicians. Such trust may not be given without scrutiny and may not be given early in the relationship, but healing will not proceed without it. Trust must exist before patients can be expected to expose themselves physically, mentally, and psychologically because trustworthiness has been promised by the professional, implicitly or explicitly.

Medical decision making is not simply technical; it must encompass moral components as well. A scientifically correct diagnosis or choice of therapy must be aligned with decisions made for the patient's good. This good is not self-evident; it is subject to definition and negotiation by the patient.

Moreover, technical medical knowledge creates obligations in those who possess it. This knowledge has been acquired with the understanding that it will be put to good use. It is obtained through the socially sanctioned privilege of a medical education. Society permits the invasion of the privacy of sick persons so that medical professionals can learn from them. These privileges could not be bought for any price but are freely given by society, which expects a commensurate return. Moreover, medical education, however costly to the student, is subsidized by society to a large extent. The monopoly on medical treatment is not to be used by physicians as private property but as a good to be held in trust. Physicians are its stewards, not its exploiters.

Finally, because the physician is the final pathway for access to treatment, he or she must be the final guardian of the patient's well being. Without the physician's complicity, nothing can be done for good or ill to the patient. Therefore, the physician cannot escape ultimate responsibility for the patient's well being.

These five characteristics require the profession to hold physicians to higher standards of effacement of self-interest than other relationships in our society. In this light, some models of the physician-patient relationship must be found wanting. At either extreme, we find the paternalistic or the libertarian model, neither of which currently has many supporters. The paternalistic model—favored by the ancient Greeks—emphasizes the physician's autonomy. Therapy is considered an act of beneficence as determined by the physician's values. The patient's agreement with the doctor's values and decisions is assumed, not sought explicitly. The more modern libertarian model emphasizes patient autonomy. In this model, the physician is regarded as a technical expert, providing information and awaiting instruction. This model is also linked to a view of preventive medicine in which individual choices of lifestyle make people responsible for their own health. Such individuals are more likely to seek healing through alternative medicine and are less likely to entrust care and decision making to a more traditional physician-patient relationship. The problems with both models are evident, and both have been rejected because of the severe imbalance they create in the relationship.

A proposed model of health care as a *business* relationship would treat health care as a commodity and the relationship between physician and patient like that between a buyer and seller. We could expect commitment and skill from a professional, but nothing more would be required. The patient would become a purchaser of services and often would be referred to as a client. The physician becomes a provider of a product, and the ethics governing the relationship would be simply the ethics of good business. People who prefer the term "health care provider" to "physician" are endorsing this model, consciously or not.

In a *contractual* relationship, the business relationship is formalized with a contract, and expectations are explicitly detailed. Doctor and patient are regarded as equal partners in a commodity transaction. Although this model is intended to empower the patient, it ignores patient vulnerability. Moreover, it is difficult to make adequate contractual demands in advance when the other party possesses most of the knowledge and skill. A contract would limit the physician's obligation to services specifically agreed upon in advance and would likely fail to meet all of the patient's needs.

Some observers have proposed a *covenant* as a model of medicine. Obligation is then placed on the patient as heavily as on the physician. Both would have a sacred trust, committing themselves to the preservation of life and health.

Pellegrino and Thomasma have revitalized the concept of a *beneficent* relationship between the patient and physician.[15] Criticisms of early variations of this model characterized it as a kind of paternalism, in which the physician diagnoses and treats according to what he or she believes to be good for the patient. In Pellegrino and Thomasma's beneficence model, the physician and the patient join in a mutual endeavor to meet the patient's needs. The physician performs a "right and good action" on behalf of the patient. The action is *right* if it is scientifically correct and medically valid. It is *good* only if it meets the needs of the patient in that particular circumstance *according to the patient's values*. Therefore, a good action by the physician is a moral action aimed at restoring health to the patient. Health, however, is regarded as a negotiable good that may move up and down a hierarchy of values as perceived by the patient. Medical treatments are neither prescribed nor withheld without consulting the patient's values.

This beneficence model makes up for the deficiencies of both autonomy and paternalism. It acknowledges the fact that patients, in their state of illness and lack of knowledge, are necessarily less than fully autonomous. It avoids paternalism by insisting on *beneficence-in-trust*. This *fiduciary* model depends on a re-emphasis on the ethic of virtue rather than the ethic of rules and rights. It recognizes that a listing of rules cannot guarantee adherence by the professional to these rules. Adherence happens only if the physician has the kind of character that disposes him or her to act in accordance with the proper principles. The beneficent relationship, grounded in trust, allows for negotiation and rests on the concept of treating the whole person, including the patient's needs and values *as defined by the patient.* This concept avoids paternalism by combining a principle of beneficence with respect for the patient's autonomy. *Beneficence-in-trust* means that physicians and patients hold in trust the goal of acting in the best interests of one another in the relationship.

The patient usually fulfills this trust by carrying out the negotiated plan for his or her health. The burden of trust weighs more heavily on the physician, who must act in the best interest of the patient under existing conditions (including social conditions). Although negotiation is important, it does not by itself establish the good of the patient. The doctor and the patient must act in the best interests of the patient by acknowledging patient preferences. Beneficence-in-trust must not override autonomy or slip into paternalism. Only in the rare case in which the physician cannot morally assent to the patient's preferences would the relationship fail. In this case, the proper response would not be to override the patient's preferences but to withdraw in favor of others who can assent to them.

In light of this careful restoration of beneficence in the physician-patient relationship and guided by the five characteristics that constitute the internal morality of medicine, we can see which actions would be reprehensible and which would be required under such a model. A virtuous physician does more than comply with the law of the land and the ethical codes of the profession. The virtuous physician does what is right and good, even at the expense of personal sacrifice and legitimate personal preferences. We see the practical effects in two different instances: the avoidance of dual obligations and the risks of honesty in the relationship.

If the doctor-patient relationship is in fact a fiduciary one, based on a commitment to the benefit of the patient, then *trust* is the bedrock on which the relationship is built. Anything affecting that trust profoundly affects the relationship. Two significant influences must be examined—one recent and one recurring.

The recent challenge to patient trust has been precipitated by the managed-care model of health care delivery. Although the practice of medicine was not free of financial incentives in fee-for-service practice, managed care organizations conspire to restrict, rather than promote, interventions—arguably to the patient's detriment. Managed care's cost-control mechanisms—guidelines and gag clauses, formularies and financial incentives, profiling and mandatory protocols—force physicians to regard the needs of the patient, the rules of the organization, and their own financial well-being as equally important. The guiding principle for the physician is no longer the patient's best interest and values but maximization of therapeutic benefit under budgetary constraints. Under managed care, the patient's needs are viewed in the context of the needs of the entire organization, including the other members of the plan. Attention to patient needs is further diverted by payment systems such as capitation, which—through incentives, withholds, and payment limits—forces the physician to act as a double agent for the organization and all its enrollees as well as for his or her patient.

Physicians and patients alike are gravely concerned by these implications. Although hard data are scarce, a recent survey shows that patients in various managed care plans doubt that their physicians will act in their best interests.[16] This perception in itself significantly damages the physician-patient relationship.

Equally challenging, though with a much longer history, is the issue of honesty between physicians and their patients. Admittedly, honesty has not always been high on the list of necessary virtues. In the days of strong paternalism, physicians did not always consider it necessary to inform a patient of a terminal diagnosis. More recently, honesty has been honored more in principle than in practice. Our problem with honesty relates to its inherent risks as well as its natural impediments. The risks seem obvious; although the impediments are more subtle, they are always present, even if they are unnoticed by the physician and the patient. One primary impediment is lack of knowledge concerning the history of the patient, the details of the diagnosis, and the proper treatment. Some uncertainty inevitably exists in medical science. This lack of knowledge is exacerbated by the time constraints that are increasingly present in current health care delivery systems. Moreover, the appearance of ignorance or indifference can lead to a loss of prestige and alter the relative status of the physician in the relationship. A simple "I don't know" may be as difficult for the physician to utter as for the patient to hear. This phrase probably should never be said without a determined promise to find an appropriate answer.

A closely related problem for honesty is the physician's lack of proficiency. No physician starts out knowing how to do a new procedure. From the early days as a medical student, each must start at the bottom of the learning curve for customary procedures, and all physicians must start over when new techniques are introduced into medical practice. This proficiency issue has always been difficult to explain to patients. Do patients really want to know how little practice their doctor has had in a proposed and necessary procedure? The doctor's need to learn must always be balanced against the patient's need for safety and efficacy in a procedure. Moreover, managed care contributes to this dilemma by pressuring primary care physicians *not* to refer patients with certain diagnoses who need specialized procedures or expert treatment, no matter what the practitioner's recent experience or current level of skill.

Honesty is not without risks. Physicians who are reluctant to admit their mistakes often cite concerns about malpractice lawsuits. This concern is probably more rationalization than justification and flies in the face of what we know about such risks. Studies have repeatedly confirmed that patients become more likely to sue not because of a physician's mistake or bad result but when they are angry and dissatisfied with the therapeutic relationship. The temptation to conceal one's mistakes may be the greatest mistake of all. Nothing is more likely to make a patient angry in the face of an unhappy result than the feeling that one is being lied to about it.

Why, then, is complete disclosure so difficult? Beyond any fear of a lawsuit, reluctance to admit one's mistakes is only natural. Such an admission detracts from our position as an authority figure or even makes us question our own competency as a physician. Moreover, as long as the medical and the legal systems focus on finding faults rather than correcting and safeguarding patients against them, impediments to honesty will continue to exist. Perhaps malpractice insurance should be replaced by some sort of "no fault" insurance for bad results, and our case review and quality assurance committees should exist not to determine guilt but to create fail-safe systems for detecting and correcting potential problems in a timely fashion.

Lest we take the honesty concept too far, we must acknowledge that any virtue taken to excess can become a vice. This tendency is certainly true with physicians who would mask their lack of empathy with the excuse that they were simply being honest. Such behavior is reminiscent of an old Thurber cartoon in which the doctor hovers menacingly over a woman's bed and informs her, "You're not my patient, you're my meat, Mrs. Quist."

It is neither surprising nor excusable when doctors are sometimes tempted to depersonalize their patients. Although some patients delight us with every visit, and we enjoy their sunny dispositions or their courage, many do not move the busy practitioner deeply. Unfortunately, a few patients can cause an inward or audible groan when they appear on the office schedule or in the emergency room. It is difficult to mask one's true feelings under these circumstances, but doctors should not confuse bluntness with honesty. We must not use these conditions as an excuse for brutal indifference or shirking of duty. With patience and compassion, we can eventually find qualities in a patient that evoke our sympathy or even our admiration. Until then, no patient should detect a lack of empathy in our actions or words.

Finally, no examination of the physician-patient relationship would be complete without acknowledging the special needs of both patients and physicians. For patients, there is a need to remember that there is a life outside the illness. Particularly with chronic, severe, or debilitating conditions, people may forget to define themselves as something more than just a *patient*. We must help them to see and maintain the other important activities and relationships in their lives. A preoccupation with illness, imagined or real, can deprive patients of the richness that can and should be present in their lives.

Physicians too must maintain a focus on their lives outside medicine. A messianic complex in some physicians leads them to regard medicine as an excuse *from* living. If they merely attend to their professional obligations, their spouses, children, and friends perforce must attend to themselves. Physicians have sometimes been enabled in this thinking from early in their careers. We go from "our studies must come first" to "our patients must come first" to the realization—often too late—that we have placed everything else second. Anyone who neglects his or her family life, intellectual life, or physical and spiritual well-being cannot be an ideal physician.

In the spiritual realm, particularly, we seem to have a poor understanding of the special needs of physicians and patients. Yet it is here that some of the most intriguing information has become available, particularly about the relationship between patients and physicians. The linkage between spiritual faith and healing is unclear but apparently undeniable. There is increasing evidence that religious faith not only promotes overall good health but also aids in recovery from serious illness. Religiously active people recover more quickly from surgery, spend less time in the hospital, and have lower mortality rates. The melding of the spiritual with the scientific and secular is not so much a "new age" fad but a very old idea that is being rediscovered. Ironically, this important connection between mind, body, and spirit may be one lesson that patients will be able to teach their doctors. This linkage would be a fitting completion of the circle of trust and beneficence in the therapeutic relationship between patients and their physicians.

NOTES

1. W. Clay Jackson, "In a Word," *Journal of the American Medical Association* 280 (1998): 493–94.
2. Benedict M. Ashley and Kevin D. O'Rourke, eds., *Healthcare Ethics: A Theological Analysis* (St. Louis: Catholic Health Association of the United States, 1989).

3. Francis W. Peabody, "The Care of the Patient," *Journal of the American Medical Association* 88 (1927): 882.
4. Glen O. Gabbard and Carol Nadelson, "Professional Boundaries in the Physician-Patient Relationship," *Journal of the American Medical Association* 273 (1995): 1445–49.
5. Lucian L. Leape, "Error in Medicine," *Journal of the American Medical Association* 272 (1994): 1851–57.
6. Timothy E. Quill and Penelope R. Williamson, "Healthy Approaches to Physician Stress," *Archives of Internal Medicine* 150 (1990): 1857–60.
7. Ralph R. Reed and Daryl Evans, "The Deprofessionalization of Medicine: Causes, Effects, and Responses," *Journal of the American Medical Association* 258 (1987): 3279–82.
8. Edmund D. Pellegrino, *Humanism and the Physician* (Knoxville: University of Tennessee Press, 1979).
9. Jackson, *In a Word.*
10. Mayday Fund, *Pain in America: Annual Report 1997* (New York: Mayday Fund, 1998).
11. Pellegrino, *Humanism and the Physician.*
12. Council on Ethical and Judicial Affairs, *Patient Responsibilities* (Chicago: American Medical Association, 1998).
13. Edmund D. Pellegrino and David C. Thomasma, *For the Patient's Good: The Restoration of Beneficence in Health Care* (New York: Oxford University Press, 1988), 101–05.
14. Edmund D. Pellegrino and David C. Thomasma, *The Virtues in Medical Practice* (New York: Oxford University Press, 1993), 42–44.
15. Pellegrino and Thomasma, *For the Patient's Good,* 32–35, 105–06.
16. Audley C. Kao, D. C. Green, A. M. Zaslavsky, J. P. Koplan, and P. D. Cleary, "The Relationship Between Method of Physician Payment and Patient Trust," *Journal of the American Medical Association* 280 (1998): 1708–14.

Friendship as an Ideal for the Patient-Physician Relationship: A Critique and an Alternative

F. Daniel Davis

The title of this collection is rich in possibilities for ethical analysis and reflection. It projects two different ideals of the health care professional: as a healer and as a friend to the patient. I have interpreted the title of this volume as a provocative challenge to explore and assess the cogency of these ideals—particularly the latter. Thus, focusing on the physician and the profession of medicine, I address two interrelated questions. First, is friendship a viable ideal for the patient-physician relationship? Second, does "being a friend to the patient" provide medical students with an appropriate ideal for their own conception, understanding, and practice of moral agency in medicine? Although both questions have significance for clinical medical ethics, the second also possesses pedagogical importance.

Although I am sympathetic to these ideals, I have reservations about their appropriateness. I acknowledge that friendship and being a friend do suggest, if not specify, certain motivations and clinical virtues that are critical to the ultimate efficacy of the patient-physician relationship. Yet I argue that these ideals are incongruent with certain inescapable realities and essential features of this relationship. Given these inescapable realities and essential features, I also argue that this relationship is more appropriately conceived as a *healing* relationship, and that the ideal of being a healer—rather than a friend—to the patient provides a more compelling guide for the conception, understanding, and practice of moral agency by medical students as well as practicing physicians.

IS FRIENDSHIP A VIABLE IDEAL FOR THE PATIENT-PHYSICIAN RELATIONSHIP?

The Friendship Ideal: Ancient Origins and Contemporary Advocates

Friendship as an ideal for the patient-physician relationship has a long history. The image of the physician as friend to the patient is prominent in the Western medical tradition—its occurrence and recurrence testimony to the enduring claims that it exerts on the moral imagination. According to Pedro Lain Entralgo, the origins of this ideal are approximately coincident with the advent of Western, rational medicine, whose epistemic and ethical beginnings are recorded in the Hippocratic Corpus.[1] That is to say, the ideal first took shape in the sociocultural milieu of classical Greece, where *philia* or friendship provided the fundamental basis of the relationship between physician and patient. In seeking out and forming their relationship, the physician and the patient were motivated by *philia*. With regard to the patient, his *philia* consisted in his faith in the efficacy of medicine in general and his physician in particular. As for the physician, his *philia* joined a love of humankind, *philanthropia*, with a love of the art of healing, *philotechnia*:

> A Hippocratic doctor's *philia* for his patient . . . was . . . love for the perfection of the human race as individualized in the patient's body: a joyfully reverent love for everything that is beautiful in nature (health, harmony) or conducive to beauty (the natural recuperative powers of the organism), and an acquiescently respectful love for the dark and terrible inevitability with which nature imposes mortal or incurable disease.[2]

Lain Entralgo chronicles the evolution of the ideal throughout the medieval period and subsequent centuries and concludes his historical account with a defense of the contemporary relevance of the friendship ideal in medicine:

> Insofar as man is an individual and his illness a state affecting his personality, the medical relation ought to be more than mere comradeship—in fact it *should* be a friendship [emphasis added].[3]

The argument that the patient-physician relationship *should* be a friendship has other contemporary proponents as well. Appealing to classical sources such as Plato, Aristotle, and Seneca, for example, Edmund Pellegrino and David Thomasma repeatedly invoke friendship as a model or ideal for "clinical interaction"—that is, the patient-physician relationship—in *A Philosophical Basis of Medical Practice: Toward Philosophy and Ethic of the Healing Professions*.[4] In an influential essay in the *Journal of the American Medical Association*—which inaugurated a special section wholly devoted to the patient-physician relationship—Ezekiel and Linda Emanuel outline four models of the relationship.[5] Each model is distinguished by a different dynamic of physician-patient interaction and "division of labor" in medical decision making. In the *paternalistic* model, the physician acts as a parental guardian; the physician decides—in an authoritative and authoritarian fashion—what should be done for the patient (whose principal role is to comply with that decision). In the *informative* model, the physician serves as a competent technical expert, recommending a course of therapeutic action but leaving the decision to the patient alone. In the *interpretive* model, the physician is a counselor and advisor who elucidates and interprets the patient's values and implements the patient's decision with regard to his or her preferred course of action. In the *deliberative* model—which the authors advocate and defend as the ideal—the physician acts as a teacher and friend to the patient, not only by informing him or her of the available therapeutic alternatives but also by attempting to persuade the patient to adopt the values that are most conducive to his or her good health.[6]

26   *The Nature of the Health Care Professional*

Friendship as a Moral Phenomenon

To appreciate the enduring appeal, as well as the limits, of the friendship ideal, it is important to clarify the meaning of friendship. In contemporary usage, *friendship* has acquired a rather elastic, protean meaning—according to Erich Loewy, "an impoverished, if not indeed an almost fraudulent meaning"—with broad applicability to relationships of varying degrees of duration, intimacy, and mutual knowledge, understanding, and care.[7] My interest, however, is in friendship as a moral phenomenon: open to and indeed demanding ethical analysis and reflection. Thus, distinctions are critical.

For this purpose, I draw primarily on Aristotle's arguments about friendship in his *Nicomachean Ethics*.[8] For Aristotle, ethics is concerned with the good, specifically the good life for humankind—that is, happiness. Happiness is possible and life is worth living, in part, because of the presence of our friends; a good life is impossible without friends. Thus, friendship is an essential, constitutive feature of the good—the moral—life for humankind.

According to Aristotle, there are three principal forms of friendship, each distinguished by a particular object. In one, the shared object is usefulness; in another, this object is pleasure. With these two forms of friendship, each friend is an instrumental means to the achievement of some egoistic end of the other:

> These two forms of friendship then are grounded on an inessential factor—an "accident"—because in them the friend is not loved for being what he is to himself but the source, perhaps of some pleasure, perhaps of some advantage.[9]

The object of the third form of friendship—the best or perfect form—is the good; by this, Aristotle means that each friend takes up the good of the other as a matter of personal concern, care, and volition. Transcending the egoistic self-interest characteristic of the other two forms, this form of friendship is distinguished by reciprocal benevolence *and* by the friends' shared awareness of this reciprocity:

> To be friends then men must have (a) mutual good will, taking the form of each party's wishing the good of the other; (b) knowledge of the existence of this feeling.[10]

And:

> . . . it is those who desire the good of their friends for their friends' sake who are most completely friends, since each loves the other for what the other is in himself and not for something he has about him which he need not have.[11]

Some commentators have criticized Aristotle's concept of perfect friendship as an artifact bound up with, if not limited to, the sociocultural context of its original formation.[12] As evidence, they cite, for example, Aristotle's argument that perfect friendship is impossible between people of unequal power and social position. Caring, concern, wellwishing, and intimacy may be characteristic of the relationships between parent and child, husband and wife, rich man and poor man, but in Aristotle's scheme, these relationships cannot attain the status of perfect friendship. Nonetheless, we can profit from Aristotle's guidance in exploring friendship as a moral phenomenon by appropriating from his thought the arguments that in true friendship, each friend takes up the good of the other as his or her own and that each is alive to and aware of this reciprocity. Moreover, this commitment to the good of the other and this shared awareness of mutual benevolence are the expressions and achievements of an intimate knowledge of each other, forged in the crucible of time and experience:

> [T]he caring within a friendship is built up on a basis of knowledge, trust, and intimacy. One understands one's friend's good through knowing him well, much better than one knows non-friends, hence much better and more deeply than one knows their good. One is more sensitive to one's friend's needs and wants than one is to non-friends. In genuine friendship one comes to have a close identification with the good of the other person, an occurrence which is generally much rarer and at a much shallower level with other people.[13]

In addition to these features—the commitment to the good of each other and the mutual awareness of this commitment—there are two other definitive elements of friendship as a moral phenomenon. First, in true friendship the moral responsibilities that each person has toward the other are equal; neither friend bears a disproportionate share of moral obligation. Second, true friendship is a relationship that is freely entered into—and can be freely dissolved—by each individual.[14]

Thus, although contemporary usage appeals to a variety of meanings of "friendship," true or perfect friendship is distinguished by the following characteristics:

- mutual, reciprocal benevolence—that is, each friend wishes the good of the other;
- shared awareness of mutual benevolence—that is, each friend is aware of the reciprocity and mutuality of this benevolence;
- knowledge and experience of each other over time—that is, friendship is an achievement of altruism mediated by an understanding, a knowledge, of each other born of experience over time;
- the free, autonomous choice of each friend to enter upon—or leave—the state of friendship; and
- mutual, reciprocal moral responsibility.

The Enduring Appeal of the Friendship Ideal in Medicine

To appreciate the enduring appeal of friendship as an ideal of the patient-physician relationship, we must consider the conceptual grounds for the sort of imperative enunciated by Laín Entralgo and other recent advocates of the ideal when they assert that the patient-physician relationship *should* be a friendship. We also must explore certain contemporary trends in medical practice and medical-ethical theory that may help to explain this model's continuing attraction.

In an essay on friendship in the *Encyclopedia of Bioethics,* Paul Wadell asserts that friendship and the patient-physician relationship do—or should—have three features in common.[15] The first feature is benevolence, the second is mutuality, and the third is a shared good. At first glance, these features appear to be constituents of that common conceptual ground between friendship on the one hand and the patient-physician relationship on the other; thus, they animate the contemporary appeal to the former as an ideal for the latter. Some of Wadell's arguments, however—especially those regarding the feature of benevolence—also suggest that friendship, in the final analysis, fails as a viable and appropriate ideal for the utterly unique patient-physician relationship, which is, as Loewy argues, "quite different from the association found in the conduct of virtually any other enterprise."[16]

Along with these putatively common conceptual grounds between friendship and the patient-physician relationship, what other factors may account for the sustained appeal of the friendship ideal in today's medicine and medical-ethical thought? One such factor is pervasive depersonalization and reductionism in modern medical practice, which often emphasizes the cure of disease rather than the care of patients. The deleterious impact of these forces on the patient-physician relationship has been intensified by recent changes in the economics, organization, and delivery of medical care. These changes have served to amplify, rather than mute, the physician's economic self-interest and to place him or her in the conflict-ridden role of gatekeeper to a system of constrained health care resources that are increasingly under the sway of the market—a system that seeks above all else to generate profits rather than to secure the good of patients. In such a context, the friendship ideal presents the potential of a moral antidote and anchor, underscoring the nature of medicine as a profession, a promise, oriented to the care and the good of the patient as a person whose health care needs are not simply biological but also psychological, spiritual, and social.

The friendship ideal offers a counter-argument to commentators who regard the broader contexts of medicine and health care as a world of "moral strangers"[17] or who argue for a contractual model of the patient-physician relationship.[18] At the same time, this ideal resonates with and provides an added stimulus to the ferment spawned by the ethics of care, by the call for a patient-centered medicine, and by the revival of a virtue ethic—all of which converge in their rejection of impartiality, detachment, and objectivity in medical practice and medical ethics and instead emphasize the moral and therapeutic significance of relatedness, care, compassion, empathy, responsiveness, and responsibility. Finally, on theoretical and practical grounds, the friendship ideal offers a secure path between the extremes of paternalism and the mythology of total patient autonomy.[19] Thus, conceptual factors and contextual aspects of the contemporary practice of medicine account for the enduring appeal of friendship as an ideal for the patient-physician relationship.

Problems with the Friendship Ideal

The friendship ideal, however, is encumbered by problems that ultimately vitiate any effort to align the patient-physician relationship with it for descriptive, prescriptive, or morally heuristic purposes. As I suggested in the introduction to this essay, these problems arise from essential features of the patient-physician relationship that are absent from friendship, for the most part. What is the nature of these essential features? They are:

> features that characterize the specific human relationship medicine entails. These are what provides medicine its moral imperatives. Taken together, these imperatives constitute an 'internal morality' of medicine—something built into the nature of medicine as particular kind of human activity.[20]

First and foremost is the "existential inequality" of the patient-physician relationship born of the ineradicable "fact of illness."[21] Illness always imposes some degree of vulnerability on the patient, who experiences this ontological assault on his or her usual state of health and wholeness. This vulnerability of the patient, coupled with the physician's knowledge and skill, results in an inequality of power—an inequality inherent in the patient-physician relationship.

As Howard Brody has argued, the physician's power has three components: Aesculapian, charismatic, and social.[22] Although all three components may ultimately engender this inequality, two are of particular significance: Aesculapian power—that is, the physician's knowledge and skill—and social power, the socially conferred authority of the physician to determine *what* counts as sickness or health and *who* warrants labeling as sick or healthy. No matter how educated patients become about health, disease, and illness, no matter how much they retain their autonomy and capacity for self-determination, some degree of inequality will remain as an essential feature of the patient-physician relationship.

Is a similar or comparable inequality of power compatible with friendship? Inequality of a sort—for example, in age or education or socioeconomic status—may characterize particular friendships; indeed, friendships can and often do transcend such differences.

Second, the imbalance of power in the patient-physician relationship is the ground of *de facto* moral obligations and responsibilities on the part of the physician toward the patient that the patient does not, in turn, bear toward the physician.[23] This analysis does not suggest that patients bear no moral responsibilities whatsoever toward the physician: For example, patients' honest self-disclosure about health-related factors in their lives—their diet, habits, hopes, and fears—is essential to the physician's ability to help them, as is patients' integrity and commitment to the good of their own health.[24] Nonetheless, the respective moral responsibilities of physician to patient and patient to physician are not mutual or reciprocal.

This situation is not the case with friendship, in which the salient qualities of the characteristic moral responsibilities *are* mutuality and reciprocity. To be sure, such mutuality and reciprocity may not define the moral phenomenology of the friendship between two individuals at all times and in all places. From time to time, one may be more dependent on the other, or one may be more faithful than the other to the moral obligations inherent in their bond. Over the long haul, however, mutuality and reciprocity are critical to the sustenance of such relationships, and the persistent absence of these qualities often warrants the dissolution of friendship.

Third, friendship is freely chosen and usually lived in a shared context that is relatively independent of social and institutional structures. This existential dimension of friendship accounts, in part, for its durability as well as its vulnerability in the face of the unavoidable contingencies of human life. By contrast, the patient-physician relationship is deeply enmeshed in social and institutional structures that impinge on both parties. Moreover, despite the rise of the notion of "consumer sovereignty" in medicine, on the one hand, and the increasingly attenuated ability of patients to select their own physicians, on the other hand, the idea that physicians and patients are unfettered in deciding whether to embark on a relationship simply does not square with the realities of medical practice. The trauma patient who ends up unconscious on a gurney in the emergency room has no choice but to submit to the care of the attending physician. Similarly, prohibitions against patient abandonment are rooted in the recognition that physicians as professionals assume profound moral and fiduciary responsibilities toward the sick and their welfare. There is, however, no explicit parallel set of obligations and responsibilities that patients assume upon their entry into relationships with physicians.

Fourth, as our Aristotelian-inspired concept of true friendship tells us, this form of interpersonal relationship is oriented to a particular good or goods: Each friend takes up the good of the other as a matter of personal concern, care, and volition. These goods, however, are left unspecified. Out of care and concern for my friend, I may assume aspirations and needs that I do not share but are, nonetheless, of critical significance to her. These goods may have to do with professional or career goals or simply with everyday life. The patient-physician relationship, by contrast, is oriented to the achievement of an end that is general insofar as it is fundamental to every such relationship and specific vis-a-vis the particular patient. This end, or good, of healing—through the restoration or maintenance of the patient's health—is of a wholly different order than that which motivates and defines friendship.[25]

IS BEING A FRIEND TO THE PATIENT AN APPROPRIATE IDEAL FOR THE CONCEPTION, UNDERSTANDING, AND PRACTICE OF MORAL AGENCY BY MEDICAL STUDENTS?

If my arguments about the appropriateness of the friendship ideal in medicine are cogent, it follows that being a friend offers an understandably appealing—yet flawed—ideal for the conception, understanding, and practice of moral agency by medical students. *Moral agency* is an individual's capacity and disposition to act habitually in a way that is morally justified. It entails a critically reflective awareness of the "internal compass" that informs and directs one's thinking and action in concrete, morally significant situations.

As a template for moral agency by medical students, friendship is a very problematic ideal. To be sure, the friendship ideal may serve to underscore the importance of clinical virtues such as compassion and empathy in the care of patients; that is, it may offer an orienting point from which to see and appreciate the link between the affective dimensions of the patient-physician relationship and the therapeutic efficacy of this relationship for the patient. Moreover, the friendship ideal offers a "ready at hand," experientially based concept of moral agency that most people have enjoyed in their lives.

Such advantages, however, are far outweighed by two key disadvantages. One of these disadvantages has to do with the pedagogical challenge of introducing medical students to the moral implications of the knowledge and skill they are acquiring through their education. Many aspects of medical school militate against the full realization by students that their accumulating knowledge and skill, along with their social status as future physicians, constitute a form of power—and that this power generates an inherent inequality within the patient-physician relationship. The sheer burden of the facts and concepts that medical students must learn, the anxieties of test-taking, and all of the inevitable difficulties that accompany their socialization as physicians-to-be often lead to doubt and fear about their ability to acquire this power, much less deploy it in a clinically effective and morally justified fashion. The friendship ideal may do more to obfuscate rather than clarify the *de facto* moral responsibilities and obligations that being a medical student and a physician entail, by encouraging misconceptions about the division of moral responsibility and obligation between patients and their physicians. In other words, the friendship ideal may obscure the nature and the weight of physician's—and medical student's—moral responsibilities and obligations to patients, creating false expectations of mutuality and reciprocity, along with an underestimation of the power inherent in their evolving role as caregivers.

The second disadvantage has to do with the ends of the patient-physician relationship. Here, too, the friendship ideal—which does little to specify the shared goods at the heart of this interpersonal relationship—may do more to confuse than to specify clearly the good at which this relationship should aim. This confusion is only compounded by the multiple, mixed messages about the ends of medicine that students often receive via the formal and "hidden" curricula, which often tend to mirror and reinforce rather than question and challenge the depersonalizing effects of contemporary medical practice.

IDEALS OF THE HEALING RELATIONSHIP AND OF BEING A HEALER

If not friendship, then what ideal fits the patient-physician relationship? Recent years have witnessed a renaissance of scholarly interest in, and practical concern for, the patient-physician relationship. Discredited and decrepit, the paternalism that was once the traditional model of the relationship has given way to competing models. Examining and assessing each of the alternative ideals is beyond the scope of this essay. Instead, I argue that we need look no further than the alternative suggested by the title of this volume. Indeed, we can find no more compelling ideal for the patient-physician relationship than that of the healing relationship. The ideals of the healing relationship and of being a healer offer all the advantages of the ideals of friendship and of being a friend—without the problems.

Pellegrino offers a valuable perspective on this healing relationship. Against the backdrop of competing and somewhat confusing definitions of medicine (e.g., in terms of its knowledge base, the goal of health, the dynamics of the patient-physician relationship), he argues that the patient-physician relationship is constituted by three elements—the fact of illness, the act of profession, and the act of healing—and that it is oriented to the end or *telos* of a right and good healing action for the particular patient.[26]

Collectively and synergistically, the three elements that Pellegrino cites define clinical medicine, distinguishing it from other disciplines and making it an intrinsically moral enterprise. We have already encountered the first constitutive element—the fact of illness—

which accounts, in part, for the imbalance of power inherent in the relationship between a physician and a patient. The second element, the act of profession, is inextricably bound up with the first. The fact of illness testifies to an ontological need, a need that is—like the fact of illness—transhistorical and universal: the need for healing. What the physician (and, indeed, every health care professional) professes and promises by her or his very presence is to heal. With the third element, the act of healing (or the act of medicine), the physician responds decisively to the patient's ontological need, fulfilling the physician's promise to endeavor not just to cure and to care but also to heal. This act of healing is a right and good healing action: It is right for the individual patient, insofar as it is consistent with the canons of sound scientific and technical reasoning and practice, and it is good insofar as it represents the patient's values (and, ideally, those of the physician).

These three elements also have pedagogical implications and significance. Consider the first element: the fact of illness. The pedagogical emphases of traditional, post-Flexnerian medical education are well known and widely criticized: Despite the curricular modifications and innovations of the past decades, the undergraduate medical curriculum continues to stress knowledge and skills for diagnosing, treating, and curing *disease.* In such a context, the fact of illness may serve to broaden the clinical and moral vision of medical students, opening their eyes to dimensions of their patients' problems that cannot be quantified or telescopically compressed into a language purged of all subjective experience. To understand the meaning of a patient's experience of illness, the physician must find access to the patient's unique story of illness—a task that draws on the physician's cognitive and affective (particularly empathic) capacities.

Helping medical students identify the strengths and limits of their cognitive as well as affective capacities should be a component of their ethical education and training, all with the aim of cultivating their capacity to address the problems of disease *and* the problems of illness. Finally, the fact of illness underscores the weight and the content of the moral obligations that physicians bear toward their patients, as well as the *de facto* nature of those obligations—particularly the obligations to respect the dignity of the patient, to be faithful to the patient's trust, and to maintain the confidentiality of the healing relationship.

The act of profession offers the advantage of exploring a cluster of ideas about medical morality, some at odds with each other. Consider the following point/counterpoint. In describing this element, Pellegrino argues, in effect, that this act of profession, this promise to heal, is inherent in the relationship of physician to patient and non-negotiable. In other words, the act of profession provides a conceptual mooring for the argument that the morality of medicine is an *internal* morality. The counterpoint, of course, is the view that this morality is negotiable, subject to the autonomous choices and deliberations of physicians and patients. How does one square this concept of medical morality with the practice of oath-taking or with the various codes of ethics promulgated by the various specialty boards and societies? How does the medical morality embodied in these codes and oaths square with the values that are ingredients of the student's and physician's own senses of medical morality?

These two questions suggest avenues by which medical students could be encouraged to explore their own sense of moral agency. (In this regard, it is interesting to note that organizations such as the American Board of Internal Medicine and the Association of American Medical Colleges have sought to move "professionalism" to center stage in all levels of medical education. These moves reflect a serious concern for the now-threatened survival of the simple but profound idea that certain motivations, obligations, and values help to define medicine, despite radical changes in the socioeconomic landscape of modern health care.) If one assumes that the act of profession is, indeed, understood as a promise to heal, "profession" can also undergird the teaching and learning of morally significant distinctions that apply to curing, caring, and healing.

Consider, lastly, the third element: the act of healing—specifically, a right and good healing action for the particular patient. If the fact of illness expresses definitively human ontological need for healing and if healing entails more than curing and caring—if it requires an empathic engagement with the patient and the ability to collaborate in restoring him or her to health—then this element offers an ideal point of entry into the often dense interweaving of the scientific, the clinical, and the moral in the person of the patient. Insofar as it is *right,* a "right and good" healing action speaks to the cognitive and skill-based resources on which healing depends; insofar as it is *good,* a right and good healing action speaks to the roles of values in the transition of physician and patient from clinical problem-solving and decision making to healing.

NOTES

1. Pedro Lain Entralgo, *Doctor and Patient* (New York: World University Library, McGraw-Hill Book Company, 1969).
2. Ibid., 23.
3. Ibid., 242.
4. Edmund D. Pellegrino and David C. Thomasma, *A Philosophical Basis of Medical Practice: Toward a Philosophy and Ethics of the Healing Professions* (New York: Oxford University Press, 1981).
5. Ezekiel J. Emanuel and Linda L. Emanuel, "Four Models of the Physician-Patient Relationship," *Journal of the American Medical Association* 267 (1992): 2221–26.
6. Ibid.
7. Erich H. Loewy, "Physicians, Friendship, and Moral Strangers: An Examination of a Relationship," *Cambridge Quarterly of Healthcare Ethics* 3 (1994):52–59.
8. Aristotle, *Ethics,* trans. J. A. K. Thomson (London: Penguin Books, 1953).
9. Ibid., 232.
10. Ibid., 231.
11. Ibid., 233.
12. Peta Bowden, *Caring: Gender-Sensitive Ethics* (New York: Routledge, 1997); D. S. Hutchinson, "Ethics," in *The Cambridge Companion to Aristotle,* ed. Jonathan Barnes (Cambridge: Cambridge University Press, 1995), 195–232.
13. Lawrence A. Blum, *Friendship, Altruism and Morality* (London: Routledge & Kegan Paul, 1980), 69.
14. Bowden, *Caring.*
15. Paul Wadell, "Friendship," in *Encyclopedia of Bioethics,* ed. Warren T. Reich (New York: Simon and Schuster, 1995): 888–91.
16. Roberta S. Loewy, "A Critique of Traditional Relationship Models," *Cambridge Quarterly of Healthcare Ethics* 3 (1994): 27–37.
17. H. Tristram Engelhardt, Jr., *Bioethics and Secular Humanism* (Philadelphia, Penn.: Trinity Press International, 1991).

18. Robert Veatch, "Just Social Institutions and the Right to Health Care," *Journal of Medicine and Philosophy* 4 (1979): 170–73.

19. Wadell, "Friendship."

20. Edmund D. Pellegrino and David C. Thomasma, *The Virtues in Medical Practice* (New York: Oxford University Press, 1993).

21. Edmund D. Pellegrino, "Toward a Reconstruction of Medical Morality: The Primacy of the Act of Profession and the Fact of Illness," *Journal of Medicine and Philosophy* 4 (1979): 32–56; Edmund D. Pellegrino, "Being Ill and Being Healed," *Bulletin of the New York Academy of Medicine* 57 (1981): 70–79; Edmund D. Pellegrino, "The Healing Relationship: The Architectonics of Clinical Medicine," in *The Clinical Encounter*, ed. Earl E. Shelp (Dordrecht, The Netherlands: D. Reidel Publishing Co., 1983), 153–72; Edmund D. Pellegrino and David C. Thomasma, *For the Patient's Good: The Restoration of Beneficence in Health Care* (New York: Oxford University Press, 1988); Pellegrino and Thomasma, *The Virtues in Medical Practice*.

22. Howard Brody, *The Healer's Power* (New Haven, Conn.: Yale University Press, 1992).

23. Pellegrino and Thomasma, *For the Patient's Good;* Pellegrino and Thomasma, *The Virtues in Medical Practice*.

24. Pellegrino and Thomasma, *For the Patient's Good*.

25. Pellegrino, "The Healing Relationship."

26. Pellegrino, "Toward a Reconstruction of Medical Morality"; Pellegrino, "The Healing Relationship."

The Dentist as Healer and Friend

Jos V. M. Welie

The dentist as healer and friend: This notion is likely to evoke cynical disbelief among many readers. Surely this must be a jest or mistake. The title of this volume itself— *The Health Care Professional as Friend and Healer*—is itself a bit implausible, but not beyond belief. The imaginative reader can probably picture an amicable, old-style family practitioner who knows inside-and-out the members of the families for whom he or she cares. If a child is ill, the physician hops in the car in the middle of the night and drives out to the farm. If grandpa has died, the doctor comforts and consoles the mourning children. The doctor listens attentively to the anxious secrets of an unfaithful neighbor and gets the insurance company to pay for a bedridden widow's home care. Of course, the physician does not consider himself or herself a true friend of his or her patients—but the patients are convinced the doctor is.

But the dentist? Although the same patients greet the dentist cordially and address him or her as "doctor," inside, they tremble when they see the dentist. The dentist reminds them of their annual check-up. They dread the thorough exams because the dentist always finds something wrong—something that requires drilling. When the dentist greets them in return, all they hear is the high pitch of the drill. Of course, many of them also remember that terrible toothache. If it weren't for the dentist's skillfulness, they would have died of pain. They are grateful for the dentist's expertise and appreciate his or her work. But a friend? Hardly.

A healer, perhaps? Dentists adamantly insist on being called health care providers. They too are doctors—doctors of dental surgery or dental medicine. They too heal patients. Many students applying for dental school (rather than medical school) do so because they believe that a career in dentistry will allow them to actually care for patients (whereas physicians are increasingly engaged in patient management and health care administration—or so dental students believe). Unlike medical specialists who spend less and less time with their patients, dentists laud the close contacts they have with theirs. Yet the idea of "dentist as healer" seems as farfetched an idea as "dentist as friend." The dentist pulls rotten molars, fills cavities, straightens crooked teeth, improves your smile. All of that has little to do with healing, however—or does it?

In view of the foregoing reflections, there seems to be little point in examining this theme of the "dentist as friend and healer" in any greater depth. Yet there is one reason—indeed, a very important reason—to take up this theme. Even if the qualifications of healer and friend seem inappropriate to characterize the dentist at first sight, they present a challenging moral ideal. Precisely because the dentist is narrowly focused on a very small part of the patient's body, there is the ever-present risk of losing sight of the patient as a person. Yet even the act of "drilling and filling" is justified only in view of the personal well-being of the patient. Moreover, because the professional relationship between the dentist and her patient often is driven by commercial interests, it is important that dentists continue to reflect on this relationship in ideal terms.

In this essay, I examine the "self-understanding" of dentistry in terms of both challenges: the dentist as healer and as friend. In the first part, I reflect on the ideal of health care as healing and review the goals of dentistry in that context. In the second part, I examine the multifaceted relationship between dentist and patient and compare this therapeutic relationship to friendship.

THE DENTIST AS HEALER

The Dentist as Fixer

Dentists generally are more likely to be characterized as "fixers" than as healers. This imagery is a relic—at least in part—of the past. Until the nineteenth century, dentists were not considered medical specialists. The trade of pulling teeth was practiced most commonly by barbers (as was, by the way, the trade of surgery). Dental treatments, more often than not, were quite successful: Yanking out a tooth tends to be an effective remedy against even excruciating toothaches. Over time, dentists developed more refined instruments to pull teeth. Yet the intervention itself does not really heal the patient; it is an effective but symptomatic treatment.

Removing carious parts of teeth and filling the resulting cavities—a treatment perfected only with the advent of high-speed drills and applicable amalgams—in some sense heals the patient. Although the original situation is not restored—and, in that sense, the patient is not really cured and made whole again—the restored tooth is functional again and the functional integrity of the human organism is restored. The same can be said of more recent dental interventions such as root canals, crowns, bridges, and veneers. In that sense, dentistry is as much an act of healing as is the removal of a cancerous segment of the intestines, the surgical insertion of a pacemaker, or a hip replacement.

There is one crucial difference, however, between dental interventions and the surgical examples. The dental patient is fully aware of the drilling, hammering, scraping, sucking, cementing, and polishing that is going on in his or her mouth, whereas the surgical patient is usually unaware of the cutting, burning, hammering, sucking, and sewing of his or her body. All the surgical patient knows is that he or she goes into the operating room as a sick person and comes out healed. The surgical patient is oblivious to the orthopedic surgeon's leaning his or her full body weight on the two-foot drill; the patient is unaware of the saw cutting off the top of his or her femur and does not see the screws that hold his or her new hip in place. The dental patient sees it all, however. His or her mouth is held open by an uncomfortable sort of spring; thick threads of floss are forced between his or her molars; rubber dams are pushed into his or her gums; the vibrations of the drill seem to reverberate through his or her jaws and head—in short, his or her teeth are being fixed.

It would be unfair, however, to base our assessment of dentistry solely on patients' perceptions. The interventions of the orthopedic surgeon are at least as manipulative as those of the dentist, even if the patient is not aware of them. In replacing an arthritic hip, the orthopedic surgeon is no more healing the patient's hip than a dentist placing a crown on a cracked tooth is healing the patient's tooth. In neither case is the part itself restored to its original healthy state. Yet the orthopedic patient who once limped badly, barely able to walk more than a few hundred feet, now is once again walking straight, even running. He or she seems truly restored to his or her old self: able to enjoy life, to work, to socialize, to engage in sports. Conversely, the fact that the dental patient returned from the dentist with a new crown will most likely go unnoticed. Unless the patient goes in with a set of crooked and strained teeth and returns with all teeth aligned, bright and shiny, a visit to the dental office seems to have little if any effect on the patient's health.

Again, however, we go off course by assessing the practice of dentistry from the perspective of bystanders. To fairly and accurately assess the role dentists play in maintaining and restoring people's health, we need to look more carefully at the goals of dentistry itself. Only if we examine the practice of dentistry can we assess the extent to which the dentist is—or is not—a healer.

The Goals of Dentistry

Pain relief. Most people visit a dentist only when they are in pain. Clearly, one of the primary goals of dentistry is to relieve toothaches. Although the solution to toothaches for many centuries was—and in many parts of the world continues to be—the unavoidably banal approach of pulling the tooth, the pain itself is not banal. Pain is a debilitating experience. Even if only part of the body hurts, the whole person suffers. Pain—certainly such severe pain as dental conditions typically cause—brings about an existential crisis. A person who is struck by a toothache is figuratively and sometimes literally brought down, knocked out, unable to live life. Such a person is a *patient* in the literal sense of that term: a person who can only be passive, who must submit to and undergo life rather than actively live life.

By relieving toothaches, the dentist allows the patient to take up his or her life again rather than passively undergoing it. Of course, once the pain is relieved and gone, the painful experience and its debilitating consequences tend to be forgotten rather quickly. Hence, the patient may not really perceive and appreciate the dental intervention as an instance of healing. Yet an instance of healing it is. Granted, the tooth had to be pulled, precluding a return to the original state of unblemished health (if such state ever exists). In terms of a person's overall health, however, the loss of a tooth is negligible compared to the existential breakdown caused by the toothache. Once again, the patient can enjoy life, albeit with one natural tooth less. In that sense, the patient is healed.

Toothaches are not the only pains caused by oral malfunction. For example, problems of the temperomandibular joint may result in headaches. A dental infection can spread to a maxillary sinus and result in excruciating facial pain. Although the patient may not consult the dentist at first, these symptoms also may require dental interventions to be relieved.

Restoration of digestive function. A toothache never goes unnoticed. Patients are acutely aware of the problem, and only the true dental phobic will hesitate to visit the dentist when in pain. Toothaches invoke immediate and virtually total debilitation, which demands a prompt response by the dentist. Treatment is often symptomatic; if necessary, a dentist will pull the tooth that causes the pain. A dentist would rather not use such drastic means, however. After all, teeth serve a vital function in sustaining the organism. Few patients are aware of this function of their teeth until they have lost so many that they cannot bite into an apple anymore or chew their food. Only at that moment do patients become aware of the functional importance of their teeth—something they had taken for granted most of their life. Indeed, the teeth are the beginning of the digestive tract. Whereas the lips help us grab food and keep in it our mouth, the teeth actually begin digesting the food by slicing and grinding it. If we did not have molars, vegetables, fruits, nuts, and other essential elements in our diet would be very hard to digest. The same holds for other parts of our oral cavity—the dentist's domain proper—such as our salivary glands, tongue, cheeks and other soft tissues, and jaws holding our teeth and enabling the actual grinding and swallowing movements.

If oral disease precludes the effective digestion or even intake of food, life itself is at stake. Granted, few dentists will ever be involved in cases in which a patient's life is actually threatened by a digestive disorder caused by an oral condition. Even the loss of all of one's teeth does not threaten life in the same acute way as an obstruction of the duodenum. Yet every dentist shares in the responsibility of preventing digestive malfunction. Indeed, the dentist shares in medicine's task of improving people's general health by protecting the digestive function of the mouth. Oral conditions that threaten this function demand a dentist's attention because they decrease the health of the person or even endanger the patient's life. By correcting misalignments, building up broken molars, or placing bridges across missing teeth, the dentist protects and restores the patient's health and thus is engaged in healing.

Fostering respiration. The mouth serves more than one physiological function. Not only is it the beginning of the digestive tract, it is also part of the respiratory tract. The arguments made in reference to digestive malfunctions apply in part to respiratory malfunctions as well. Edema of the tonsils may cause dyspnea; loose objects (including fractured dental prosthetics) can obstruct the airways; a stroke-induced loss of control over one's oral movements can result in inhalation of food, resulting in pneumonia. Again, life-threatening respiratory conditions caused primarily by oral diseases are rare; even less common are life-threatening respiratory conditions to be treated by a dentist (rather than a pulmonologist, otolaryngologist, or oral surgeon). By virtue of his or her skills, however, the dentist shares in medicine's burden of preventing such conditions altogether and improving respiratory functioning generally.

The dentist as diagnostician. The oral cavity is an intrinsic part of the human organism. The mouth is part of the respiratory and digestive tracts. Outer skin and internal epithelium meet in the oral cavity. The anatomy of the oral cavity involves bone, soft tissues, glands, blood vessels, and nervous tissue. In short, many diseases of the body can affect the oral cavity or reveal themselves in the oral cavity. Even if these conditions require treatment by a medical specialist, the dentist may well be the first to notice such conditions in an incipient stage. Whereas a family physician may inspect a patient's mouth only once every other year when the patient has a persistent cold, the dentist is likely to see the same mouth twice a year during regular dental check-ups.

The vigilant dentist may spot a small oral cancer before it becomes life-threatening. Leukoplakia of the mouth may be an early sign of AIDS. Asymmetry in tongue movements may indicate nerve damage or a stroke. Changes in the oral cavity may be symptoms of vitamin deficiencies, hematological disorders, or infections. Moreover, psychiatric and psychosomatic conditions may become visible in the patient's mouth. For example, acidic damage of a young woman's enamel is indicative of anorexia or bulimia, and attrition of teeth may point to anxiety disorder-induced bruxism. In fact, dental conditions (such as fractured teeth) may indicate serious social disorders in the patient's life.

The dentist as speech therapist. Probably the most important existential function of the mouth is speech. Human beings are essentially communicative beings. Although we communicate with one another in many ways, speech is undoubtedly the most important. The inability to speak clearly constitutes a major hindrance to the fulfillment of human life. Poor speech can be a source of significant unhappiness and even grave suffering.

Conditions of the oral cavity can impede clear speech. Though many speech impediments demand the interventions of a professional speech therapist, at times the causes are structural and require the services of a dentist. The orthodontist may have to realign a patient's teeth by means of braces; a lost tooth may have to be bridged or a diastema closed; sometimes, even more radical surgical corrections of the jaws are indicated.

The inability to communicate clearly and the resulting social withdrawal and loneliness are potentially even more serious threats to a human being's well-being and integrity than the most serious of organic diseases. In conjunction with other specialists (e.g., speech therapists, otolaryngologists, or clinical psychologists), the dentist can help patients regain confidence in themselves, along with a sense of ability and wholesomeness.

A matter of taste. There is yet more to the mouth. It allows us to savor the world more fully because it is through our mouth that we can taste the world's bounty of flavors. We do not usually value this sense as much as we value sight, hearing, and touch. (Note that babies only master the sense of touch by way of their mouths; note, too, that our lips continue to do much of our daily touching in life.) Yet the most important social events of our lives—meals—are predicated on our ability to taste. The loss of taste constitutes an important existential loss. Most of the aforementioned diseases, from caries to oral cancer, not only threaten our biological health. They also impede the full enjoyment of our meals. By reversing these diseases, the dentist allows us once again to savor our meals and enjoy a dinner in good company.

The dentist as sex therapist. We express and embody our love for one another via our lips and, more intimately, our tongue and teeth. Almost universally and at all times, the kiss is the most clear and convincing form of lovemaking. Any impediment of the mouth that hinders the act of kissing is therefore a genuine hindrance to the realization and fulfillment of human happiness. By removing impediments from bad breath to painful gingiva, the dentist restores the patient's ability to enjoy the erotic side of human life.

Keeping up appearances. Finally, the mouth is an intrinsic part of the human face. The face is the single most important feature that identifies us for the world. Others recognize us primarily by our face. Our face is copied to identification cards. It is our face—rather than our minds and hearts—that people read and interpret. Although people's reactions to our more peculiar facial characteristics are more indicative of their own emotional and mental immaturity than of our facial imperfections, in the end we may suffer severely as a result of their responses.[1]

The Dentist as Healer

The foregoing reflections suggest that the dentist is not simply catering to patients' wishes. The dentist is truly engaged in healing the patient. Note that in all of the aforementioned examples—pain, disease, speech impediment, loss of taste, inability to kiss, unattractive appearance—it is *not* the peculiar wishes of the patient that constitute the moral obligation on the part of the dentist to treat the underlying conditions. The conditions themselves and the resulting suffering evoke the moral obligation to care and treat. In other words, there are dental "goods" that can be determined independently from patients' subjective and idiosyncratic wishes (even though, as should also be clear from the examples, it will generally be very difficult to discern and specify what those goods exactly are without the patients' input). Although dentists may be tempted—and sometimes give in to the temptation—to cater to patients' preferences, the practice of dentistry is itself a practice of meeting patients' objective needs and hence of healing patients.

THE DENTIST AS FRIEND

A Definition of Friendship

This essay examines two possible characterizations of dentists: the dentist as healer and the dentist as friend. In the preceding section, I have argued that a case can be made for the characterization of the dentist as healer—irrespective of the traditional, and in part justifiable, imagery of dentists as fixers. The dentist as friend, however, is a far more challenging characterization.

We generally dread a visit to the dentist, even though it is for our own good—which would certainly not be true of a visit to our friend. We go because we have no choice (lest we suffer even more). We certainly don't go to please the dentist—which suggests once more that the dentist is definitely not our friend. The dentist does good work, and we appreciate his or her efforts, but the best dental visit is a painless one that lasts five minutes or less. In fact, even the dentist is most satisfied when his or her patient has no need for her services. The shorter the visit, the better for all parties involved. Again, this characterization would not be true of genuine friendship. In sum, it seems paradoxical on all accounts to even consider the dentist as one's friend.

Before we embark on the seemingly pointless task of probing the characterization of the dentist as friend, it should be noted that there is a real problem with characterizing any health care provider—not merely the dentist—as a patient's friend. The problem is twofold:

It is unclear what exactly friendship is, and it is even less clear whether a health care provider can properly be characterized as a friend.

In *A Philosophical Basis of Medical Practice*, Edmund Pellegrino and David Thomasma argue that the clinical interaction between the health care provider and his patient is, among others, a relationship of friendship (p. 64).[2] Pellegrino and Thomasma quote Plato's dialogue devoted to friendship, the *Lysis*, in which Socrates has his partners-in-dialogue agree to the seemingly obvious hypothesis that "The sick man . . . is the friend of the physician" (§218). When the dialogue continues, however, we find that this line of argumentation runs amok, and the dialogue ends with the admission that they have yet to discover what friendship is (§223).[3]

For the sake of argument, I make two assumptions about friendship. First, a friend is another human being who is cherished and held dear because of a familiarity as well as affinity with that person's character and personality. Second, because friendship rests on familiarity and affinity, it is generally mutual. Whereas one person can love another person without the latter loving the former, it would be implausible to say that X is a friend of Y, but Y is not a friend of X. Although true friendship can exist between very different people—rich and poor, old and young, men and women—in most such cases the friendship does not exist because of those differences but in spite of them. Friendship is based on equal respect and respectful equality.

The Therapeutic Relationship

If we grant this definition of friendship, it is immediately evident why the relationship between a health care provider and a patient is unlikely to be one of friendship proper. Because the patient is diseased, sick, vulnerable, dependent, and in need, whereas the caretaker is healthy, able, powerful, independent, and needed, a relationship of true friendship is not really possible.

Codes of medical ethics have prohibited care providers from entering into erotic relationships with their patients for 2,500 years—with good reason.[4] Patients are too dependent on their caregivers and hence too vulnerable to resist advances by their physicians. Moreover, patients must be confident that the most private information they share with their physicians will be used for diagnostic and therapeutic purposes only. Patients also must reveal the most private parts of their bodies to their physicians. If a physician is attracted to his or her patient so much so that the physician cannot resist the temptation to explore an erotic relationship, the therapeutic relationship must be terminated.

Friendship usually does not involve erotic behaviors. Yet friends certainly share life in a much more intimate manner than mere acquaintances or neighbors. Sometimes, friends confide secrets to one another in order to obtain advice—much as they may consult their physician. At other times, we call on our friends simply to be there for us, to listen to our secrets, fears, and pains. Shared sorrow is lessened sorrow. Conversely, shared joy is augmented, so we celebrate the joyful moments of life with our friends. Neither would be true of our physician. We consult the physician because he or she is a medical expert who may be able to give us the kind of specialized advice a layperson cannot. We do not expect from a physician the kind of compassion we expect from our friends; we expect sound, scientific advice. In fact, if our physician becomes too involved in our sorrows, he or she will no longer be able to give us the kind of scientific advice a compassionate friend cannot give. A therapeutic relationship demands a certain emotional distance between patient and caregiver.[5]

This emotional distance is maintained in a variety of ways. Although patients confide their secrets to their physician, a physician—unlike a friend—will not confide his or her secrets to a patient. A physician may share a past personal experience with a patient in an attempt to counsel or console the patient, but patients would feel very uncomfortable if their physicians suddenly were to confide their own ongoing trepidations. Paradoxically, the physician's complete abstention from sharing private information with patients makes the latter sufficiently comfortable to share their own private information with their physician.

This absence of mutuality raises the question how patients come to trust their physicians so that they are willing to confide (i.e., to share in trust) their secrets to their physicians. We trust our friends because they trust us. Mutual trust between true friends grows as they share more of their private lives with one another. Patients, however, continue to share very private things with physicians even though the latter never share even the smallest of private moments with them. In fact, patients confide very private information to physicians they have never before met—total strangers on all accounts. Indeed, the basis of a patient's trust in his or her physician is not the personal familiarity between the two; it is the fact that the physician is a representative of the profession of medicine. The relationship between patient and physician is not one of close friends; it is a distantial relationship between a suffering human being and a professional healer.

A second token of the distance between patient and physician is the bill. Unlike in a friendship, patient and physician are always also related to one another as agents in an economic exchange. The physician does not heal the patient out of the goodness of his or her heart; the physician bills the patient for his or her services. Granted, at times physicians will offer their services for free to indigent patients who cannot afford their expert assistance. Such *pro bono* work, however, is the exception that confirms the rule. Likewise, at times friends will pay one another for a service rendered. As a rule, however, they help one another for free. Not only is the patient the only one volunteering private information while the physician remains a closed book; the patient actually has to pay the physician to listen to those private secrets. Clearly, then, the relationship between patient and physician is a therapeutic relationship, not friendship—let alone love.

If this description is true of the relationship between physician and patient, it should be true *a fortiori* of the dental relationship. Few patients will ever have to confide very sensitive secrets to their dentist. Admitting one's failure to floss daily may be a bit embarrassing, but it is not like admitting that one's gonorrhea was caused by an extramarital affair. Of course, dentists treat AIDS patients; they counsel patients who feel ashamed about their smile (or the lack thereof); and occasionally they may run into cases of physical abuse. As a whole, however, the practice of dentistry is much more distantial than the practice of medicine, nursing, or counseling. Patients do not expect a personal rapport and mutual openness between themselves and their dentists. Among the manifold patient-caregiver relationships, the dental relationship is possibly the clearest example of an economic exchange: The dentist provides a therapeutic service, and the patient pays the bill. Little, it seems, could be gained by recasting this relationship in terms of friendship.

Friendship Versus Professional Altruism

My emphasis on the economic aspects of the patient-caregiver relationship in general and the dental relationship in particular may evoke some frowns. Is it fair and correct to characterize the dental relationship as an economic exchange? Isn't there an element of altruism at the core of this relationship? After all, dentists, like other health care providers, profess to direct their practices at their patients' interests, not at their own interests. By doing so, dentists voluntarily commit themselves to a moral standard that differs from the standard of other, economically motivated service providers.

Indeed, dentists are held to a different standard (even if they do not publicly profess to be[6]). Notwithstanding an increasing emphasis on individual freedom and autonomy on the part of patient and dentist, dentists do not enjoy the kind of liberties other service providers enjoy. Consider the single most important and influential dental-ethical principle: the patient's right to respect for his or her autonomy. Under this right, the dentist is obligated to obtain consent from the patient for proposed treatments prior to intervening. Moreover, the consent to be obtained by the dentist is not simply a freely given consent; it is supposed to be *informed* consent.

At first glance, dentists may not seem too different from other service providers in this regard. Waiters, salespersons, movers, builders, beauty consultants, hair dressers, and interior decorators also must obtain a client's consent prior to providing a service. These service providers, however, are not obligated to inform their customers about the less attractive aspects of their products, cheaper alternatives, or limitations in their own expertise or skillfulness. They certainly are not obligated to give advice *against* using their services or buying their products when they know that their customers don't really need them. They also are not obligated to make referrals to colleagues who may serve their customers better. At times, it may be prudent for a salesperson to suggest a cheaper alternative; it could increase the customer's satisfaction and lead to profitable repeat visits. If the customer is a tourist who will not likely be back, however, the salesperson may recommend the more expensive item. We generally agree that this behavior is ethically justifiable as long as the salesperson does not lie, cheat, or otherwise deceive the customer. The relation is governed by a widespread acceptance that the buyer must "beware."

However, we do not condone a dentist trying to sell the most expensive dental treatment to a patient, particularly not when this patient is a tourist in sudden need of dental care. Apparently, dentists are obligated to look after their patients' best interests by fully informing them even if in doing so they may end up making less money or losing the patient altogether. The altruistic obligation to benefit the patient first and foremost supersedes any and all economic aspects of the patient-dentist relationship.

The practice of dentistry is intrinsically geared toward patients' well-being. Dentistry is not a morally neutral technique that can be applied to any number of goals, catering to the desires of those who pay for these services. Dentistry is necessarily aimed at restoration of the patient's health. Dentists are morally obligated to foster their patients' best interests—not because they are contracted by patients to do so but because such care and concern are at the heart of dentistry.

Dentists are *called to care*. Dentists who—like the priest or the Levite in the parable of the Good Samaritan—simply disregard the needs of their fellow human being, minding their own business instead, actually are not minding their own business. The business of dentistry *is* caring for patients. To be a dentist is to be concerned for people with dental needs.

It seems, then, that there could be some validity in characterizing a dentist as a patient's friend. An essential part of being someone's friend is that one cares for that other person and offers prompt help whenever needed. There is a fundamental difference, however, between the altruistic friend and the altruistic dentist.

All human beings are morally obligated to assist their fellow human beings in need.[7] Friends, however, are morally obligated to make an extraordinary effort on behalf of their friends because such extra effort is part of the definition of being a friend. One cannot be a true friend and not make an effort to give assistance in times of need, regardless of the kind of need. Even if a friend is not capable of relieving those needs effectively, the friend is obligated to stay with his or her friend. After all, *assisting* a person is all about *staying with* or *close by* that person.

As human beings, dentists are called to care for needy fellow human beings. Like any human being, the dentist is called to make a reasonable—not necessarily extraordinary—attempt to assist his or her fellow human being in need. The situation changes, however, if the patient's needs are dental. One is obligated to rescue a drowning person only if one can swim oneself; conversely, the expert swimmer is obligated to also attempt the more difficult and risky rescue operation. Likewise, because of his or her scientific expertise and particular skills, the dentist is morally obligated to offer dental assistance to those in need of such care, whereas the layperson is under no such obligation.

In short, whereas the extraordinary obligation of friends to assist each other is founded on their being friends, it is the dentist's expertise that creates an extraordinary obligation. This extraordinary obligation of dentists exists only to the extent that those in need of assistance have dental needs.

Altruism and Justice

The difference between the altruistic obligation of friends and that of dentists can be further clarified in reference to the principle of justice. Friends are called to make extraordinary efforts to assist their friends precisely because they are friends of one another. In other words, this obligation is always specific for certain people: Friends only have to make an extraordinary attempt to assist their friends, not their enemies. Dentists, however, are obligated to treat even their enemies. This obligation exists because such an extraordinary effort does not depend on a mutual relationship; it depends on the qualities of the dentist. By virtue of being able to effectively heal another person's toothaches, the dentist is obligated to provide that person such help.

If dentists were only obligated to treat their friends, many people would go without dental care. If dentists were obligated to treat only the people they love, even fewer patients would be healed. Dentists are obligated, however, to assist anybody in need of their expert services—their "own" patients, as well as those who are new to the dentist's office but in bad pain.

Of course, that obligation is not absolute and unlimited. Dentists have only two hands and limited time. As a practical matter, it is impossible to treat anybody and everybody in dental need. A dentist's primary obligation is toward his or her own patients. If a dentist has started to treat one person, the dentist may not abandon that patient to treat a new patient even if the latter patient is in greater need or would benefit more from the dentist's care. Such abandonment would undermine the fiduciary relationship between dentists and patients. On the other hand, dentists may not devote all of their time and resources to a select number of patients and completely disregard the dental interests of other patients. If an all-out investment in a select number of patients leaves other patients without even basic dental care, dentists have failed properly to balance their obligations to those in need.

The dentist's duty to treat persons in need, irrespective of *whose* patients they are, is properly understood as a professional duty. Dentists are jointly responsible to assist patients in need of dental care. This burden would become unbearable if only a minority of dentists end up with all the indigent patients. In fact, those few dentists would go bankrupt very quickly. Dentists are jointly responsible to guarantee that all of their fellow human beings in need of basic dental care, not just their friends, have access to such care; at least, dentists must jointly strive towards that ideal.

Dentists have an obligation to treat patients in need even if they pose an economic risk. In fact, dentists carry an even heavier burden. They also have to treat patients who pose a health risk to their own health. Although dentists are not expected to sacrifice their lives for the good of their patients, they are expected to accept a certain degree of risk to their own health. A dentist may not refuse to treat patients suffering from infectious diseases such as tuberculosis, hepatitis, or HIV merely because they pose a risk to the dentist's own health.

Once more, this obligation at first sight seems perfectly analogous to the duty of friends to come to the rescue of their friends when the latter are in need, even if such rescue entails risks to their own health and well-being. Friends are expected to take such risks because that is what beings friends is all about. Again, however, friends are expected to do so only for their friends, not for anybody in need. On the other hand, the dentist is required to assist anyone in need, including the HIV-seropositive patient. (Rather, dentists are jointly responsible to take care of HIV-positive patients and others who pose a health risk to their caretakers.) This professional obligation is shared by all dentists.

Although every dentist is obligated in principle to treat every patient in dental need—except when such treatment poses an unusually severe risk to the dentist's own health, life, and well-being—the duty to treat is an obligation shared by all dentists. Dentists are jointly responsible for the health of patients, so they must each assume an equal burden. If some dentists begin to refuse to treat infectious or indigent patients, their colleagues end up with a disproportionate risk.

The Dentist as Friend Revisited

The foregoing reflections lead us to conclude that the analogy between the dental relationship and friendship is flawed for the most part. The duties of dentists toward their patients are not grounded in a personal and mutual relationship. Rather, they are grounded in the needs of the patient on the one hand and the expertise of the dentist on the other. Only if a dentist retains a certain distance (as opposed to friendly affection) toward the patient can the dentist be an effective healer. Moreover, the friendship analogy could suggest that dentists carry responsibilities toward their "own" patients only: patients they have selected because they like those patients. The friendship model, therefore, is at odds with the principle of justice: Dentists carry a shared responsibility to care for all patients in need, not simply those they like.

Conflicting Roles for the Dentist

The dentist relates to the patient as a professional care provider, not as the patient's friend. In this regard, the differences between dentists and other health care providers are probably quite small. There is, however, one aspect of the dental relationship that is much more pronounced and deserves our attention. Unlike most physicians and nurses, dentists tend to work as sole practitioners or in small group practices. Although the days of a simple fee-for-service payment system are over for most dentists—as they have been long since for physicians—dentists tend to operate (and have to operate) their professional practices as private businesses.

The economic aspect of the caregiver-patient relationship does not necessarily undermine a professional, fiduciary relationship. It does entail a conflict of interest for the dentist. If the dentist's material well-being (and that of the dentist's family) depends on whether the dentist treats (or, in case of capitated payment, does not treat) the patient, the dentist's clinical decision making is inevitably influenced by those economic considerations.

As a professional healer, the dentist will be most satisfied when his or her patients do not or no longer require the dentist's interventions. The dentist is supposed to heal patients, not create needs. As a businessperson, however, the dentist must maximize profit margins by selling his or her services. Many dentists will not shy away from actually creating needs—not by harming patients and then healing them but by persuading patients that a particular imperfection should be treated. Indeed, treatment for purely esthetic reasons constitutes an increasing part of many dental practices.

In and of itself, a commercial relationship is not necessarily unfair, provided both individuals in such a relationship are able to relate to one another as commercially motivated and astute business partners. Patients, however, do not relate to dentists as free buyers of an optional service or good. Dental patients are in need—in very serious need, indeed, if they suffer from a toothache. They do not have the liberty of shopping around for the best deal, postponing treatment, or even forgoing the service altogether. They depend on their dentist. The dentist holds all the cards.

As professional healers, dentists are obligated not to abuse their competitive advantage over their patients. In an increasingly competitive world, however, the temptation to sell dental services that patients really do not need becomes hard to resist. If all other dentists in town take the entrepreneurial route, what choice does the individual dentist have but to become an entrepreneur as well? Limitations on entrepreneurship that were once enforced by the profession of dentistry itself are disappearing. In recent decades, several countries have lifted bans on advertising by dentists. In the late 1970s, the American Dental Association was forced to withdraw its ban on advertising when the Federal Trade Commission deemed that such a ban hindered competition—which, of course, it was intended to do all along.

Many authors have pointed out that a commercial model of dentistry is at odds with a professional model; at the very least, combining both models into one harmonious practice is a very challenging task for dentistry—and even more for the individual dentist.[8] If there is any role for friendship in the dental relationship, it may be to serve as a bridge between the two models. Neither commercial relationships nor professional relationships are analogous to friendships. Consequently, substituting either model with the friendship model, or merging the two into a friendship model, is not likely to be successful and effective. Nonetheless, when the dentist's professionalism leads him or her toward unjustified paternalism, the friendship paradigm may remind the dentist of the importance of communication and interaction with the patient, while keeping the dentist from embracing a purely commercial model (as if commercial relationships are the only interactive relationships). Conversely, if the dentist's commercial interests tempt the dentist to put his or her own needs ahead of those of the patient, the friendship paradigm may remind the dentist of his or her altruistic calling, yet also keep the dentist from embracing a purely professional model (as if only professionals are called to care). Dentists and their patients are not friends, but the therapeutic relationship can be strengthened and enriched by drawing from that marvelous human virtue called friendship.

EPILOGUE

The conclusion seems inevitable: The dentist is not the patient's friend. At first, this conclusion seems very unfortunate. To be a non-friend seems to be the same as being unfriendly—that is, uncaring. I hope to have shown that the latter equation does not hold. Dentists are not their patients' friends, even though they have their patients' interests at heart, because the model of friendship does not do justice to the essence of the therapeutic relationship between dentist and patient. The dentist is a healer—but not a friendly healer. The dentist is a professional healer.

NOTES

1. Jos V. M. Welie, "'Do You Have a Healthy Smile?' Ugliness as a Medical Indication for Dental and Surgical Cosmetic Treatment," *Medicine, Health Care and Philosophy: A European Journal* 2 (1999): 169–80.
2. Edmund D. Pellegrino and David C. Thomasma, *A Philosophical Basis of Medical Practice* (New York/Oxford: Oxford University Press, 1981).
3. Plato, *Lysis,* trans. B. Jowett, in *The Dialogues of Plato* (Chicago/London: Encyclopedia Britannica Inc., 1952).
4. American Dental Association, *Principles of Ethics and Code of Professional Conduct* (Chicago: American Dental Association, 1999). Although the ADA's present *Code of Ethics* does not prohibit such relationships, this is a serious and undesirable void. The modern relationship between dentist and patient continues to be one of unequals, the principle of respect for autonomy notwithstanding.
5. Pellegrino and Thomasma, *Philosophical Basis of Medical Practice,* 86–87. Pellegrino and Thomasma discuss Plato's *Lysis* to prove that there is a necessary link between medicine and friendship. Presumably, healing takes place by means of a friendship or *philia*. It seems to me, however, that Plato's reference to medicine in the *Lysis* is ontological rather than ethical in nature. Socrates is trying to discover the logical object of friendship. He invokes medicine as an analogical example: A diseased body needs health; health is the

object of medicine; hence medicine (or physicians impersonating this practice of healing) is dear to us. It is in this ontological sense that the physician (or rather, medicine) is
the friend of the sick man (or rather, the diseased body).

6. Unlike graduates of medical schools, many dental school graduates do not swear a public oath underscoring professional altruism.

7. Jos V.M. Welie, *In the Face of Suffering: The Philosophical-Anthropological Foundations of
Clinical Ethics* (Omaha, Neb.: Creighton University Press, 1998).

8. David T. Ozar, "Three Models of Professionalism and Professional Obligations in Den-
tistry," *Journal of American Dental Association* 110 (1985):173–77; David T. Ozar and
D. J. Sokol, *Dental Ethics at Chairside: Professional Principles and Practical Applications*
(St. Louis: Mosby, 1994).

Learning through Experience and Expression: Skillful Ethical Comportment in Nursing Practice

Patricia Benner

Nursing practice is a public extension of the ordinary care of family and self in everyday life.[1] When people are critically and gravely ill, family members can become overwhelmed by the emotional and physical labor of caregiving, and nurses can support and extend the caregiving resources of the family. During times of transition such as birth or the care of an elderly parent or ill partner, nurses can assist with the new adaptations to caregiving required.

Florence Nightingale envisioned the work of the nurse as placing the body in the best condition for repair and recovery.[2] In the West, nursing has developed as a moral tradition within the Judeo-Christian tradition of the Good Samaritan or compassionate stranger.[3] Nursing has also developed as a public extension of women's role of caregiving in the home for family members and neighbors. Institutional care was given special impetus during the industrial revolution in the United States, when men migrated to jobs, ahead of their families (women caregivers), and lived in crowded tenement houses—where the environment itself was hazardous to health.[4]

Nurse-philosopher Kari Martinsen, drawing on the work of philosopher Knud Logstrup, claims that caring for others is a response to the fundamental or sovereign life expressions of trust, mercy, solidarity, love, frankness, and fidelity given at birth.[5] This position does not regard human will or ethical decision making as primary moral sources or motivation for responding to the other; but it asserts that a fundamental trust is given and demanded of all human beings as central to being human by reason of their birth. Trust is more basic than mistrust. This is especially evident during times of illness and vulnerability, when one must surrender his or her life into the care and trust of others. No one escapes the necessity of trust in human existence.[6] This position bears a resemblance to the work of Levinas, who points to the human face and to touch as primordial demands to respond to the other.[7] Such a vision places knowing and meeting the other as a central condition of being human.

This essay focuses on nurses' experiential learning of *phronesis* (clinical and ethical reasoning about the particular across time), moral agency, relational skills of involvement, and the capacity to make qualitative distinctions. The position I take on experiential learning draws on eight years of research into the clinical learning and knowledge of a total

sample of 205 critical care nurses.⁸ I also address philosophical questions about how skillful
ethical comportments in particular helping relationships can be taught or learned.

Nursing work has been transformed as advances in medical science have required
new caregiving skills and new social and physical environments to render technical cures
safe (e.g., hospitals, surgical suites, intensive care units, homes, schools, and other community sites). Nurses extend the practice of medicine; they also translate and bridge the gap between prescribed cures and the working out of those cures in daily life. With the advent of
surgical procedures and life-sustaining medical technologies, caregiving has become more
technical and complex, requiring more knowledge of medical sciences. Yet this technical
medical knowledge can never replace daily caregiving sustenance of the self and family,
however constituted. The goal of medicine and nursing is to make the person independent
of technical interventions. In this way, it returns the person to the usual daily care required
for health and sustenance. A maxim of intensive-care nurses is that "if you are not helping
with mechanical ventilation, you are almost always hurting."⁹ Through the work of Florence Nightingale and other less well-known nurses, nursing has developed within the bureaucratic institutions of the hospital, the church, and the military tradition of caring for
the sick and wounded in battle. The current trend in our market-driven health care system
is increasingly moving technical care into the home.

Caregiving may be considered a public and private practice, where practice is defined as a socially organized set of skills, intents, and relationships with internal notions of
good.¹⁰ Caregiving as a practice is embedded in a moral community of practitioners who
must learn relational and technical aspects of caring for particular persons or communities.
Nursing practice requires both *phronesis* and *techné*. The demands of *phronesis* encompass
practical judgment and wisdom about action and relationship in the particular situation
across time. *Techné* refers to the skill and technique of applying medical and nursing technologies. Consequently, skillful ethical comportment in nursing requires the development
of emotional attunement, discernment, and relational skills with particular patients/fami-
lies/communities, as well as astute clinical judgment about the administering of highly
technical medical interventions.¹¹

Because the ultimate goal of nursing is to restore the person to his or her usual level
of independence and repair the disruptions caused by the illness or injury, nursing's goal
cannot be defined as making things or "achieving" health.¹² Nursing practice cannot be
broken down into techniques to be applied through rational calculation; it must be delivered in an engaged, thinking way to enable the nurse to act creatively and responsibly in
particular caregiving relationships. This is the distinction between *techné*, the making of
things, and skillful ethical comportment in a practice. As Dunne points out:

> When a craftsperson "acts" on suitable materials in order to produce an artifact
> which is comfortably within his or her proficiency, there is a predictability about
> success which is commensurate with this proficiency itself. However, when one's ac-
> tions are not imposed on materials but are directed toward other persons, such mas-
> tery is not attainable. One cannot determine in advance the efficacy of one's words
> and deeds. Efficacy turns out to be a form of influence; it lies not so much in one's
> own operation as in the cooperation of others. The nature and extent of this cooper-

ation cannot be counted on beforehand, and even afterwards one cannot be sure just what it has been.[13]

Caregiving relationships may open possibilities, or close them down. Even with the best intent and comportment, however, the person being cared for may not be able to respond to care. "Outcomes" in caregiving relationships are necessarily interdependent and mutual. Moreover, not all types of influence are morally acceptable. Manipulation, coercion, or misuse of professional influence in persuading a patient to accept a treatment are unethical. Consequently, when things go well, and the patient or family is able to respond to caring practices, the practitioner cannot attribute the good outcome solely to the efficacy of some technique he or she may have used.

The current focus on "prespecified outcomes" and identifying and evaluating nursing outcomes (case management) is based on the premise that only technique is involved in health care—that one knows the outcomes to expect and that all things can be "fixed." The situation is further complicated by institutional resources or constraints to good caregiving. Meeting and responding to the other may clash with the bureaucratic goals of care for the many in the most cost-efficient manner. For all these reasons, developing moral agency and skills of involvement presents ongoing demands for experiential learning and character development. Viewing nursing as a basic human encounter and as a practice requiring *phronesis* has major implications for nursing education and the moral development of practitioners.[14]

The ethical demands of excellent nursing practice entail that the other be met as an individual, family, or community. From an "outside-in" perspective, or the perspective of learning reliable techniques, the teacher and learner of such a practice are confronted with the impossibility of imagining all the skills and virtues that might be required for all possible nursing care relationships. In philosophy, this problem is called the limits of formalism—the problem of making explicit and elemental aspects of common sense everyday skillful comportment in complex worlds.[15] From a de-situated philosophical world, one imagines that the person is a container and possessor of knowledge that is gathered up and applied in specific situations.

In traditional Western philosophy, virtues and knowledge possessed by the individual are applied to the particular situation, and only this thoughtful, willful use of knowledge qualifies as knowledge and virtue. Such a causal model is static; it cannot account for the possibilities created by emotional attunement, relationship, and skilled action. A technical view of character holds that it is possessed by the individual and carried to the passive situation where it is applied.[16] This technical view of virtue and knowledge overlooks how one perceives and encounters the particular situation with its particular demands and possibilities. How one learns and teaches skillful ethical comportment in a variety of particular situations gets off to pretentious and abstract beginnings because everyday skilled ethical performance is overlooked.

The teacher and learner assume that the learner will recognize when a situation calls for virtue X and knowledge Y and Z and that the learner can choose from an internal virtue menu—or a decision-supported infrastructure—the wisdom and compassion required by the situation.[17] The focus is on justifying decisions, adjudicating between right choices. Relationship, attunement, skillful comportment, moral perception, and action take a back seat to decision making, rational calculation, and justification in this school of moral teaching and learning. Curiously enough, even the "problem-solving process" focuses on solving pre-identified problems in moral dilemmas or clinical case studies. Sorting out which problems are most salient, problem perception and identification, and making qualitative distinctions within the problem tend to be deemphasized in favor of procedures of classifying the relevant principles or identifying the relevant knowledge and virtue components in the identified problem.[18]

An alternative perspective is a thinking-in-action or skill-oriented approach that draws on everyday skilled ethical comportment. This approach focuses on experiential learning. Experiential learning opens new possibilities for nurses to meet and care for the other, so that nurses literally see new issues and concerns as they develop in their practice. Nursing is so thoroughly a practice discipline that even *techné* (that which can be rationally calculated) depends on *phronesis*—reasoning about the particular across time through transitions in the nurse's and patient's understanding and through transitions in the patient's or family's condition.[19] *Phronesis* also depends on a caring relationship. Caring sets up the conditions of possibility for meeting the other so that identification and expression of concerns and possibilities can occur.[20] This approach is similar to the Kierkegaardian[21] and Rosensweig[22] "common sense" approach:

> The thinking subject is not an abstract being; mind and consciousness cannot be understood mathematically. Common sense regards individual human existence with utter seriousness. Here the "thinking individual" is personally involved both in the question and in the answer; his thinking does not concern his mind only but has an existential relevance.

Birth, suffering, sickness, recovery, and dying are human experiences laden with existential relevance. Sickness causes a rupture in the familiar human world. The social, sentient, skillful embodied person dwells in habits, skills, practices, concerns, and relationships that constitute and respond to a life-world. The embodied person also may fall ill or be injured, making the familiar world fall away. The familiar human world pulls and beckons the ill person toward recovery. Caregiving in nursing entails recognition practices that support the patient's or family's recovery of familiar worlds and the repair of ruptured meanings. In a pluralistic society, this practice requires that the nurse recognize the patient's or family's particular life-world. Caregiving works within the possibilities already inherent in the person's embodiment and world. Caregiving practices include physical comfort care and nurturance for growth and recovery; these practices are relational. Thus, nurses' clinical judgments and interventions cannot be separated from notions of good drawn from the patient's and family's life-world. Therefore, skillful ethical comportment in nursing requires relationships, skills of involvement, and moral agency that enable the nurse to meet and respect the patient and family in particular illness and life situations.

THE DEVELOPMENT OF SKILLS OF INVOLVEMENT AND MORAL AGENCY

Skills of interpersonal involvement and problem engagement reflect the emotional labor of nursing. Nurses must be able to engage with the patient's plight to be with suffering patients, advocate on their behalf, or engage in pain infliction caused by technical procedures. In Kant's traditional view, moral agency deals with will and intellect to make uncoerced free choices. Perception, relationship, action, embodied skilled know-how, and sentience are all but left out of a Kantian view of agency. However, it becomes clear that capacities for moral agency in particular situations depend on the person's ability to meet and acknowledge the other. It is clear from observing nurses' practice and from reading first-person accounts of clinical practice that the capacities for moral agency change with experiential learning.

What the nurse discerns as possible depends on experientially learning the skills of interpersonal involvement and problem engagement. For example, the novice nurse experiences practice as a task world. The nurse's skills of involvement may be poorly adjusted to the emotional labor and demands of nursing practice, so that the nurse over-identifies or under-identifies with the patient's situation. The beginning nurse uncritically and unreflectively brings skills of involvement from his or her everyday life. These skills of involvement must be critically examined, and the role of the compassionate and intimate "stranger" must be learned experientially from patient and family encounters and from reflection on practice.

The interpersonal skills of engagement may be understood spatially as standing too close or too far away in a particular patient/family situation. For example, nurses learn to be available without being intrusive, presumably by seeing or engaging in emotional availability or openness and emotional unavailability. This approach is illustrated in one nurse's account of caring for a dying man and his family in the intensive care unit. The patient is unconscious and dying, and his wife is lying next to him, holding him as he dies:

> I stayed just outside the room most of the time, but I'd come in to see, just to touch the wife and put a wet washcloth on her forehead. She had asked that the rest of the family come in, but not to stay, so I went to get them and brought them and asked them not to stay for too long because she wanted this time pretty much alone with him. Yet once they got there, it seemed like the proper thing to do. They didn't want to leave right away, so they stayed longer. But they finally pulled themselves together and went out and left her alone with him. But then they came back and they hung out in the hallway. But I always was within sight of her and sound of him. And I'd come in and out. . . . She had a lot of support, but she wanted a lot to be alone with him, so people just sat back and were quiet mostly until afterwards. . . . If they could, they [nurse managers] create nursing time to be able to do that, which to me is real important. It's just as important as a code or anything else. It all goes together. I don't know how to explain how you know. I just know that she didn't really want me there all the time at the bedside, but that she appreciated that if there was anything she needed I would have gotten it for her.[23]

Historically, nursing literature shows changing patterns in emotional expression and labor. For example, with the advance of surgical and medical interventions at the beginning of the twentieth century, the pendulum swung to professional detachment and objectivity as a sign of expert knowledge.[24] During the past thirty years, the nursing literature has increasingly pointed to the centrality of emotional engagement and the emotional labor of nursing practice. In research my colleagues and I have found that developing the skills of involvement determined whether the nurse could go on to develop expertise.[25] This finding is logical because skills of interpersonal involvement and problem engagement determine the nurse's perceptual acuity and possibilities of developing nurse-patient relationships.

Nurses talk about the importance of knowing the patient, following the body's lead, and protecting a patient's life.[26] The particular historical relationship with the patient sets up possibilities. This factor is illustrated in the following nursing narrative:

> We had a patient who was having unstable angina. He had multiple M.I.'s [myocardial infarctions] and a poor ejection fraction, and he came in with chest pain and unstable angina. He was totally mentally alert and coherent for two days. And he was being tended to by a loving family, very giving. On Sunday night he had deteriorated and required a lot of lasix for flash pulmonary edema. He got an A-line, he was on nitro (nitroglycerine), and doing fair. I came in on Monday morning, and there was a new nurse who was on and I was asked to back her up. So I went in with her after I had done the assessment of my patient; I'd gone in with her and was helping her get organized for the day. She was busy calculating her drips and looking at her A-line and pressure tubing and everything. And I attended to the patient. And I brushed his teeth and his dentures and washed his glasses, and he asked me for some toast and tea, and I went and got that. When I came back, he said, "Before I have this, will you get my shaving kit?" And I got his shaving kit, and he had a prayer in there that he said every day, and he said, "I want to say my prayer." I knew the prayer, and I said it with him. And he thanked me and said, "I have been saying this prayer every day for a long time, and I've been saying it even more frequently now that I know that I'm very sick." And he was sharing that he was not really afraid of death and he felt strong even though he was very sick. That day he went into flash pulmonary edema and required intubation, so . . . he was not doing very well. He was very agitated with his endotracheal tube and required fentanyl and he wasn't pavulonized [paralyzed], but he did require a lot of fentanyl and ativan. Then I was off for a couple of days, and by the time, two days later, when I came on duty, the same nurse was taking care of him and I was asked again to back her up. And he was still intubated, but by this time he was made a DNR [do not resuscitate]. I guess his family and he had extensive talks [about death] prior to this admission but didn't really realize how imminent it was. And so he was a DNR and that day I helped the other nurse in the morning. And she was doing all her drips and everything. And I pulled out his shaving kit, and I got his prayer and I said his prayer to him. And he was lucid enough to know that I was saying it. He held my hand, and he obviously couldn't say it with me because he was still intubated, but he held my hand and nodded his head when I was finished. And that day he died. And it was just very moving to know that on his last day I prayed with him.[27]

This nurse-patient relationship is particular and historical. The nurse does what she sees and understands. Logstrup has pointed out the problem of making ethics a matter primarily of decisions rather than action and relationship.[28] The ethical decision, for example, to withdraw heroic therapies has no more moral import than the actions and care that surround the actual withdrawing of therapies. The relationship sets up the conditions of possibility for action and decision. All three aspects—relationship, decision, and action—are of equal moral import.

PHRONESIS AND CLINICAL REASONING ACROSS TIME ABOUT THE PARTICULAR

The development of *phronesis* (skills of practical reasoning and wisdom in concrete clinical situations) is experientially learned. Consequently, the actual or effective moral agency of the nurse necessarily differs for beginning and expert nurses. Another way to say this is that the nurse's actual moral agency can never be beyond experiential learning and acting in concrete clinical situations. This stance differs from the Kantian vision of moral agency as the intentional and free will of the moral agent.[29] Bringing action and relationship into the moral equation requires an examination of actual moral agency embedded in the particular relationship and situation. Consideration of the particular can reflect an instantiation of commonly held notions of good, as well as living out instances of rights and responsibilities. Because engagement and action in particular encounters are central to good practice, teaching context-free principles and rational calculation about entitlements, responsibilities, and rights, though helpful, are not sufficient. Practice of engagement in particular nurse-patient relationships and opportunities to reflect on the skills of engagement and ethical responses to suffering and vulnerability are necessary for learning excellent caring practices and ethical comportment.

The following nursing narrative, written by a graduate nursing student in a class about ethics and nursing theory, illustrates the use of narrative to capture experiential knowledge and to articulate notions of good in practice:

The Courage to Love, by Anne Tsolinas

When I returned from my house calls that day, the referral was on my desk: "Nineteen-year-old, unmarried primipara [first-time mother] living with the father of baby and raising his two sons ages six and four . . . gavaging breast milk, supplies at home." I remember thinking, "nothing unusual" and continued reading. Then I saw the diagnosis. "Anencephaly, mom wishes to have the baby die at home."

My head was spinning. How could this be? I was used to getting the referrals for high-risk infants and mothers, since that was my specialty, but the prospect of caring for this child left me shaken.

Gathering myself, I quickly left a message for the obstetrician to call me. I then called the nurses in the postpartum unit to get their sense of the situation. Those directly involved in the case couldn't be reached, and those not directly involved had kept their distance. I needed to get answers—and to get my bearings. I needed something, anything, to guide me in the awful task at hand. Yes, I had already decided it would be an awful task.

I was able to locate the pediatric resident, and asked him what I could expect. Since he didn't know this infant, he advised me about all the possible physical deformities I *might* encounter. Perhaps the infant would have eyes in the wrong place or one eye or none. He couldn't advise me, though, on how to care for the child in the home setting. We were in uncharted territory.

I waited until the last possible moment to call to make the appointment for the following day. When I spoke to the child's mother, she was pleasant. She told me she just had some questions about breast milk and feedings. I was relieved that she had questions for which I had answers, but what about the questions that might arise for which I would have no answers?

That night I read everything I could find on anencephaly. Unfortunately, all the information ended at birth in the hospital. I had no pictures to prepare me. How would I cope with a terribly deformed infant? What could I do to help? What if the parents found out I didn't have all the answers? The unknown scared me.

The next morning, before I knocked on the family's door, I uttered a quick prayer, asking that they be protected from my inadequacy and that I somehow be of help. I knocked; a moment later I was greeted by a darling young woman with a clear, bright smile. This must be Jennifer, the baby's mother. She was radiant, as are many primiparas. She told me the baby was asleep, and we had time to talk. I was relieved. I could get to know Jennifer and ease myself into the assignment. As we talked, I observed her appearance and looked for anything unusual. I found nothing and surmised she was in denial. Now I had a handle on it, a path I could follow.

Then she said, "And, oh, yes, her exposed brain is really starting to smell awful. What can I do?" I had surmised wrong. She wasn't in denial. Where was my path now? As the words "Well, let's take a look and see what we can do" came out of my mouth, I wished I could run and be anywhere else.

Jennifer brought out baby Emily, beautifully dressed and groomed except for the smell. Jennifer cuddled her, kissed her, then handed her to me, saying, "She doesn't look so bad, does she?" And in that moment, as I held this baby, who was loved and cared for, she really didn't look so bad. Her mother's love made her lovable. One person taking the chance, brave enough to love Emily, opened the doors. What would this drama teach me? I was still in uncharted territory.

I examined Emily. Much of her body was abnormal, and she had a high-pitched, weak cry, but she responded like any other baby to her mother's tender touch and voice. She rooted when her cheek was stroked, and she grasped with her one functional hand. She accepted the gavage feedings and made feeble attempts to suck. Jennifer cared for Emily with the attention and compassion any mother in love would. But this wasn't any baby. This was a baby with an exposed, rotting brain that smelled bad.

I went off to search through the supplies I kept in the trunk of my car to devise some sort of dressing. (Somehow, with my head buried in the trunk, I usually could gather my thoughts enough to tackle problems for which there were no clear solutions.) I returned composed, with Neosporin, normal saline, and plenty of Kerlex in hand, ready to dress the brain.

In the days to come, I dealt with Emily's physical needs as they arose. Her exposed brain still smelled. One day I remembered that honey applied to particularly foul decubitus ulcers [bedsores] had reduced their odor. Would it work on a rotting brain? We tried it.

Jennifer had physical needs as well. She was one week post-vaginal delivery and pumping breast milk. The stress began to take its toll; her episiotomy didn't hold, and she developed mastitis. She was sleep-deprived and emotionally spent. She didn't smile as easily, and her radiance was waning. Her spirit, however, was sustained by her desire to take in every precious moment she might have with her daughter. She knew time was running out.

As Emily's condition declined, the activity in the household increased. The two young boys acted out their feelings. Emily's dad didn't say much. Friends and family came and went, eager to be supportive but not knowing what to do. And in the midst of this commotion, Emily was dying.

I searched my mind for all the nursing knowledge and expertise I had acquired. I dealt with the family's physical and emotional needs. I offered advice on issues relating to the children. I made referrals and directed willing volunteers into purposeful activity. I discussed with Jennifer and her partner what to do when Emily died, who to call, and how to arrange for the funeral. Although I had much nursing knowledge to offer this family, the family had much to offer me. I was the student in a place I had never known before in either nursing practice or life. I watched and listened as this young mother taught me what I did not know.

Amid all the activity, Jennifer began to tell me her story. She told me about the thrill she felt on learning she was pregnant. She recalled her feelings of devastation when the obstetrician told her, in her fourth month of pregnancy, that her baby had anencephaly and her sadness when the physician scheduled an abortion. And she told me about the wonder she felt when, a week later, Emily kicked for the first time. At that moment, she decided to have the child. "I didn't think the baby would be able to move, but when I felt her kick, I knew she was alive. After that, I just wanted to give her a chance to live and experience her mother's love."

Jennifer spoke of her frustration with the medical profession, beginning with her obstetrician's negative reaction to her desire to continue the pregnancy. The obstetrician told her, "You are going through a no-headed pregnancy. There is no hope, and I won't do it." It was a reaction she experienced again and again as she searched for someone willing to support her decision. Only one physician would take her as a patient; she admired him for that.

Jennifer described the sense of "abandonment" she felt when, after giving birth to Emily, the postpartum nurses cloistered her and the baby in a single-patient room. Jennifer felt that the nurses didn't know what to do for her or Emily because, unlike most infants with anencephaly, Emily lived. She hadn't planned to bring Emily home, but she couldn't leave her daughter in the hands of nurses who seemingly didn't care. She couldn't bear the thought of her daughter dying alone and unattended in a hospital bassinet. Jennifer would care for her daughter at home until the end. Emily's last moments on earth would be filled with her mother's love.

Meanwhile, the honey was working. Emily's brain didn't smell as bad. However, her diaper hadn't been damp in days. We weren't sure if she was experiencing any discomfort, but to be on the safe side, we gave her Tylenol suppositories around the clock. She wasn't crying anymore.

I marveled at this young mother's courage to love and keep on loving in the face of her daughter's certain death. Peace seemed to come over little Emily when she was in her mother's arms. Now in her tenth day, Emily had lived far longer than anyone ever imagined possible. But Jennifer knew their time together was short and wanted a lock of Emily's hair. At the nape of Emily's neck was a small tuft of strawberry-blond hair. I helped Jennifer wash and cut the tiny tuft of hair, the one physical piece of her daughter she could keep. We then preserved it in Emily's baby book.

The call to my home came at 2:30 in the morning. It was Emily's father; she had died. I could hear Jennifer wailing in the background. "She is holding her and rocking her," the father said. "Can we have more time with her before the mortuary picks her up?" In the wee hours of the morning, I made the necessary arrangements.

A few weeks later, Emily's unique story hit the local papers. Jennifer shared with the reporter facts about her pregnancy and Emily's birth. She explained her wish to take the baby home. There was no mention in the article about Emily's ten days at home or the effort it took to allow her to die there. It only noted that it was Emily who sustained Jennifer during that time. And though it wasn't mentioned in the article, it was Jennifer's love and Emily's response that made my nursing care possible.[30]

This narrative demonstrates experiential learning and ethical comportment. Dilemmas might be raised, but not without considering the notions of good encountered in the narrative. The concrete and particular relationship supplants the abstract. Moral imagination is created as Ann Tsolinas responds to Jennifer and Emily. This particular narrative was selected for presentation to the whole class and with the author's became part of the text of the class; it also was published in the *American Journal of Nursing*.[31] In the process, we learned that knowledge development occurs in the practice of nursing, not just in textbooks.

PHRONESIS IN EDUCATION

My colleagues and I have used nursing narratives from particular situations that contained ethical demands for meeting and responding to the other person; we structure the classroom discussion around these open-ended, unfolding narratives.[32] We ask students to bring in relevant aspects of the assigned readings to bear on the unfolding situation being discussed. Even though the student is able to read ahead and find out the outcome to the narrative, this approach allows for a discussion of inherent ambiguities in the actual situation and encourages identification of ethical concerns in the unstructured situation. Students can identify the nurse's moral agency in the particular situation and expand their own moral imagination about the ethical issues arising from the particular situation.

In addition to the pre-selected nursing narratives we use to structure the seminar discussions, we ask students to generate their own narrative examples from their nursing practice. The teachers read these narratives; then, with any needed clarification—and with permission from the students—they are duplicated for the whole class to read. This method encourages students to generate texts of their own experiential learning. Students are taught to reflect on the narratives using an "inside-out" or inductive approach. They identify the concerns that organize the story and the notions of good depicted by the narrator, along with knowledge and skill evident in the narrative. The goal is to make the process of experiential learning more visible and valued. The ethical concerns and notions of the good inherent in the story guide their reflections. This approach allows for an internal critique of the narrative, from the perspective of the narrator. When moral lapses, or character flaws in the actors, are discovered, the focus is on the experiential learning required to better instantiate or actualize the ethical concerns in the particular situation.

The goal of this approach is to avoid an obsessive reflective moralism in which the focus is forever returned to (or turned in on) character strengths or weaknesses of the individual actor rather than the issues or ethical concerns at hand in the situation.[33] Likewise, in considering the skills of interpersonal involvement, the goal is to refrain from engaging in sentimentalism or focusing on the emotional plight and risks of others as if they were one's own, rather than respecting the other as separate and unique and allowing emotional responses to guide action and involvement or disengagement.[34] Moralism and sentimentalism tend to displace concern and attentiveness from the issues at hand in favor of the emotional responses of the helper (e.g., in moralism, shame and blame, and in sentimentalism, sensationalism, or self-absorption).

We also encourage students to present "paradigm cases"—clinical situations and nurse-patient relationships that opened new possibilities for them as nurses. These paradigm cases gather meanings that are common to many clinical situations because they are told in their particularity with the concrete nurse-patient or family relationships and historical unfolding of events and responses. They represent what Logstrup calls singular universals.[35] Rather than seeking universal expression through decontextualization and abstraction, universal human concerns and experience of the human condition (e.g., finitude, embodiment, vulnerability, suffering, love, fear) are expressed in particular events, relationships, and life-worlds.

We also emphasize valuing of clinical experiential learning in clinical sites, where students are asked to reflect in similar ways on their experiential learning, skills of clinical inquiry, and action in particular patient-nurse encounters. The goal is to avoid the academic tendency to freeze learning into abstract assignments about ideal situations; instead, we focus on actual learning and action in real clinical situations.

Bourdieu notes the importance of context and contingency in teaching teamwork in sports.[36] Teaching team members to coordinate their actions with one another without focusing on the teamwork generated by playing an opposing team will not teach the most relevant teamwork. The goal of reflecting on practice is to teach *phronesis* by articulating the links between ethical and clinical reasoning in actual clinical situations. Soon the practitioner learns that action and judgment are guided by the patient's and practitioner's notions of good in particular situations. Practice in articulating relational and ethical concerns along with action and clinical judgment increases the likelihood that the clinician will develop sensitive moral perceptions in actual clinical situations. In fact, naming the concerns of particular clinical situations mimics the everyday practical logic of practitioners.

MAKING QUALITATIVE DISTINCTIONS

Qualitative distinctions are at the heart of discernment and judgment. Distinctions are qualitative when context, tone, transition, meaning, or other qualities are required for understanding and acting in the situation.[37] The qualitative distinction may be clinical, as in distinguishing between emotional responses—such as a patient's psychological withdrawal as distinct from a decreased level of alertness resulting from an organic cause such as sepsis. I noted above the qualitative distinction between being available without being intrusive. A qualitative distinction may be about what Charles Taylor calls strong evaluations, such as the religious distinction in "double effect" theory between adequate pain medication given to a dying person primarily to alleviate suffering (but which may also hasten death), versus giving pain medication as a way of hastening death (as in euthanasia).[38] This "strong evaluation" is also embodied because it depends on the agent's intent, skill, and action in making the distinction in administering and titrating pain medicine and comfort measures. Making qualitative distinctions is central to ethical comportment—for example, discerning when a patient or family denies the implications of a proposed therapy, or simply has not received an adequate explanation, or chooses not to know all the details about the therapy. Each of these possibilities has distinct ethical implications about informing the patient and family and working with their concerns and fears; each refers back to the agent's intent and relationship to the patient or family.

Taylor points out that reasoning through transitions allows one to take into account what has improved or impeded action or understanding.[39] This historical understanding may be crucial to making qualitative distinctions. Keeping track of changes in the patient's condition and one's clinical understanding across time allows the clinician to judge progress, relapse, or clinical grasp.[40] Information systems and decision supports are useful only to the extent that the clinician has a good grasp of the patient's particular condition, and this requires attentiveness over time.

DEVELOPING AN ACTION-ORIENTED NARRATIVE PEDAGOGY THAT ENCOURAGES EXPERIENTIAL LEARNING

In nursing and medical education, knowledge increasingly is reduced to what can be rationally calculated. The problems of nursing and medicine are presented as problems of managing information gained from research (evidenced-based medicine and nursing).[41] Attention is placed on the aggregate, the standard, the patient population. This approach assumes that this knowledge of the aggregate can be transferred and applied directly to the individual. This shift radically affects the nurse, who is pressured to have an individual patient conform to a standard critical pathway. The logical assumptions of this focus are many—for example, that aggregate data can be applied sensibly in the particular case and that thinking about the patient's condition can be reduced to single points in time at which data are interpreted and appropriate knowledge applied. What this picture leaves out is the life-world of the patient, the ambiguities and artfulness inherent in developing a diagnosis, the clinical trajectory of the particular patient, and an ongoing assessment of the particular patient's response to therapies. Consequently, case studies and problem-based learning increasingly point to predefined problems. The ambiguities involved in encountering particular patients across a trajectory of illness are overlooked.

As Jane Rubin points out, making decisions can appear to be a process of weighing objective evidence and applying it to the particular situation.[42] Judgment is reduced to rational calculations; perceptual acuity in recognizing signs and symptoms are ignored, and the possibility of making qualitative distinctions and evaluating the meaning of a symptom or the patient's response in the particular context is obscured or ignored in favor of weighing objective evidence, reducing judgment to an evaluation of cause and effect. Rubin suggests that to teach qualitative distinctions, nurses will need to focus on goods specific to excellent nursing practice and on developing the skills and discernment that allows a nurse to recognize when those goods are at issue in practice.[43]

CONCLUSION

Aristotle concludes that in cases of statesmanship and ethical inquiry, *techné* or procedural knowledge is insufficient for action.[44] The civic leader needs experience, character, and judgment. Dunne argues that without experience, character development is impossible.[45] One cannot become an excellent practitioner without experiential learning. Experience is defined as active learning; changing perceptions and understanding are the minimal qualification for experience, not just passage of time or repetitive practice.[46] Experiential learning that attends to worthy ends or notions of good practice is essential for character development. Experiential learning not only improves technique, it transforms the practitioners' perceptual field, sense of salience, skilled know-how, and attunement to the situation or person. Dunne emphasizes that experiential learning and *phronesis* are connected:

> . . . *phronesis* is a habit of attentiveness that makes the resources of one's past experience flexibly available to one and, at the same time, allows the present situation to "unconceal" its own particular significance—which it may do comfortably within the terms of one's own experience or else only evincing as insight which, while it could not occur without one's past experience, still transcends, and so enriches it. . . . This level is not that of *techne* or *episteme*, however. For these latter include reference to the particular only as abstractly represented in general rules, formulae, definitions, and demonstrations which can be taught, whereas the higher level reached when experience becomes *phronesis* must be continually renewed in one's insightful dealings with particular situations, and is a hexis, a formed disposition, only insofar as one is capable of such repeated renewals.[47]

Character development and ethical comportment are better regarded as learning skills of engagement, emotional attunement, and thinking-in-action rather than sedimented traits and habits of will and intellect alone. It is characteristic of expert nurses to see the unexpected and subtle changes in a patient's condition. Seeing the unexpected is possible for expert nurses because of the way they take up and use their background experiential knowledge about the usual recovery or treatment-response trajectory. Tacit expectations based on prior experiential learning become a background for noticing the unusual or unexpected. Without openness to experience and insight, the usual could dull attention and produce rote, rigid responses. Openness to experience, having one's expectations turned around, or the ability to see the subtle and the unusual are hallmarks of experiential learning, ongoing skill acquisition, and character development.

A primer that my colleagues and I recently created on ethical and clinical reasoning and action in nursing describes two pervasive habits of thought and action: clinical grasp (reasoning across time about the particular through transitions in the patient's clinical condition and the clinician's understanding) and clinical forethought (anticipating likely eventualities and immediate futures).[48] The book is further organized into common clinical situations, complete with their clinical goals and ethical and clinical concerns. For example, if the practical situation is one of managing a patient who is hemodynamically unstable, the logic of this patient's care is likely to be ordered by this major concern. Recognizing that the global concerns and situation guide the ethical and clinical (practical) reasoning, narrative examples of nurses' experiential learning in particular situations assist in articulating notions of good and ethical concerns about rights and responsibilities. The particular examples reveal relationship, chronology, and context, complete with the ambiguities inherent in the original situation.

Good experiential learning is not innate; it is cultivated within a practice and a tradition that strives to make the experiential learning of the members cumulative and collective. The excellent practitioner continues to learn experientially from practice—extending, comparing, and remembering paradigm cases that open and articulate new practice possibilities and moral concerns within the practice. These paradigm cases reflect particular universals: examples of the human experience of vulnerability, sickness, recovery, dying. In the midst of particular life-world concerns and practices, the human condition that we hold in common becomes more visible.

NOTES

1. Aristotle, *Nicomachean Ethics,* trans. T. Irwin (Indianapolis: Hackett, 1985).
2. F. Nightingale, *Notes on Nursing: What It Is and What It Is Not* (Philadelphia: J. B. Lippincott, 1969).
3. P. Benner, "When Health Care Becomes a Commodity: The Need for Compassionate Strangers," in *The Changing Face of Health Care,* ed. J. F. Kilner, R. D. Orr, and J. A. Shelly (Grand Rapids, Mich.: William B. Eerdmans, 1998): 119–35.
4. A. MacIntyre, *After Virtue: A Study in Moral Theory* (Notre Dame, Ind.: University of Notre Dame Press, 1981).
5. K. Martinsen, *From Marx to Logstrup* (Oslo, Norway: Tano Publishers, trans. in progress); K. E. Logstrup, *The Ethical Demand* (Notre Dame, Ind.: University of Notre Dame Press, 1997), and *Metaphysics, Volume I,* trans. R. L. Dees, (Milwaukee, Wisc.: Marquette University Press, 1995): 140–41.
6. Logstrup, *The Ethical Demand.*
7. J. E. Lynaugh, *The Community Hospitals of Kansas City, Missouri, 1870–1915* (New York: Garland Publishing, 1989).
8. P. Benner et al., *Clinical Expertise in Nursing Practice, Caring, Clinical Judgment and Ethics* (New York: Springer, 1996); P. Benner, P. Hooper-Kyriakidis, and D. Stannard, *Clinical Wisdom and Interventions in Critical Care: A Thinking-in-Action Approach* (Philadelphia: Saunders, 1999).
9. Benner et al., *Clinical Expertise in Nursing Practice,* 165.
10. Aristotle, *Nicomachean Ethics;* P. Benner and J. Wrubel, *The Primacy of Caring: Stress and Coping in Health and Illness* (Menlo Park, Calif.: Addison-Wesley, 1989); P. Benner,

"The Role of Articulation in Understanding Practice and Experience as Sources of Knowledge," in *Philosophy in a Time of Pluralism: Perspectives on the Philosophy of Charles Taylor*, ed. J. Tully and D. M. Weinstock (Cambridge: Cambridge University Press, 1994), 136–55.

11. Benner, "The Role of Articulation"; P. Benner, *From Novice to Expert: Excellence and Power in Clinical Nursing Practice* (Menlo Park, Calif.: Addison-Wesley, 1984); P. Benner, "A Dialogue Between Virtue Ethics and Care Ethics," in *The Influence of Edmund D. Pellegrino's Philosophy of Medicine*, ed. D. C. Thomasma (Boston: Kluwer Academic Publishers, 1997): 47–61; Benner et al., *Clinical Expertise in Nursing Practice;* E. D. Pellegrino and D. C. Thomasma, *The Virtues in Medical Practice* (New York: Oxford University Press, 1993); S. Reverby, *Ordered to Care: The Dilemma of American Nursing: 1850–1945* (Cambridge: Cambridge University Press, 1987); J. Dunne, *Back to the Rough Ground, Practical Judgment and the Lure of Technique* (Notre Dame, Ind.: Notre Dame University Press, 1997).

12. H. Gadamer, *The Enigma of Health: The Art of Healing in a Scientific Age* (Stanford, Calif.: Stanford University Press, 1996).

13. Dunne, *Back to the Rough Ground*, 359.

14. Nightingale, *Notes on Nursing;* Pellegrino and Thomasma, *The Virtues in Medical Practice.*

15. H. L. Dreyfus, *What Computers Still Can't Do: A Critique of Artificial Reason* (Cambridge: Massachusetts Institute of Technology Press, 1992); H. L. Dreyfus and S. E. Dreyfus, *Mind Over Machine: The Power of Human Intuition and Expertise in the Era of the Computer* (New York: Free Press, 1986).

16. A. Tsolinas, "The Nurse as a Wise Compassionate Stranger: The Courage to Love," *American Journal of Nursing* 97 (1997): 27–34.

17. Dreyfus, *What Computers Still Can't Do;* Dreyfus and Dreyfus, *Mind Over Machine;* H. L. Dreyfus, S. E. Dreyfus, and P. Benner, "Implications of the Phenomenology of Expertise for Teaching and Learning Everyday Skillful Ethical Comportment," in *Expertise in Nursing Practice, Caring, Clinical Judgment and Ethics,* ed. P. Benner, C. A. Tanner, and C. A. Chesla (New York: Springer, 1996): 258–79.

18. J. Rubin, "Impediments to the Development of Clinical Knowledge and Ethical Judgment in Critical Care Nursing," in *Expertise in Nursing Practice: Caring, Clinical Judgment and Ethics,* ed. P. Benner, C. A. Tanner, and C. A. Chesla (New York: Springer, 1996): 170–92.

19. C. Taylor, "Explanation and Practical Reason," in *The Quality of Life,* ed. M. Nussbaum and A. Sen (Oxford: Clarendon, 1993): 208–31; Benner, "A Dialogue Between Virtue Ethics and Care Ethics"; Benner et al., *Clinical Expertise in Nursing Practice.*

20. Benner, "The Role of Articulation"; Benner, Hooper-Kyriakidis, and Stannard, *Clinical Wisdom.*

21. Rubin, "Impediments to the Development of Clinical Knowledge."

22. N. N. Glatzer, "Introduction," in *Understanding the Sick and the Healthy,* trans. N. N. Glatzer (Cambridge, Mass.: Harvard University Press, 1999): 24–25.

23. Benner, Hooper-Kyriakidis, and Stannard, *Clinical Wisdom*, 273.

24. J. Rubin, *Too Much of Nothing: The Self and Salvation in Kierkegaard's Thought* (unpublished doctoral dissertation, University of California, Berkeley, 1984); MacIntyre, *After Virtue.*

25. Benner et al., *Clinical Expertise.*

26. Benner, "The Role of Articulation"; Benner, Hooper-Kyriakidis, and Stannard, *Clinical Wisdom.*

27. Benner, Hooper-Kyriakidis, and Stannard, *Clinical Wisdom,* 290.
28. Logstrup, *The Ethical Demand.*
29. I. Kant, *Critique of Practical Reason,* trans. L. W. Beck (Indianapolis: Bobbs-Merrill, [1788] 1956).
30. Tsolinas, *The Courage to Love.*
31. Ibid.
32. Benner, Hooper-Kyriakidis, and Stannard, *Clinical Wisdom.*
33. Benner, Hooper-Kyriakidis, and Stannard, *Clinical Wisdom;* Logstrup, *The Ethical Demand.*
34. Logstrup, *The Ethical Demand.*
35. Ibid.
36. P. Bourdieu, *The Logic of Practice,* trans. R. Nice (Stanford, Calif.: Stanford University Press, 1980, 1990).
37. Taylor, "Explanation and Practical Reason."
38. C. Taylor, *Human Agency and Language: Philosophical Papers Vol. I* (Cambridge: Cambridge University Press, 1985); C. Taylor, *Sources of the Self: The Making of the Modern Identity* (Cambridge, Mass.: Harvard University Press, 1989).
39. Taylor, "Explanation and Practical Reason."
40. Benner, Hooper-Kyriakidis, and Stannard, *Clinical Wisdom.*
41. D. M. Frankford, "Scientism and Economism in the Regulation of Health Care," *Journal of Politics, Policy and Law* 19(4): 773–99.
42. Rubin, "Impediments to the Development of Clinical Knowledge."
43. Ibid.
44. Aristotle, *Nichomachean Ethics.*
45. Dunne, *Back to the Rough Ground.*
46. H. Gadamer, *Truth and Method,* trans. G. Barden and J. Cumming (New York: Seabury, 1975).
47. Dunne, *Back to the Rough Ground,* 305–06.
48. Benner, Hooper-Kyriakidis, and Stannard, *Clinical Wisdom.*

Engendering Trust in a Pluralistic Society

Marian Gray Secundy and Rodger L. Jackson

Trust originates not from a neutral starting point devoid of social attribute and ethical meaning, but from concrete historical circumstances.[1]

Trust on the part of a patient may be the central requirement of the fiduciary relationship between patients and health care providers.[2] The ideal situation occurs when a patient places himself or herself—or is placed by others—in the hands of the caregiver with complete trust. The reality is that such complete trust seldom exists. We must accept the reality that in today's climate, limited levels of trust are likely to exist. Health care professionals must learn how to maximize the possibility of that trust wherever the opportunity exists.[3] We ought to welcome moral and cultural disagreements and differences, and we should refuse to believe in unequivocal moral truths when they conflict with the beliefs and cultural mores of persons from cultures or subcultures other than our own. In appreciating all that we and our patients hold in common, we may be able to regard "difference" from a more appropriate perspective.

Dealing with issues of engendering trust in a pluralistic society presents an interesting research challenge. Our research and writing focuses primarily on physicians in training and the doctor-patient relationship. Recently, however, responsibility for a new multidisciplinary course in the health sciences has required us to turn our attention to issues that other health care professionals face. The course requires that we examine differences and similarities in the ethical concerns facing each discipline.

What difference does trust, or lack of trust, make in the operating room, for example, when patients and nurses confront one another? We wondered just how much contact patients and nurses actually had in that environment. A nursing colleague laughed and remarked, somewhat cynically, that trust—or the lack of it—probably made no difference until an African American patient looked up from the operating room table and saw no black faces among the group of nurses gazing down. This colleague—an African American woman from Alabama—reminded us of her own recent experience after an automobile accident. She found herself—a highly qualified nurse educator with impeccable academic credentials—in the emergency room of a local suburban hospital and recalls her panic at looking up and realizing where she was. She remembers with great embarrassment seeing one black face and thinking to herself, "Well, I guess I'll be alright as long as he is here." She

65

next recalls waking up again in a semi-conscious state and not seeing that black face—at which point she screamed aloud, "Bring me back that black man!" She could not overcome her basic primal fear and distrust, despite years of education and positive interactions with white Americans; her distrust was grounded in the historical legacies and collective consciousness of most African Americans.

Most of us understand that a patient must have some level of trust in his or her doctor to gain the maximum benefit from medical treatment. Patients must trust the floor nurse to experience a meaningful level of comfort. Perhaps less understood and appreciated is how essential trust is. There must be trust not only in the entire health care enterprise but in all of the situations one might encounter. The levels of trust needed may vary with the duties and tasks performed. A cumulative effect exists that most likely influences the course of the patient's illness and recovery, especially within hospitals.

When a patient speaks of trust in a health care setting, he or she is essentially speaking about a comfort level, a feeling of safety, a belief that he or she can rely on people with power not to hurt or exploit him or her. Maximization of those positive feelings on the part of the patient is essential to optimal recovery. Such positive feelings can ensure appropriate cooperation and compliance during the course of an illness. When such feelings are absent or ambivalent, the patient's behavior can influence outcomes negatively. There are several areas in which trust is relevant: The patient can trust or distrust the system of health care itself, the specific institution or setting in which health care services are being delivered, and the person or persons providing service or care.

In the African American experience, obstacles to trust take many forms. Although similar obstacles exist for Americans from other ethnic groups, some obstacles may be considered universal. Universal obstacles often result from the experiences of illness itself. Most of our observations, however, address issues of particular relevance to African Americans.

To the extent that nurses, as health care providers, comprehend the nature of such obstacles, they can increase the likelihood of overcoming them. For it is the nurse who has the most hands-on, moment-to-moment contact and interaction with patients. Often the nurse is the first person a patient encounters; sometimes, as in the case of surgical procedures, the nurse may be one of the last—if not the last—person the patient sees before losing consciousness.

Obstacles to trust include but are not limited to the following:

- historical violations
- alternative beliefs/explanatory meanings
- language/semantics
- lack of knowledge/inadequate information
- negative/hostile encounters

HISTORICAL VIOLATIONS

A book by Spencie Love about the life and death of noted surgeon and blood plasma pioneer Charles R. Drew provides interesting insights.[4] The story of Drew's death in an automobile accident in the South has become apocryphal. The common folklore alleged that Drew was refused treatment in a white hospital and therefore bled to death. The truth is that all efforts were made to save him. Curiously, the myth of his death lingers and has taken on a life of its own. In a review of Love's book, James Goodman observes that "truth has many levels, that sometimes false stories can be true. . . . For the people who tell the story and believe it, the story is true because it makes a meaningful statement about the world Drew lived in and the world they live in today." Goodman goes on to note that the persistence of the myth is tied to the reality of the lives of those who have kept it alive—noting that in the 1950s, every black American knew someone who had suffered from separate and grossly unequal medical care. Many knew someone who had died after being denied care.[5] There is a vast amount of literature describing such violations, as well as rich commentary about the ways in which black people have coped with and managed their lives in the face of those violations. One way, of course, has been to develop a distrust and suspicion of white caregivers that is protective, yet at times dysfunctional.

Alice Walker states, "I belong to a People so wounded by betrayal, so hurt by misplacing their trust, that to offer us a gift of love is often to risk one's life, certainly one's name and reputation. . . . I belong to a people, heart and mind, who do not trust mirrors . . . our shame is deep, for shame is the result of soul injury."[6] Black people remember the words of Frederick Douglass, who stated in his autobiography, "The Motto which I adopted when I started from slavery was this . . . trust no man. I saw in every white man an enemy and in almost every colored cause for distrust. . . . "[7]

John Gwaltney recounts conversations with African Americans about their health and health care. Gwaltney describes a sixty-one-year-old woman living in Harlem who told him:

> We are, by reason of the lives we have led, a suspicious people. We are the children of suspicious people. . . . We think white people are the most unprincipled folks in the world, but everybody bears watching. . . .[8]

Of course, white people are not the only people that African Americans do not trust, for black Americans also have a significant amount of self-hatred. This self-hatred causes many of them to have very little confidence in other blacks in professional roles. It is not surprising that such disregard should exist when one has been taught—or, as some believe, programmed to think—that all blacks are inferior. How does it make sense to entrust one's very life and health to them? The task of engendering trust is not as simple as replacing a white health care provider with a black one.

ALTERNATIVE BELIEFS/EXPLANATORY MEANINGS

Acceptance of western medicine's methods and procedures varies; it depends on prior experiences, educational, and class status, and so forth. Each ethnic group has its own ways of explaining illness and symptoms of illness. This observation is not novel, but it reminds us of the importance of paying attention to how alternative beliefs and competing explanatory meanings of illnesses or symptoms influence responses to providers, compliance with regimens, and whether patients trust or distrust. The relationship between memories and/or myths of historical violations and alternative beliefs and explanatory meanings is significant as well.

Loudell Snow's *Walkin' Over Medicine* is one of the most comprehensive descriptions of belief systems of predominantly lower-class and rural African Americans.[9] Snow's anecdotes and ethnographic work provide major insight into the lives and minds of many patients. Snow found an ongoing interrelationship between how one feels about doctors, hospitals, nurses, and other caregivers and the various explanations and beliefs one holds about whatever malady one may have, as well as any explanations one has for treatments to which one may be subjected.

We know that many people, regardless of ethnic background, rely first on friends and informal support systems for diagnosis and treatment of illnesses. We have less awareness and understanding about the underlying beliefs that inform those friends and support systems.

Within the African American community, a rich history of traditional medicine reflects numerous continuities with African cultures. Regional adaptations of those cultures and inclusion of beliefs of other cultural groups (e.g., native American, Hispanic, Caribbean, Haitian, and Appalachian) result in a complexity of split beliefs and split loyalties. Sometimes these beliefs work together; sometimes they work separately, manifesting in noncompliant behaviors.

African American traditional medicine incorporates naturalistic and personalistic views. One is likely to find attitudes toward the natural world that differ greatly from attitudes of non-ethnic patients. In this sphere, the spiritual world, nonanimate objects, and the role of ancestors take on special meaning. This perspective incorporates beliefs about the etiology of health problems and disease that bear little relationship to our understanding of scientific medicine. Particularly among uneducated persons, for example, one is likely to encounter beliefs in healers ordained by the spirit world or now in the spirit world, in psychics and faith healers.

Patients often find it difficult to discuss these beliefs with health care providers trained in Western medicine because they are fearful of ridicule or criticism. Yet positive outcomes in reaching appropriate diagnostic and treatment plans can occur only to the extent that reconciliation of the conflicting issues occurs. If patients believe that medicines are designed to hurt them, they will not take them. If they believe that their tumors, for example, are the result of divine punishment or the negative activities of a *"root"* doctor, they are less likely to respond to other interventions.

For example, an elderly midwife spoke of the fears of patients, noting, "They was afraid of doctors givin' 'em a dose of something just because they was black . . . they may give me the black bottle . . . means poison. . . . "[10] Another patient in 1970 discusses similar fears: "You learn about the black bottle just from growing up. Me, I was kind afraid to go to a hospital man, you know, cause when the nurse come around say, 'Eddie take your medicine,' I'd look around and wait till she'd leave, you understand, and I'd pass it on to my friends and say—hey man, try some of this here, you know, and I'd watch and see what its gonna do to him, see?"[11]

The strong spiritual beliefs of most African Americans also must be understood and respected to build cooperative and trusting relationships with patients and their families. These beliefs can and do manifest themselves in the absence of any organized or formal church affiliations. These ideas are usually there, sometimes just beneath the surface of highly sophisticated exteriors. One woman told Loudell Snow, "See now, if you have cancer, the doctors can't cure cancer! But if they go prayin' for you, and you have lots of faith, the Lord will cure that cancer!"[12]

LANGUAGE

Although we share a common language in this country, our ability to understand one another depends on the extent to which we understand various accents, colloquial expressions, dialects, and slang. Vocabularies differ regionally and are influenced by our experiences and our educational exposures. Loudell Snow reminds us that

> the potential for misunderstanding is very great when outsiders hear a linguistic style that is unfamiliar. . . . But it may also be true when speaker and listener speak the same language . . . ; because they share a common vocabulary they may not recognize that they are failing to communicate. . . . Words or phrases that are familiar to both parties may have entirely different meanings: "Fell out of *what*?" I heard a resident say impatiently one afternoon, after a mother reiterated her concern that her small son "fell out twice yesterday.'" The mother was referring to a fainting spell. The resident assumed that little Johnnie must have fallen out of a window.[13]

Snow's assessment of high blood pressure as a concept is illuminating. She notes that high blood pressure in traditional belief differs from the biomedical model in a number of ways: "If asked to define 'high blood' or 'high blood pressure,' someone subscribing to the traditional view might suggest that it means (a) having too much blood, (b) having blood located high in the body, and/or (c) having blood that is too sweet."[14] The interrelationship between language and explanatory meanings of illness is fascinating. Implications for accurate medical diagnosis, appropriate management plans, and treatment are awesome. The burden on caregivers, particularly nurses, to clarify and interpret is apparent.

Alice Walker makes a compelling case for all situations in which humans must interact. She observes that "it is language more than anything else that reveals and validates one's existence, and if the language we actually speak is denied us, then it is inevitable that the form we are permitted to assume historically will be one of caricature, reflecting someone else's literary or social fantasy." The message for health care providers is the need to attend to what people are saying to actualize them as real people, real patients. For all of us, Walker states, "the language is an intrinsic part of who we are and what has, for good or evil, happened to us."[15] The challenge is for us to learn to understand and communicate with the patient on his or her own terms. Such a responsibility does not reside with the patient.

LACK OF KNOWLEDGE/HEALTH INFORMATION

Fundamentally, the interrelationships among issues of trust/distrust, explanatory meanings, and language all manifest in levels of health information and knowledge possessed by patients. Of course, education and socioeconomic class are central determinants; these factors, however, are greatly influenced by the ways in which patients relate to health care providers and the ways in which health care providers relate to them.

If I trust, I am more likely to accept the diagnosis and proposed management plans presented to me than if I am suspicious. This trust allows for the possibility that my explanation and understanding of what ails me and why may have other explanations that are equally valid if I believe that I am valued and understood. If my health care providers can understand and communicate with me accurately, I am more likely to receive appropriate care.

Many patients must be convinced that there are other valid explanations for their illnesses, as well as other valid treatments than those with which they may be most familiar. Basic information about the body and how it works is essential, of course, to this process and cannot be assumed. The capacity to correct such misunderstanding without disrespect is an art.

Health care providers themselves must be open to new information, remain nonjudgmental, and express a willingness to collaborate with alternative plans if they are not explicitly harmful. We must never underestimate the influence of social and cultural history as the definer of perspectives, beliefs, and what we think of as knowledge. In acknowledging the possibility of more than one way of doing things and explaining phenomena, we do not deny other realities; therefore, we are more likely to encounter cooperation instead of resistance. The truly effective nurse or physician possesses the ability to place himself or herself in the patient's body, if you will, and to understand the illness experience as the patient understands it. Empathic skills are crucial.

CURRENT ISSUES

According to Sissela Bok, if one is not trusted, one has greatly decreased power.[16] This statement is true at all levels within the health care system. We must not minimize the importance of recognizing that trust violations or perceived violations can and do negatively affect the ways in which many ethnic Americans view the world and radically reconstruct the ways in which they interact with others. Judith Sklar's discussions of trust in this context are useful.[17] The psychological effects of illness are complex. Because of this complexity, the capacity to trust others becomes even more important. The extent of illness determines the amount of physical vulnerability, as well as one's sense of psychological vulnerability. Clearly, when that reality is combined with the sense of being at the mercy of a person and/or health care system that cannot be trusted to take care and to protect one's well-being, one is likely to be resistant, combative, or passively uncooperative.

Often, it is difficult for Americans who are not persons of color to appreciate the extent to which historical circumstances shape the attitudes and behavior of patients today. Health care providers of differing backgrounds must suspend disbelief and themselves trust in the validity of information they are given in this regard.

Actual past violations are retold, often with additional embellishments. More recent violations to personal dignity have given way to exaggerated accounts of greater infractions. The social and political climate lends itself to rumors and conspiracy theories that patients often bring into the clinical encounter. Requirements for "cultural competence" among health care professionals include acknowledging the existence of these theories and understanding how and from where they may emanate.

Cultural competence also requires a desire and capacity to learn and use strategies and information to better influence patients. For example, many African Americans approach health care settings, particularly hospitals, with a belief—albeit irrational and not credible—that they are merely sacrificial guinea pigs. Again, the burden of proving otherwise falls upon the provider. AIDS, genetic technologies, and various drug therapies are viewed with fear and suspicion. Organ donation requests and compliance with requests for advanced directives are viewed as ways to obtain easy access to body parts; many African Americans believe that such requests are likely to result in improper treatment and premature death.

Today's organizational structures in health care delivery often create additional problems of trust. Long waiting periods, limited accessibility, episodic care, and disrespectful treatment encourage the continuation of suspicion on the part of many Americans of color. Cultivation and maintenance of trust in a depersonalized, contractual health care system such as that in current managed care environments represent an enormous critical challenge to all health care professionals.

RECOMMENDATIONS

Professionals in health care must first suspend disbelief and not resist the validity of claims of distrust. Considerable denial and defensiveness often surface when these subjects are introduced. Basic skills of observation and listening will allow professionals to begin to realize the possibility of mastering strategies that acknowledge difference, distrust, and anger on the part of some ethnic American patients. Such acknowledgment presents opportunities for skill development, new information, and self awareness that assist in increased competency in working with patients in more effective ways. Sensitivity training sessions and workshops that focus on cultural competency and enhanced communication skills are recommended. Ongoing support groups where patients are seen within the health care system are essential. Expansion of the health care team to include persons who are knowledgeable about specific cultural differences and alternative belief systems is helpful. Central to this discussion is the responsibility of the health care professional to understand the interrelationship of history and social and political conditions to illness behavior. Beyond cultivating understanding is the obligation to emerge as a meaningful change agent.

SUMMARY

No amount of theoretical knowledge can substitute adequately for basic respect of persons as individuals. Appreciation of difference does not mean that we should make assumptions without attention to that individuality and special personhood of each of our patients. In meeting the challenge to engender trust in this pluralistic society in which we live, our acquisition of skills, attributes, and knowledge constitute a fundamental requirement. Most of all, as Pellegrino and Thomasma note, "Truthfulness and probity are absolutely essential to effective healing. Justice, tolerance and trust enhance the provider-patient relationship without detracting from it. They are not absolutely necessary for the healing relationship to occur, yet they can often impede it if absent and enhance it measurably when present."[18]

NOTES

1. Edmund D. Pellegrino, Robert Veatch, and John Langan, eds., *Ethics, Trust, and The Professions: Philosophical and Cultural Aspects* (Washington, D.C.: Georgetown University Press, 1991), 47.
2. Ibid., 49.
3. Peter Johnson, *Frames of Deceit* (Boston: Cambridge University Press, 1993), 68.
4. Spencie Love, *One Blood: The Death and Resurrection of Charles R. Drew* (Chapel Hill: University of North Carolina Press, 1966).
5. James Goodman, "The Death of a Legend," *Washington Post Book Review,* 14 July 1996, p. 14.
6. Alice Walker, *From the Same River Twice: Honoring the Difficult* (New York: Washington Square Press, 1997), Preface.
7. Frederick Douglass, *Narrative of the Life of Frederick Douglass, An American Slave* (New York: Signet, 1968), 126
8. John Gwaltney, *Drylongso* (New York: Vintage Press, 1980), 7.
9. Loudell F. Snow, *Walkin' Over Medicine* (Boulder, Colo.: Westview Press, 1993).
10. Ibid., 266. See also Vivian K. Cameron, "Folk Beliefs Pertaining to Health of the Southern Negro" (Master's thesis, Department of Sociology, Northwestern University, 1930).
11. Snow, *Walkin' Over Medicine,* 267.
12. Ibid., 57.
13. Ibid., 263.
14. Ibid., 119.
15. Alice Walker, *Living by the Word: 1973–1987* (New York: Harbrace Press, 1989), 58, 65.
16. Sissela Bok, *Lying: Moral Choice in Public and Private Life* (New York: Vintage, 1979).
17. Judith Sklar, *Ordinary Vices* (Boston/Bellknap: Harvard University Press: 1984), 114.
18. Edmund D. Pellegrino and David C. Thomasma, *For the Patient's Good: The Restoration of Beneficence in Health Care* (New York: Oxford University Press: 1988), 110.

PART II

The Moral Basis of Health Care

Internal and External Sources of
Morality for Medicine

Robert M. Veatch

Edmund D. Pellegrino's call for integrity in the professional practice of medicine has been powerful and prophetic. Among physicians of the second half of the twentieth century, none has more clearly challenged practitioners to eschew roles assigned to physicians that have the potential to corrupt the practice. Pellegrino has challenged the use of the physician as economic gatekeeper,[1] mercy killer,[2] illicit accomplice in nuclear war,[3] tool of state ideology,[4] and reliever of unwanted pregnancy.[5] He has reminded his physician colleagues—as well as persons who practice medicine in one of the other health professions or only as lay people—that there are ways that medicine ought not be practiced and behaviors no one has a right to ask of a physician.

Pellegrino has not been content merely to be a prophetic voice when medicine is exposed to abuses in various nonmedical social programs. He also has contributed to building the theory of the healer's role. He has distinguished between *internal* and *external* sources for morality in medicine, arguing that the proper norms for the practice are internal to the profession and can be derived from a proper understanding of the very purpose or end of medicine as a practice.[6]

In appreciation of Edmund Pellegrino's many crucial contributions to the field of medical ethics—and to my own thinking as one who came after him in the field of medical ethics and at the Kennedy Institute of Ethics—I attempt in this essay a systematic reconstruction of Pellegrino's views about how the morality of medicine is *internal* and can be derived from a proper understanding of the meaning of medicine's purpose. After attempting to restate his views, I then press further, particularly over the question of whether the bare notion of the concept of medicine can do the work he assigns to it without relying on some more fundamental systematic and integrated religious or philosophical world view (such as the Roman Catholicism to which he most faithfully subscribes). In the end, I ask whether the claim that medicine's morality is intrinsic or internal to it is not incompatible with a more fundamental affirmation of various religious or secular world views to which each of us professes loyalty. In short, I ask whether the "internal morality of medicine" thesis is compatible with being a good Catholic (or a good Jew, or a good believer in feminism or liberal political philosophy).

THE CASE FOR A MORALITY INTERNAL TO MEDICINE

Several theorists—almost all physicians—have made the claim that the morality of medicine is "internal" to the profession.[7] Although some physicians may not know it, these references seem to trace back to the work of Alasdair MacIntyre. More sophisticated physician-theorists, including Pellegrino[8] and Brody,[9] cite MacIntyre's influential work, *After Virtue*.[10]

MacIntyre's Notion of Ends Internal to a Practice

MacIntyre's effort to reassess the place of virtue in morality includes the pivotal notion of what he calls a *practice*. He defines a practice as

> . . . any coherent and complex form of socially established cooperative human activity through which goods internal to that form of activity are realized in the course of trying to achieve those standards of excellence which are appropriate to, and partially definitive of, that form of activity, with the result that human powers to achieve excellence, and human conceptions of the ends and goods involved, are systematically extended.[11]

As examples of practices, MacIntyre gives football, architecture, farming, physics,[12] and—crucial for our purposes—medicine.[13] The essential point for physicians who claim that the ends of medicine are internal to it is that there are two kinds of goods that any practice can yield. First, there are *external* goods—that is, goods that are contingently attached to the practice and could be obtained by means independent of the practice. In the example of chess playing, MacIntyre suggests that prestige, status, and money—all of which are contingently related to being a champion chess player—are external goods.[14] These goods could be obtained by other means.

On the other hand, MacIntyre says, there are goods that can be obtained in no other way than by playing chess. Presumably, the joy of making a brilliant chess move or becoming a chess champion would qualify. He goes on to claim that these goods are *internal* for two reasons: because "we can only specify them in terms of chess or some other game of that specific kind and by means of examples from such games"[15] and "because they can only be identified and recognized by the experience of participating in the practice in question. Those who lack the relevant experience are incompetent thereby as judges of internal goods."[16]

MacIntyre builds his conception of internal goods by citing an example from Aristotle. Aristotle suggests that a man living well is analogous to a harpist playing the harp well.[17] MacIntyre suggests that, likewise, a watch would be considered a good watch only if it kept time well.[18] In general, any phenomenon is a *good* exemplar of its kind if, and only if, it manifests well the purpose for which its kind is characteristically wanted. By analogy, persons and actions are *good* manifestations of their kind to the extent that they manifest their purpose or function. Thus, just as a watch is a good watch to the extent that it keeps time accurately, a physician is a good physician to the extent that he or she carries out the purpose or end of medicine well.

Pellegrino's Formulation of The Good Physician

This Aristotelian understanding of the relation of the good to the end being pursued provides the basis for Pellegrino's conception of the good physician and the ends of medicine. If Pellegrino can determine the end internal to the practice of medicine, he can establish the characteristics of the good physician. Moreover, he will have done so in a way that will shield professional practitioners of medicine from those who would use medicine for the pursuit of external goods: managed care managers who want physicians to help pursue profits, states that want psychiatrists to assist by institutionalizing political dissidents, lay people who would have physicians solve nonmedical problems through abortion or euthanasia. If these external ends are incompatible with the internal ends of medicine, they cannot be part of the practice of the good physician.

Pellegrino—often writing with his colleague, David Thomasma—began the quest for the proper formulation of the ends of medicine even before MacIntyre popularized this pursuit.[19] In 1977 and 1978, Pellegrino was analyzing the meaning of relevant concepts, including *illness* and *profession*.[20] By 1981, he and Thomasma were probing the "end of medicine" and had come up with their standard formulation. In this formulation, the end of medicine was "a right and good healing action for a particular patient."[21] In a more recent essay, Pellegrino has elaborated his most current and complete formulation.[22]

Distinguishing Goals from Ends

First, Pellegrino makes a sharp linguistic distinction between the *goals* and the *ends* of medicine. The ends (*telos*) are

> . . . tied to the nature of medicine, to its essence. Ends serve to define medicine. Without certain ends, the activity in question does not qualify as medicine. The ends of medicine distinguish it from other arts and sciences which have different ends. To convert the ends of medicine to the purposes of economics, politics, or professional prerogative, transforms medicine into economics, politics, or professional preference.[23]

To use the earlier language, the ends of medicine are *internal* to it. Pellegrino further contrasts medicine with medical knowledge, which can be put to uses other than medicine. Medical knowledge is used for medicine only when it is used to pursue medicine's ends, which he restates as activity that meets the needs of a particular patient, to "cure, care, help, or heal."[24]

By contrast, *goals* or *purposes* "are not formally tied to the essence of medicine."[25] Medical knowledge can be used for "torturing political prisoners, genocide, 'cleansing' society of the unfit or handicapped, participation in state-ordered executions, making political converts, punishing political dissidents or managing medical care for non-medical purposes."[26] These goals are *external* to medicine's *telos*.[27]

Essentialism Versus Social Constructionism

Second, Pellegrino distinguishes between what he calls *essentialist* and *social constructionist* views of medicine's ends and goals. The *essentialist* approach is grounded in the nature of medicine taken as a reality, an essential end independent of what society would like to use medical knowledge for. This approach defines medicine by reflecting on its *internal* end. Pellegrino contrasts this view with the *social constructivist* view of medicine, in which each community sets the goals and defines medicine's mission in terms of its own values and its own perceptions of reality.[28]

The Substance of the Essentialist Conception: Curing, Caring, Helping, and Healing the Individual Patient

The essentialist view is given content, according to Pellegrino, by proper understanding of the critical terms of medicine—terms such as *healing* and *profession.* To understand what it means to heal a person in need of healing is, according to Pellegrino, all one needs to understand medicine's proper ends. There is a single, univocal, proper understanding of what it means to be a *medical professional.* To be a medical professional is to profess the end that is internal to the very concept of medicine: to cure, care, help, and heal. All other agendas for the use of medical knowledge are goals that are *external*—a piece of some socially constructed project that may be important to a particular culture but is not essential to medicine. Although such socially constructed projects may be consistent with the *practice* of medicine, they also may be quite incompatible with such a practice.

A CRITIQUE OF MORALITY INTERNAL TO MEDICINE

The view that one can discern the proper ends of medicine and the morality appropriate to the physician's role by reflecting on the concept of medicine is not without its problems. Several of these problems are worth considering. Pellegrino manages to avoid some; others pose the potential for serious difficulties, especially for those less capable than he at avoiding them.

The Epistemological Claim of an Internal Morality

MacIntyre calls the goods of certain practices "internal" for two reasons: The goods can be specified only in terms of the practice and they can be identified only by persons experienced in the practice. The first reason could be called *conceptual*: The very concept of the practice specifies the good. The second could be called *epistemological*: Competence, or being experienced in the practice, gives one epistemological expertise in knowing the goods of the practice.

This second claim has long been recognized as controversial in medical ethics. The idea that only members of the professional group—those with professional expertise—can know the goods, the ends, or the norms of a practice dominated the Hippocratic school of medical ethics. Hippocratic physicians reflected the view that knowledge was inherently esoteric, that it could be known only by those inside the group, and that leaking the esoteric secrets of the cult to outsiders was potentially dangerous. Hence, the Hippocratic Oath requires the physician to swear to keep the secrets of medicine from outsiders. In modern medical ethics, this view leads to the now oft-challenged claim that only members of the medical profession can know what is ethical in the practice of medicine. In fact, for many years, two of the defining characteristics of a profession were believed to be internal self-regulation and the creation of its own code of ethics.

Of course, contemporary critics of professional medical ethics have rejected the claim that a profession can generate its own code or be self-regulating. Critics have long suggested that there is no evidence that experience in medicine gives one an added or special insight into the norms of medical practice.[29] In fact, the case has been made that being an expert in a professional field can make one uniquely biased in understanding the nature of the norms for the practice. There is substantial evidence that members of a professional group view the ends, norms, and principles for their profession differently from outsiders. Even from an essentialist perspective such as that of Pellegrino, there is no *a priori* reason to assume that professionals—those with some unique set of beliefs and values that lead them to specialize in a profession and lead them to absorb a special way of seeing the world—are systematically more right in conceptualizing the role they assume. In the end, the claim that a practice has a morality internal to it in the first sense—in the sense that the ends are entailed in the very concept—seems to be independent of the claim that persons with expertise in the practice are better at knowing what those ends are.

Pellegrino has been a forceful leader among medical professionals in rejecting this epistemological claim. He thereby departs in an important and insightful way from MacIntyre. Pellegrino has always been in the forefront in affirming that lay people are potentially capable of reflecting on a concept such as medicine or healing and understanding the ends internally implied. He states this view explicitly:

> This line of reasoning does not assume that defining the ends of medicine as intrinsic to medicine necessitate that physicians are the arbiters of those ends. . . . They can make, have made, are making, and will make errors in defining those ends. . . . Physicians have no epistemological sovereignty in defining the ends of medicine.[30]

Pellegrino recognized at the earliest stages of contemporary medical ethics the danger of claiming that professionals in a practice have epistemological authority in articulating the ends of that practice.[31] The American Medical Association (AMA) itself—long a defender of professional arrogance in claiming that the profession must define the norms of the practice—has now acknowledged the increasing necessity of lay participation in specifying norms for both the lay and professional roles (although the AMA has been reluctant to say this very loudly to the public).[32] Among physician medical ethicists, Pellegrino's affirmation of public participation in furthering the understanding of the professional role has been forceful.

Social Constructionism Versus Essentialism: Some Potential Problems

A second area of potential concern in the "internal morality" thesis is the suggestion that the social constructivist view about formulating the ends of medicine necessarily leads to the conclusion that there are no ends *intrinsic* to medicine.[33] Pellegrino understands social constructivism to be the view that practices are nothing more than the invention of a culture:

> An influential approach today in the definition of reality and morals is through social construction. The foundation of this approach so far as goal setting goes is that there is little likelihood of agreement on such things as essences, definitions, or ethical norms. In consequence, there can be no universalizable ends. . . .[34]

This analysis suggests that social constructivist attempts to define the nature of medicine are relativist. They could produce a different formulation for each culture and make medicine the servant of some of each society's other goals.

There is no doubt that some social constructivist accounts are relativist, but not necessarily all are. A wise Jesuit priest/philosopher/physician has referred to some versions of social constructivist accounts as "value-dependent realism."[35]

A realist account of social construction holds that although there is one reality "out there" to be described, human capacities for observation and human language permit an unlimited number of correct partial descriptions (as well as many clearly incorrect descriptions that conflict with that reality). Each culture may emphasize different aspects of the reality being described and use concepts available to that culture to attempt to convey the account of the reality being described. There are many finite ways of giving true, if partial, accounts of reality. Different cultures will give somewhat differing accounts, each dependent on cultural concepts, values, and linguistic capacities. It is therefore possible for several of these accounts to be correct, if incomplete. Of course, some other accounts may be just plain wrong.

The bottom line is that the mere fact that human accounts of reality must be socially constructed does not mean that these accounts are fabricated independent of some underlying reality. Some of the accounts may turn out to be correct social constructions of some aspect of reality. Pellegrino cites sociologists of knowledge Peter Berger and Thomas Luckmann when he suggests that there can be no universalizable ends or purposes in a social constructionist world,[36] but elsewhere Berger makes clear that the social constructionist view does not rule out the possibility that there is a reality underlying such accounts and that some of them may be more correct than others.[37]

This line of argument leads to the suggestion that even if human groups do construct accounts of the ends of medicine, the social constructionist view is not in complete opposition with the essentialist view. If there is one essential, correct understanding of the ends of medicine, as Pellegrino would have us believe, one or more of the socially constructed accounts may get it right—or at least close to right. The key distinction is not so much between essentialist formulations and social constructions. All accounts of the ends of medicine are social constructions—including the social constructions that more or less accurately reflect the essence of medicine (should such an essence exist).

How the Terms Medicine and Healing Are Essentially Ambiguous

This reformulation of the essentialist/constructivist distinction still leaves us with a crucial problem. Is it possible, even in theory, to deduce the ends of medicine or the morality for the various roles associated with medicine from reflection on critical concepts such as *medicine* or *healing*, independent of some broader socially constructed system of belief and values and some broader account of reality external to medicine?

Pellegrino's approach is to reflect on core concepts such as *medicine* and *healing* to determine their essence and the ends and moral constraints they contain. I have argued that every such reflection will involve social constructions—including social constructions that might accurately reflect some underlying reality. The core problem with the Pellegrino approach is that any effort to determine the proper normative content of these concepts will necessarily rely on some broader conceptualization of the ends of human life. The point here is not that one must appeal to a human social conceptualization of these ends. All conceptions of the ends of human life are social constructions, even if they perfectly mirror reality or some important part of it. The point is that it is impossible to give any content to critical concepts such as *medicine* or *healing* or *health* without going well beyond medicine to some system of belief and value that is external to medicine.

Consider Pellegrino's formulation: The end of medicine is to meet the needs of the individual patient—that is, to cure, care, help, and heal.[38] Each of these terms is terribly ambiguous. In fact, they are so ambiguous that a physician might have almost no idea what is called for from the bare terms standing by themselves.

Understanding What Help Means Requires Standards External to Medicine

Consider *help* first. The idea that the physician is to help the patient does not necessarily imply limiting help to the medical sphere. Perhaps that limit is implied, but many of the more famous codes of medical ethics for physicians do not impose such a limitation. The Hippocratic Oath, the Oath of a Muslim Physician, Percival's *Medical Ethics*, and the code of the American Nurses Association all give the mandate in very broad terms such as working for the patient's *benefit* or *welfare* or *interests;* other codes—such as the Declaration of Geneva and the code of the American Pharmacists' Association—use much narrower language, limiting the health professional to concern about areas such as *health* or *safety.* Even among those that limit the end of medicine to the health of the patient, there are enormous differences in what is included in *health.* Conceptions of *health* range from the World Health Organization's all-inclusive "physical, mental, and social" well-being to very narrow organic conceptualizations. In the end, the claim that "help to the patient" is "internal" to the concept of medicine leaves us with enormous ambiguity about what is really called for.

This ambiguity simply cannot be resolved by thinking harder and harder about the concept of *medicine* without reference to the culture's linguistic categories. Some cultures will have more finely divided social-professional roles; others may have fewer. For certain traditional cultures, helping done professionally for all manner of spiritual, psychological, and social problems remains undifferentiated: The task is assigned to the "medicine man." In early Christianity, for example, the categories of health and healing were not differentiated from spirituality and psychotherapy. To this day, it is not always clear whether psychiatrists, psychologists, and psychotherapists are engaged in the practice of *medicine.*

Differentiating Between "Helping" and "Hindering" Requires Standards External to Medicine

Even more critical is the ambiguity in deciding whether an action counts as a "help" or a "hindrance." Presumably, only actions that improve the lot of the patient are helpful (others are neutral or harmful). Is relieving a woman of the physical burden of pregnancy by aborting her pregnancy helpful to her physical well-being? Is withholding extraordinarily burdensome treatment helpful or harmful if the result is an unintended but foreseeable shortening of life? If the end of medicine is to help (presumably in the organic sphere) improve one's well-being, the physician will need to know what counts as a benefit and what as a harm. Once again, there is no way that bare reflection on the concept of medicine will tell us which interventions that change a patient's organic state are helpful and which are harmful. Some effects may be sought by some patients and dreaded by others, and in either case the outcome may or may not conform to the human's proper *telos*.

I assume that Pellegrino, the essentialist, shares my view that at least some of these value judgments may really be right or wrong. The problem, however, is that one must move beyond medicine to a more general theory of the ends of life to know which judgments about outcomes are right and which wrong. Mere reflection on the concept of *medicine* will not do the job. A more comprehensive system of belief and value—a religious world view or its secular substitute—that goes well beyond medicine must be incorporated. That system of belief and value must be external to medicine and more fundamental.

Understanding What It Means to Heal, Cure, and Care Requires Standards External to Medicine

Similar ambiguities arise with the other terms. *To heal* is so ambiguous that it is used for all manner of improvements in a person's state, from setting a broken bone to Paul's miraculous restoration of sight. We can heal relationships, marriages, pets, and plants, yet presumably most are not in the physician's mandate. On the other hand, psychic healing may not be excluded altogether from the mandate. At least, we take a dim view of physicians who narrowly limit their gaze to the organic. Likewise, to label a behavior as producing a *cure* or manifesting *care* requires some external standard. Even if we can agree that the end of medicine is to "cure, care, help, and heal," those labels are contentless without some broader framework of beliefs and values that define the proper end of life. That framework is necessarily external to medicine.

Resolving Conflicts Among Medical Ends Requires Some Standard External to Medicine

Most critically, there are times when these ends of medicine are in conflict with one another. Relieving suffering may require withdrawing a burdensome treatment that will remove any chance of a cure. Preserving health may require reordering priorities so that less time and energy is available for curative medicine. In the ideal world *cure, care, help,* and *healing* can all come together—and all parties will agree that these labels apply—but in most medical encounters, this is not likely to be possible.

Some broad view about the ends of life, some broad system of beliefs and values, will be necessary to specify just which actions count as healing actions. What counts as a major medical success according to one world view may be an utter failure in the next. Simply deciding that medicine implies the ends of cure, care, help, and healing may tell us almost nothing. What fits one of these terms in one world view will fail to satisfy the other terms using that world view, and the proponents of another world view may have an entirely different assessment of whether some or all of these terms apply to a physician's action.

I cannot fully develop in this essay the claim that what counts as healing in one major tradition of belief and value may utterly fail to count as that in another. The essential claim here is that even if one is an essentialist, one must turn beyond medicine to more fundamental and inclusive systems of belief and value to understand what the real ends of medicine are.

The key point here is that figuring out what counts as curing, caring, helping, or healing simply cannot be done by means of naked, isolated reflection on some all-purpose concept of medicine. To know what counts as medicine, one has to know what counts as curing, caring, and so forth—but to know these things, one must move beyond medical knowledge and medicine. One must move to some integrated world view that includes within it an understanding of the ends of life.

The Possibility of Many Medicines

In fact, it may turn out to be a mistake to suggest that there is a single entity called *medicine*. There may be as many different *medicines* as there are world views. Each will have a different account of what counts as meeting the needs of the patient. Imagine an Orthodox Jewish physician, a militant feminist physician, a Roman Catholic physician, a Marxist physician, and a Nazi physician, all trained in Western allopathic medicine. They may have greater differences than similarities in their understanding of what counts as healing the patient. In fact, the militant feminist might not even accept the word *patient* because of its implications of passivity and subordination. These practitioners, even assuming they have the same metaphysical beliefs about medical science, will have such radically different ideas about what constitutes help or healing that they can be said to be practicing different medicines.

These world views may be religions; they may be secular surrogates for religion, such as Marxism, Nazism, secular liberalism, libertarianism, or feminism. Each will have its own peculiar conceptualization of the proper ends of human living, of what makes humans flourish. What counts as *medicine* for one will fail utterly for another. To know what medicine is, one must necessarily go beyond medicine. The morality of the practice, the end to be pursued, cannot be internal to the practice itself. It must come from beyond medicine—from some integrated world view about the meaning and purpose of life.

Is There Only One Correct or "True" Account of Medicine?

From the foregoing discussion, one should be able to see that the question of whether there is one and only one "correct" or "true" way to conceptualize medicine remains open. Clearly there are many accounts of the ends of medicine—one for each religious or secular world view about the ends of human life. That situation leaves open the question of whether one or more of these accounts is essentially true. To use Pellegrino's language, the question of whether one or more of the social constructions essentially corresponds to reality remains open.

Whether there is one, or more than one, correct account of medicine will depend on whether there is one, or more than one, correct world view. Bluntly put, to know whether there is one true medicine, one must first determine whether there is one true religion.

Clearly there are many social constructions of religious systems. Each will have implications for an understanding of the proper norms for the practice of medicine from the perspective of that system. What is less clear is whether one and only one of these social constructions reads reality correctly. It is possible that one world view—say, some formulation of Roman Catholicism or Marxism—will turn out to understand the true ends of human existence. In that case, there will be one true "religion," and from that foundation we should be able to figure out what true way to practice medicine. The correct understanding of the practice of medicine would be the pursuit of the ends of human existence—presumably constrained to the organic or organic/psychological sphere—as articulated by the correct world view. That conclusion would imply that many other possible pursuits of physicians are not good medicine.

The key point, however, is that to know what good medicine is we must look outside medicine. We must understand morality and the ends of life outside medicine to know how medicine is to be practiced. Hence, if one accepts the religious/metaphysical position that Roman Catholicism understands the ends of human life correctly, then one would expect that the Roman Catholic belief system could be used to articulate the ends of medicine as a practice within that tradition. One cannot know what good Catholic medicine is until one knows what good Catholicism is. (A similar claim would be made for holders of each and every belief system.)

CONCLUSION

This analysis leaves me with a final puzzle. How can it be that Edmund Pellegrino—who certainly has not hidden his deep, faithful commitment to a particular religious tradition, who seems clearly to understand how far physicians can stray from the Catholic conception of the ends of life—would not insist that one can only understand the practice of medicine by turning outside medicine to understand first the ends of life as articulated by the religious tradition to which he affirms loyalty? It would seem that only then—as a subsidiary, derivative task—would he be able to turn to matters of medicine and ask what the ends of medicine should be. It seems that Pellegrino should be saying that it is impossible to know the norms, ends, and morality for the practice of medicine until one turns to standards external to medicine, to one's religious or philosophical system of belief and value.

NOTES

1. Edmund D. Pellegrino, "Managed Care at the Bedside: How Do We Look in the Moral Mirror?" *Kennedy Institute of Ethics Journal* 7, no. 4 (1997): 321–30.

2. Edmund D. Pellegrino, "Doctors Must Not Kill," in *Euthanasia: The Good Patient,* ed. Robert I. Misbin (Frederick, Md.: University Publishing Group, 1992), 27–42.

3. Edmund D. Pellegrino, "The Physician, Nuclear Warfare, and the Ethics of Medicine," in *Nuclear Weapons and the Future of Humanity: The Fundamental Question,* ed. Avner Cohen and Steven Lee (Totowa, N.J.: Rowman and Allanheld Publishers, 1986), 341–58.

4. Edmund D. Pellegrino, "Guarding the Integrity of Medical Ethics: Some Lessons From Soviet Russia," *Journal of the American Medical Association* 273 (May 24/31, 1995): 1622–23.

5. Edmund D. Pellegrino and David C. Thomasma, *The Philosophical Basis of Medical Practice* (New York: Oxford University Press, 1981), 185.

6. Edmund D. Pellegrino, "Toward a Reconstruction of Medical Morality: The Primacy of the Act of Profession and the Fact of Illness," *Journal of Medicine and Philosophy* 4 (March 1979): 32–56; Pellegrino and Thomasma, *The Philosophical Basis of Medical Practice* (especially chapters 8 and 9—the latter of which is a revised version of Pellegrino's 1979 article); Edmund D. Pellegrino and David C. Thomasma, *For the Patient's Good: The Restoration of Beneficence in Health Care* (New York: Oxford University Press, 1988) (especially pages viii, 78, and 116); and Edmund D. Pellegrino, "The Goals and Ends of Medicine: How Are They to be Defined?" in *The Goals of Medicine: The Forgotten Issues in Health Care Reform,* ed. Mark Hanson and Daniel Callahan (Washington, D.C.: Georgetown University Press, 1999) (hereafter cited as *GEM*).

7. Howard Brody, "The Physician's Role in Determining Futility," *Journal of the American Geriatrics Society* 42, no. 8 (1994): 875–78; Lawrence Schneiderman, Nancy S. Jecker, and Albert R. Jonsen, "Medical Futility: Response to Critiques," *Annals of Internal Medicine* 125 (October 15, 1996): 669–74.

8. Pellegrino and Thomasma, *For the Patient's Good,* 115.

9. Brody, "The Physician's Role in Determining Futility," 877.

10. Alasdair MacIntyre, *After Virtue* (Notre Dame, Ind.: University of Notre Dame Press, 1981).

11. MacIntyre, *After Virtue,* 175.

12. Ibid.

13. Ibid., 181.

14. Ibid., 176.

15. Ibid.

16. Ibid.

17. Ibid., 56, citing Aristotle's *Nichomachean Ethics,* 1095a 16.

18. MacIntyre, *After Virtue,* 57.

19. Because several of Pellegrino's most sustained efforts appear as books co-authored by Thomasma, I want to make clear that I am here attributing the views in those joint works to each of them and thus will cite them as Pellegrino's views for purposes of this article.

20. Edmund D. Pellegrino, "Humanistic Base for Professional Ethics in Medicine," *New York State Journal of Medicine* 77 (August 1977): 1456–62; Edmund D. Pellegrino, "The Fact of Illness and the Act of Profession: Some Notes on the Source of Professional Obligation," in *Implications of History and Ethics to Medicine—Veterinary and Human,* ed. Laurence B. McCullough and James Polk Morris, III (College Station: Texas A&M University, 1978), 78–89.

21. Pellegrino and Thomasma, *The Philosophical Basis of Medical Practice,* 219.

22. Pellegrino, *GEM*.

23. Ibid.

24. Ibid.

25. Ibid.

26. Ibid.

27. Ibid.

28. Ibid.

29. My earliest effort to make this case appeared as Robert M. Veatch, "Medical Ethics: Professional or Universal," *Harvard Theological Review* 65, no. 4 (October 1972): 531–39.

30. Pellegrino, *GEM.*

31. Edmund D. Pellegrino, "Toward an Expanded Medical Ethics: The Hippocratic Ethic Revisited," in *Hippocrates Revisited: A Search for Meaning,* ed. Roger J. Bulger (New York: Medcom Press, 1973), 133–47, *especially* 144.

32. James S. Todd, "Report of the Ad Hoc Committee on The Principles of Medical Ethics [of the American Medical Association]" (unpublished, 1979).

33. Pellegrino, *GEM.*

34. Ibid.

35. William E. Stempsey, "Fact and Value in Disease and Diagnosis: A Proposal for Value-dependent Realism," Doctoral dissertation, Georgetown University, 1996.

36. Pellegrino, *GEM.*

37. Peter Berger, *The Sacred Canopy* (Garden City, N.Y.: Doubleday, 1967), appendix II, pp. 179–88.

38. Sometimes there are internal variations in Pellegrino's formulations. On page 21 of *GEM,* for example, he states that the end of medicine is to "heal, help, care, and cure, to prevent illness, and cultivate health." I take the addition of "prevent illness and cultivate health" to be significant: It adds preventive medicine and perhaps even holistic health to the agenda. I ignore these variations in the unpacking of the ends implied in the concept of medicine at this point in my analysis, however.

Doctoring and the (Neglected) Virtue of Self-Forgiveness

Jeffrey Blustein

SELF-FORGIVENESS: A CHALLENGE FOR PHYSICIANS

Self-forgiveness has received little attention in the philosophical literature on moral psychology. Few papers are devoted to the subject,[1] and most discussions of forgiveness do not mention it at all. Others take it up, but only within the context of a discussion of interpersonal forgiveness and not as a topic in its own right.[2] In these papers, the interpersonal cases are taken to be the paradigm cases; against this backdrop, the authors raise the question of whether we can properly speak of self-forgiveness at all.

One view is that however natural the phrase "self-forgiveness" may appear to be in certain situations, the term must be taken metaphorically. Its literal sense refers to something precisely like the interpersonal kind, except that it occurs within one person. This usage, however, generates the moral paradox that a self-forgiver is both innocent (as the one who forgives) and guilty (as the one who is exonerated). Another view is that although talk of forgiving oneself is admittedly anomalous, there are enough similarities between that which applies to self and that which applies to others to justify stretching the term "forgiveness" to encompass intrapersonal cases. This analysis accepts the concept as a version of forgiveness, not a different concept by the same name.

Given this general lack of philosophical interest in the topic of self-forgiveness, it may not be surprising that this topic also has been neglected by writers on medical ethics—even by those who have turned to virtue ethics as a corrective to principle-based approaches that have not been sufficiently attentive to the importance of character in defining the responsibilities of physicians. Edmund Pellegrino and David Thomasma, for example, have written at length on the virtues of the good physician,[3] pointing out that what we prize in a good physician is not just the physician's outward conformity to moral prescriptions but his or her characteristic motivational structures. The good physician, Pellegrino and Thomasma claim, is one who puts the good of the patient before his or her own good and practices virtues such as compassion, benevolence, honesty, fidelity to

I thank Rita Charon, Bart Collopy, Hilde Lindemann Nelson, Ronald Salzberger, and William Ruddick for helpful comments on earlier drafts of this paper.

promises, and, at times, courage. There is no mention, however, of the role of self-forgiveness in the physician-patient relationship, nor any discussion of its place within a conception of the good physician.

This omission would not be serious if self-forgiveness were not a virtue or if there were no particular reason to include it among the virtues specific to the good physician. Quite obviously, not every instance of self-forgiveness is deserving of moral praise; one may forgive oneself indulgently for things that oughtn't be absolved or do so prematurely without having honestly confronted one's wrongdoing and taken full responsibility for it. Sometimes one shouldn't absolve oneself—at least, not yet or not in this way. On the other hand, sometimes one should or at least try to do so, lest one be gratuitously self-punitive. Furthermore, persons may have *characteristic* ways of dealing with self-forgiveness—that is, their acts or omissions may be caused by or give expression to tendencies that are actualized in repeated occurrences of the same type. A person who is disposed to work toward forgiving himself or herself when it is appropriate to do so and in an appropriate manner has this virtue; with respect to that element of character, at least, this person is a better person than one who is prone to self-indulgent, premature, or obstinate withholding of self-forgiveness.

It remains to be shown why it is good to be disposed to self-forgiveness, but even if we grant that this virtue is a beneficial trait, it may not be apparent why it is important for the *physician* to possess it. Alasdair MacIntyre's account of the virtues provides a framework for addressing this question.[4] According to MacIntyre, virtues have inherent and instrumental worth—the latter deriving from their relationship to what he calls "practices." Practices are complex and demanding activities with standards of excellence and goods "internal" to them, and medicine is a practice in this sense. To realize the goods internal to a practice, practitioners must submit to the rules of the practice and align themselves with the historical tradition that has given rise to its canons of excellence. In MacIntyre's account, a virtue is a learned human quality without which one cannot attain these goods. From this perspective, the virtues of the physician are acquired traits of character that are necessary to realize goods that are internal to medicine and should be cultivated for this reason.

To explain why the virtue of self-forgiveness is a virtue of the good physician, therefore, two things are required: first, an account of what the practice of medicine calls for one to do and second, an explanation of why the physician must possess this virtue if he or she is to do it.

Medical ethicists have addressed the first issue under the heading of "the ends of medicine," and it will be sufficient for my purposes to note agreement on the following: "Restoring the health of sick individuals, relieving suffering, ameliorating ill health when health cannot be achieved, and caring for the sick" (in Ezekiel Emanuel's formulation);[5] or in a slightly more elaborate formulation, "the restoration or improvement of health and, more proximately, to heal, that is, to cure illness and disease or, when this is not possible, to care for and help the patient to live with residual pain, discomfort, or disability"—or "healing and helping," for short (in Pellegrino's and Thomasma's version).[6] Some of these ends are defined independently of any virtues, and some seem to incorporate motivational elements, but I am more interested here in how the virtue of self-forgiveness relates to the overarching end of the patient's good. In particular, I argue that this virtue is one of the traits of character that dispose the physician to act in a way that advances and enriches the ends of the medical relationship.

Why is cultivation of the virtue of self-forgiveness on the part of physicians instrumentally valuable? What are the consequences for patients if this virtue is not cultivated? Answers to these questions explain why self-forgiveness is one of the virtues that make for a good physician. Moreover, they provide the basis for ethical criticism of a range of contemporary medical practices. Not only has self-forgiveness not been a topic of *theoretical* interest among medical ethicists; it has also been ignored as a *practical* matter in the education and socialization of physicians: Little is done to encourage appreciation of its value, and much is done to discourage it. Self-forgiveness is a particularly sensitive issue for many physicians, partly because of the personalities of those who are drawn to the profession of medicine and, perhaps to a greater extent, because of the way the culture of that profession shapes and reinforces their characters and self-conceptions.

Self-forgiveness, especially when one has seriously injured another, can be one of the most daunting tasks a person confronts. It can take years to accomplish if there is no help from others or if a person does not work very hard at it, and at times it must not be accomplished at all. For some people, including many practicing physicians, self-forgiveness presents special challenges. Beginning in medical school and continuing in residency training and beyond, physicians are socialized to expect of themselves a kind of omnipotence that sets them apart from virtually everyone else. The message is clear, if largely implicit, and its incorporation into the physician's internal self-regulation is difficult to resist and dislodge: The physician is a healer who is engaged in an aggressive war against death and disease, and anything less than victory is second best: a proof of failure. There is also a powerful emphasis on perfection in diagnosis and treatment.[7] Role models in medical education reinforce the notion of infallibility, and the organization of medical practice—particularly in the hospital—perpetuates it. As a consequence, anything short of perfection tends to be viewed by the physician as a failure of character.

Cultivating a norm of high standards among physicians is highly desirable, of course. This cultivation is the counterpart of a fundamental goal of medical education—namely, developing the physician's sense of responsibility for the patient. A commitment to high standards of professional practice expresses and underscores the seriousness of the physician's vocation, its ethic of serving the sick and protecting their vulnerability against exploitation. However, the processes that motivate physicians to maintain excellent standards of practice do not include an emphasis on the cultivation of humility—with the result that many physicians, particularly early in their careers, are prone to overestimate their capabilities. Needless to say, the belief in physician infallibility and omnipotence that medical training and socialization instill and sustain are unrealistic, and the standards they set for the physician are impossibly high. Inevitably, these beliefs will collide with evidence of the physician's limitations and shortcomings, and if the physician acknowledges these shortcomings, he or she will either have to rethink those beliefs or remain in a state of inner conflict and cognitive dissonance.

A person who possesses the virtue of self-forgiveness is able to discern when feelings of self-reproach are appropriate and has the psychological resources to deal constructively with them. Traditional medical training and practice, however, do not foster development of the skills, attitudes, and traits needed to accomplish these tasks. As a result, standards of professional excellence tend to engender unreasonable expectations in physicians of perfection and control over death and disease—and patients have been conditioned to accept no less. Failures to meet these expectations occur and may cause the physician enormous distress, but the opportunities to discuss them in a supportive environment are limited. The one forum in which physicians can talk candidly about their mistakes—the mortality and morbidity conference—is designed more to promote group solidarity and reinforce medical hierarchy than to encourage participants to openly discuss their mistakes and their emotional responses to them.[8] In some cases, because of the lack of social supports to mitigate stress, the physician may be plagued by recurring self-doubt or lapse into neurotic behavior to deal with his or her anxiety and guilt.[9]

The emotional impact of perceived wrongdoing can seriously disrupt the physician's professional and personal life. Self-forgiveness does not insulate the physician from all such bad feelings—nor should it. Rather, it enables the physician to cope better with those feelings by regulating and modulating them. Self-forgiveness can benefit the physician's patients as well. The good physician does not hold himself or herself to standards that demand a degree of control or flawless performance that exceeds what most people would find reasonable. If the physician possesses this virtue, his or her feelings of self-reproach are responsive to reasonable beliefs about his or her fault and the faultiness of his or her conduct. The physician does not persist in blaming himself or herself when it is inappropriate to do so— which has important implications for the physician who is caring for patients who are beyond the physician's ability to cure. In other situations, when it is appropriate for the physician to blame himself or herself the physician does so, but he or she knows how to manage these feelings constructively. The physician addresses his or her lapses honestly and courageously; a critical part of this process is taking responsibility for his or her mistakes and disclosing them to patients and/or patients' families.[10]

The neglect of self-forgiveness that is rooted in the very culture of medicine provides the context and much of the impetus for the investigation that follows. Specific recommendations for how to introduce this topic into the mainstream of medicine are beyond the scope of this essay. My task is to establish a conceptual and ethical framework for thinking about self-forgiveness and to show how the ends of medicine are furthered when it is treated as a central goal of physician education and socialization. This essay is divided into three main sections. Section II provides an account of interpersonal forgiveness and uses it to structure a conceptual analysis of self-forgiveness. Section III examines the conditions under which the disposition to forgive oneself can properly be considered a *virtue* and the reasons for regarding it as such. Section IV returns to the physician-patient relationship and offers some reasons for thinking that self-forgiveness is a particularly important virtue in that context.

THE CONCEPT OF SELF-FORGIVENESS

We cannot sensibly discuss the virtue of self-forgiveness and its application to the physician-patient relationship without first understanding the nature of self-forgiveness. The following several subsections take up this conceptual task.

Preliminary Comparison with Interpersonal Forgiveness

The model of interpersonal forgiveness provides a potentially illuminating analogy. Yet we should not expect these two concepts to be analogous in all respects, nor should we require them to be so. The expression "self-forgiveness" refers to a set of related phenomena that are analogous to interpersonal forgiveness in some but not all ways.

The following analysis of forgiveness (I do not endorse all of its particulars) can help structure our thinking. According to Joram Haber, S forgives an agent X for her act A if and only if S "represents as true" that:

1. X did A;
2. A was wrong;
3. X was responsible for doing A;
4. S was personally injured by X's doing A;
5. S resented being injured by X's doing A;
6. S has overcome his resentment for X's doing A or is at least willing to try to overcome it.[11]

To what extent do these conditions provide a satisfactory analysis of self-forgiveness if S is replaced by X, thereby making the forgiver and the forgiven the same person? Conditions 1–3 seem relatively unproblematic: In cases of self-forgiveness, the agent has committed a wrong for which she holds herself responsible. However, if *wrong* is understood to mean wrong done to another—as it normally is—arguably we can properly speak of self-forgiveness even when such injury has not occurred. That is, if we interpret *wrong* in this way, condition 2 need not apply to self-forgiveness. Condition 4 tells us that in self-forgiveness the agent must (also) have done herself some personal injury (because S = X) by her wrongdoing. We can think of some obvious examples in which this happens: She may have ruined her career, tarnished her reputation, or lost a valued friend. Or she may suffer personal injury in the sense that she imaginatively identifies with the harm she caused another. We also speak of self-forgiveness when none of this occurs, however. What kind of personal injury, then—if any—is presupposed by self-forgiveness? Moreover, even if some sort of personal injury must be suffered in all cases, in many instances the injury we have done to ourselves is not and should not be the focus of our concern. When we have wronged another, it is chiefly this harm about which we should feel bad and for which we should work to forgive ourselves, if self-forgiveness is morally appropriate at all.

Conditions 5 and 6 require that the wrongdoer experience self-directed resentment that she then tries to overcome. Some readers may object that talk of self-directed resentment is anomalous: Resentment is typically regarded as an emotion that is directed toward another person—though resentment does not preclude acknowledging, of course, that one is partly to blame for this mistreatment. Even if we grant that self-resentment is a viable moral psychological concept, it is only one of the emotions that can prompt self-forgiveness.

Thus defined, the analogy between forgiveness of others and self-forgiveness is imperfect. Perhaps a single account of forgiveness could be constructed that provides a unified explanation of interpersonal and intrapersonal cases, but that task would take this essay too far afield.

Self-Forgiveness as Condoning?

According to R. S. Downie, "self-forgiveness" is a misnomer. Downie claims that infliction of injury is a necessary condition of forgiveness properly so-called; he argues that because we do not make injury to self a condition of using the expression "self-forgiveness," this concept is not forgiveness at all but the different notion of *condoning*. Properly understood, Downie argues, forgiving oneself for what one has done is condoning that behavior—that is, excusing it, overlooking it, or treating it indulgently. We can adopt this attitude without having been injured ourselves, and it masquerades as self-forgiveness. "When we say, 'I cannot forgive myself,'" Downie asserts, "we mean that we cannot let ourselves off lightly or find any excuse for treating our own failure with indulgence."[12] By the same token, when we say, "I forgive myself," we mean that we have found such an excuse or are prepared to overlook what we have done.

Admittedly, we sometimes say we forgive ourselves when what we have done is trivial, harmless, or of no importance or when we admit that what we did was wrong but excuse ourselves for it. Strictly speaking, however, use of the term in such cases is idiosyncratic.[13] If we collapse self-forgiveness into condoning and deny the former an arena of its own, we would have no basis for claiming that sometimes it is condoning rather than forgiving and sometimes forgiving rather than condoning—that is, the appropriate response to what we have done. Nor could we sensibly make the observation that condoning is frequently used as a morally inferior substitute for self-forgiveness because it is often psychologically easier to condone the injury by playing down its extent than to face up to it honestly and engage in the process of self-forgiveness. Yet we do distinguish between self-forgiveness and condoning in terms of the gravity of what we have done and our responsibility for it. If self-forgiveness were only a matter of excusing or ignoring or denying, as Downie claims, we would need another label for the often long and difficult process that goes by the name of self-forgiveness. This revisionist move seems awkward and counterintuitive, however. We speak of self-forgiveness precisely in cases in which we *cannot* condone what we have done; any credible account of self-forgiveness must be able to accommodate such cases, instead of denying that they exist.

The Wrong That Self-Forgiveness Addresses

Concerns about self-forgiveness are often occasioned by wrongdoings or mistakes that cause injury or harm to other persons. In some cases, the wrongdoing is particularly pernicious in that it involves damage to what Norman Care calls the "moral personality" of another, which "centrally involve[s] the various capacities that allow one to develop and enjoy self-respect and to be capable of respect for others."[14] Persistent wrongdoing suffered by persons whose self-image and self-respect depend on the way they are treated by the offender is likely to be of this sort. Injury that damages the moral personality of another is not the only way one can seriously injure another, however, and it does not frequently occur in the cases that interest me.

The actions that occasion self-forgiveness may be wrong in either of two senses: wrong other things equal (i.e., *prima facie* wrong) or wrong all things considered. In some instances of moral conflict, moral wrongdoing may be inescapable, even though all things considered we are justified in acting as we do. As Michael Stocker notes, "One can be justified in doing an act that ineliminably has a part it would be wrong to do on its own—and more importantly for us, which remains a wrong, albeit a justified wrong, when done in doing what is right."[15] In these cases, one might feel the need to forgive oneself for the *prima facie* wrong one is responsible for having committed, and this feeling might not be misguided. In other cases, the wrong we do is not part of an overall justified act; here too, one might seek self-forgiveness.

In addition to distinguishing between types of wrong in this way, the usual understanding of wrong needs to be amended, at least if we want to maintain an analogy between self-forgiveness and forgiveness of others. Although the wrongs with which self-forgiveness is concerned are most commonly done to others, we also have to include reflexive wrongs that do not entail others. To be sure, recent philosophers tend to discard the idea of wronging oneself as a conceptual confusion on the grounds that wrongdoing is essentially a social or interpersonal phenomenon. The issues that this objection raises are too complex to examine here, but everyday discourse at least is not so exclusionary. Thus, we often say of a person who has allowed herself to be demeaned or degraded by others, for example, or who has behaved in ways that are contemptible in her own eyes that she has wronged herself.

The Self-Inflicted Injury in Self-Forgiveness

Usually one does not speak of forgiving or not forgiving oneself unless one's actions have injured one's self-respect—that is, one's sense of one's inner worth as a person. If the actions resulted in injury to others for which the agent holds himself or herself responsible and the agent is a morally sensitive person who recognizes that he or she stands in certain relations to other people, the agent's self-respect is bound to be injured. Less commonly, as H. J. N. Horsbrugh notes, we might also speak of self-forgiveness when no other person has suffered injury because "one's moral image can sustain a severe fracture"[16] as a result of actions for which one blames oneself even in these cases. In neither type of situation, however, is this injury to self-respect the wrong for which the agent has to forgive himself or herself. What has to be forgiven is either the injury to others or, when others are not injured, "the weak or vicious actions that resulted in the injury"[17] to self. In other words, we should be careful not to confuse a *necessary condition* of the proper use of the term "self-forgiveness" with the *object* of self-forgiveness.

The injury to self-respect can be explained in different ways, depending on how we understand having a sense of worth as a person. There is a kind of self-respect that involves the belief that, whatever others might think, one has an equal status in a system of moral rights. Thomas Hill's examples of the overly deferential wife and the extremely self-deprecating person illustrate an absence of this type of self-respect.[18] These individuals submit to denial of their basic rights, and this pattern of acquiescence may be something for which they are right to hold themselves responsible and blameworthy, at least to some extent. Under these circumstances, concerns about self-forgiveness may arise quite appropriately for them.

Another type of self-respect involves developing and living by commitments and attachments that ground a set of personal standards by which the individual judges his or her self-worth. These standards may or may not be ethical ones, and the individual may or may not criticize others or all others for not having the same ones: As the individual sees it, these standards may apply only to himself or herself or only to others in the same profession. The standards implicate the individual's sense of self-worth because the commitments and attachments are constitutive of his or her self and because it is impossible to have constitutive commitments and attachments without having some view of what is expected or required to sustain them. This view need not be very articulate and may only become so under special circumstances, but if the individual fails to live up to these self-imposed expectations, he or she fails to be himself or herself. On this view, to have a conception of self-respect is to have a sense of one's constitutive commitments and attachments, and one has self-respect to the extent that one is disposed to act in accordance with that conception.

An interesting question is whether we can also speak of self-forgiveness when one's actions have injured one's *self-esteem*, where self-esteem is distinguished from self-respect and one suffers a blow to self-esteem without at the same time suffering an injury to self-respect. Gabriele Taylor distinguishes between self-respect and self-esteem as follows:

> The person who has self-esteem takes a favorable view of himself, while he who lacks it will think of himself in unfavorable terms. . . . There is a connection between self-esteem and emotional pride: the person who is proud of this or that enjoys, at the time of feeling proud, an increase in his self-esteem; he can now take a more favorable view of himself (in some respect). . . . For a person to have self-respect does not mean that he has a favorable attitude towards himself, or that he has any particular attitude towards himself at all. Nor is self-respect connected with emotional pride.[19]

Pauline Chazan also argues that self-respect and self-esteem are distinguishable from one another: Self-respect involves "aspects of a person which are experienced by her as essential parts of what she is," whereas self-esteem, like pride, involves "evaluations of some aspect or aspects of the self"[20] that may belong to one merely contingently. To be sure, as both writers point out, self-respect and self-esteem are not unconnected: A lack or loss of self-respect will adversely affect how one feels about oneself, and retaining self-respect is always a ground for self-esteem. A lowering of self-esteem does not necessarily undermine self-respect, however, and lowering of self-esteem may be sufficient for self-forgiveness to be possible even if self-respect remains intact.

Physicians who meet the minimum requirements for competency may esteem themselves for doing so, and if Stephen Darwall is right that "whatever qualities ground our self-esteem are qualities of which we are proud,"[21] they then have reason to feel pride as well. They might also feel proud of their skill in situations that surpass what is normally expected, in which case they will enjoy an increase in self-esteem. Whatever qualities ground their self-esteem, that self-esteem is diminished if they come to evaluate themselves less favorably in some respect. Injury to self-respect, by contrast, necessarily has a larger impact because self-respect concerns what is constitutive of one's selfhood.

Although there is a tendency to think that self-forgiveness only has application when there has been an injury to one's self-respect, it would be a mistake to insist that actions resulting only in loss of self-esteem cannot be possible objects of self-forgiveness. Against this view, one might argue that "self-forgiveness does not come about easily"[22] and that the difficulty of self-forgiveness is best explained by an injury to self-respect and not merely a blow to one's self-esteem. An injury to self-respect strikes deeper than a blow to self-esteem, and self-respect will be more difficult to recover. Yet this conclusion is not invariably true. A blow to self-esteem might strike quite deep for a person who is inordinately vain and who cares more than he or she should about self-esteem.

The Emotion(s) Overcome by Self-Forgiveness

Self-forgiveness involves overcoming a range of negative emotions on the basis of certain considerations. Learning to live with these emotions is not sufficient. *Overcoming* them is required because self-forgiveness, like forgiveness of others, is primarily a matter of changing the way one feels about a person—either oneself or another. I do not forgive another if I continue to harbor hostile feelings towards that person but simply do not outwardly display them; similarly, I do not forgive myself if I do not let go of self-hatred and other painful emotions engendered by my past behavior.

.How are we to understand this process of "letting go"? It does not involve canceling the judgment that I have culpably wronged another or failed to act in accordance with my core commitments. Forgiveness—of others as well as of self—does not involve overcoming the judgment that a wrong has been done and that some punishment or compensation would therefore be appropriate. Rather, one "lets go" of the bad feelings that tend to accompany the judgment. Letting go, it should be emphasized, is not the sole or main motivation of self-forgiveness; if it were, self-forgiveness would be no different morally from going to a psychotherapist to have the bad feelings taken away, or forgetting what you have done, or talking yourself into a better frame of mind by telling yourself that you did nothing wrong. The primary point in seeking self-forgiveness, as in forgiveness of others, cannot be the desire to be rid of these bad feelings.

One plausible way of explaining how this "overcoming" is possible is Robert Roberts' proposal that we think of emotions as "perceptual" states analogous to the ones we are in when we view the gestalt figures in certain psychology books."[23] On this view, not feeling hatred and the like is a matter of not seeing oneself or another as "bad, alien, guilty, worthy of suffering, unwelcome, offensive, an enemy, etc.,"[24] and of focusing on reconciliation and "harmonious relationship."[25] This perception is compatible with retention of the initial judgment of wrongdoing.[26]

Someone who is struggling with self-forgiveness may feel shame or guilt acutely or chronically. Shame has an especially close connection with self-respect; in light of the relationship between self-forgiveness and self-respect, shame has particular importance in the analysis of self-forgiveness. Thus, according to Gabriele Taylor, occasions for loss of self-respect and occasions for feelings of shame coincide, and the prospect of experiencing shame inhibits one from doing things that would injure one's self-respect:

> To respect the self . . . is to do that which protects the self from injury or destruction. . . . And shame is the emotion of self-protection: It may prevent the person concerned from putting himself into a certain position, or make him aware that he ought not to be in the position in which he finds himself.[27]

Guilt may not be *the* emotion of self-protection, but here too there are frequently connections with self-respect. A serious violation of a rule can both engender guilt and do damage to one's self-respect, if adherence to that code of conduct is among one's core commitments.

THE VIRTUE OF SELF-FORGIVENESS

Self-forgiveness for wronging *another* may appear to be morally suspect because it deflects attention from the victim and what the offender must do vis-a-vis the victim to mitigate the offender's guilt. If I have committed a wrong against you, I cannot simply remove the guilt at will. I may be able to rid myself of guilty feelings, but I cannot render them unwarranted at will. To suppose otherwise, Richard Swinburne argues, is to fail to "take seriously the fact that the act is an act by which you are wronged, and in the wiping out of which you ought therefore to have a say. One consequence of my harming you is just that it is in part up to you whether my guilt is remitted."[28] Often the victim will require at least some minimal atonement, such as an apology and an effort to make reparation. Alternatively, the victim may, out of generosity or compassion, forgive the offender even if repentance is not forthcoming—and sometimes it is good that the victim should do so. Whatever the victim chooses to do, the remission of guilt depends in part on his or her willingness to forgive the offender.

The victim's power to determine what the offender must do before he or she may be forgiven is limited, of course. If the offender has repented and atoned in such a way that a reasonable person would grant forgiveness, then arguably the offender should no longer feel guilt, even if the victim refuses to grant forgiveness. Sometimes, when the offender's efforts to gain the victim's forgiveness are rebuffed or deemed insufficient, the offender may nevertheless be justified in forgiving himself or herself as a kind of second-best alternative to forgiveness by another.[29]

In principle, the victim's forgiveness is not required to validate self-forgiveness. In fact, however, objective verification that self-forgiveness is appropriate is often required to ensure that one is not deceiving oneself about having met the conditions for self-forgiveness.

Self-forgiveness is warranted only when considerations favoring forgiveness by the victim obtain. If some suitable atonement by the wrongdoer is necessary for forgiveness to be appropriate, and if the wrongdoer's atonement is inadequate to the offense or perfunctory or insincere, the offender should not be forgiven—and should not forgive himself or herself, either. In general, the disposition to forgive oneself regardless of whether a reasonable person in the victim's position would forgive can hardly be considered a virtue. Self-forgiveness should not routinely substitute for or bypass the often painful task of seeking forgiveness from those we have wronged. In this sense, forgiveness by the one wronged functions as a constraint on forgiveness of self. As theologian Paul Tillich succinctly observes, self-forgiveness in a vacuum "is simply a self-confirmation in a state of estrangement"—which is "just the opposite of what forgiveness means."[30]

Seeking forgiveness from others is a humbling undertaking that we typically approach with some degree of trepidation and anxiety, in part because of the possibility that the victim will reject our offers of atonement. We may be tempted to disavow our dependence on the victim to remit guilt, limited though this dependence is. Thus, it should come as no surprise that rather than face their victims and plead for forgiveness, wrongdoers take the path of least resistance and grant themselves the forgiveness they have not sought from others. Taylor observes:

> It seems quite possible for a generous person to forgive a wrongdoer who does not show much sign of a change of heart without thereby being indifferent to whatever wrong he may have committed. . . . But in the case of self-forgiveness such generosity would hardly be in place; it would suspiciously look like being indulgent towards oneself and making matters too easy for oneself.[31]

The suspicion that the self-forgiver is "making matters too easy" for himself or herself may lead us to question whether self-forgiveness is a virtue at all. According to Aristotle, virtues are about what is *difficult,* and one might think that self-forgiveness is all too easy because the offender is the judge of the adequacy of his or her own atonement: He or she is like the criminal pardoning himself or herself. This analysis would be a mistake, however. Genuine self-forgiveness can be one of the most difficult tasks a person faces. Like seeking forgiveness from others, it is humbling. Moreover, there is a virtue of self-forgiveness in part because self-indulgent generosity toward oneself is a common temptation. Genuine self-forgiveness is a virtue for the same reason that Philippa Foot claims courage and temperance are virtues: That is, it is a "corrective disposition" that is "standing at a point at which there is some temptation to be resisted."[32]

Similar points can be made about self-forgiveness in cases in which no other person has suffered injury. Here too, one may make matters too easy for oneself by turning attention away from the failure to sustain one's constitutive attachments and commitments, or by self-deceptively denying that one has failed to do so.

If what Taylor describes as making matters too easy for oneself is an *excess* of self-forgiveness, being too hard on oneself can be a *deficiency.* Self-forgiveness, we might say, is an activity in which one can engage too much, too little, or to the proper degree. There is a better way to explain the vices of self-forgiveness, however, in terms of a continuum of self-regard. Self-love and self-hate are the extremes on this continuum and proper self-criticism the mean; these emotions underlie excessive, deficient, and appropriate self-forgiveness, respectively.[33] In cases of excess and deficiency, there is a lack of proper self-regard, which can be exhibited in one's life generally or only in some specific area or role. Because of temperament or upbringing or training or a combination of these factors, some individuals may find it exceedingly hard to let go of negative moral emotions such as shame and guilt. Such persons see themselves as having done things that the person they took themselves to be would not do. Whereas almost anyone on occasion feels that he or she has been a failure in a particular instance, self-depreciation is deep and long-lasting for such individuals.

A difficult question that arises in connection with the appropriateness of self-forgiveness (but would take me too far afield to examine here) is whether there are some acts for which one should not forgive oneself. Suppose one is not too easy on oneself. That is, one recognizes and acknowledges the wrong one has done, takes full responsibility for it, confesses one's flaws, and makes some attempt to make amends.[34] Might there nevertheless be some acts for which it would be wrong to forgive oneself because of the enormity of the wrong? In light of the way in which interpersonal forgiveness functions as a constraint on self-forgiveness, we can pose the following question: Are there some acts that a reasonable person would not forgive, and hence for which the offender should never forgive *himself or herself*? Arguably there are acts of this sort.[35] There may be acts of such gravity that forgiving oneself would be incompatible with respect for one's victim(s). If there are such acts, a person who possesses the virtue of self-forgiveness would not forgive himself or herself for them, no matter how conscientiously he or she works through the process of addressing past wrongful behavior.

The person who is too unself-forgiving is so not because he or she is unwilling or unable to forgive himself or herself for unforgivable wrongs (assuming there are such wrongs) but because he or she is unwilling or unable to let go of self-reproach even when a reasonable person would judge it appropriate to do so. It may be that this person does not begin the process of self-forgiveness or ends the struggle before accomplishing the tasks that are needed to make self-forgiveness complete. Beverly Flanigan characterizes the psychological state of persons who have not achieved self-forgiveness as one of conflict with the "enemy within"—conflict that is "ended, at least where peace is the result, through self-forgiveness. . . . When we forgive ourselves, we make peace with ourselves. We restore trust in ourselves."[36] This idea of making peace with oneself, of mending a rift in one's relationship with oneself, helps us to understand better what makes self-forgiveness a virtue.

The characterization of self-forgiveness as a process of seeking reconciliation with the "enemy within" has a parallel in cases of interpersonal forgiveness. The practice of forgiveness, Robert Roberts claims, is "at home in an ethic of community or friendship—one underlain by a sense of belonging to one another." Forgiveness is motivated by a desire for "reconciliation—restoration or maintenance of a relationship of acceptance, benevolent attitude, and harmonious interaction."[37] The virtuous person seeks reconciliation because he or she tends to feel uncomfortable with the anger he or she feels toward the offender and with the alienation from the offender that this anger engenders. Reconciliation is not all that matters to the virtuous person, of course. He or she is open to seeing the offender in a different light, as one with whom a harmonious relationship can be (re)established, but he or she will not seek reconciliation in ways that betray his or her self-respect.

Similarly, basic to the virtue of self-forgiveness is a dispositional concern to live in peace with oneself. As with interpersonal forgiveness, however, reconciliation is not the only thing that matters to the virtuous person. The concern for a harmonious relationship with oneself springs from a discomfort with being self-alienated, but the virtuously self-forgiving person is not willing to do whatever it takes to overcome this alienation. He will not avoid a thorough examination of his wrongdoing and accountability; she will not be willing to achieve inner peace by downplaying her culpability and denying that she deserves some punishment or reprimand for her wrongdoing. Self-reconciliation achieved this way betrays a lack of self-respect and a lack of respect for one's victims.

Achieving self-forgiveness is good for several reasons. First, it offers *psychological benefits*. Chronic feelings of dejection and unworthiness may undermine self-confidence; sap one's interest in people, things, or activities; and engender desperate and futile appeals for reassurance of one's goodness to counteract self-hate. In psychoanalytic theory, the inability to forgive oneself is explained in terms of a failure to attain an integrated realistic view of oneself that contains good and bad aspects.[38] Individuals who are capable of self-forgiveness and who embark on this task draw on their resources of self-love and attempt to come to terms with debilitating feelings that interfere with their enjoyment of life.

Second, self-forgiveness benefits the individual by making possible the *recovery of agency.* Norman Care clarifies this notion as follows:

> What this recovery is of (viz., "agency") is then lots of things, including a sense of one-self as intact in a way that allows responsible forward-looking action, plus a measure of self-worth, and perhaps even the capacity to find in oneself interests and enthusi-asms with enough strength to give meaningfulness to certain of one's activities.[39]

Self-forgiveness, as I have characterized it, is motivated by a desire to repair a breach in one's relationship with oneself. If this breach is serious enough, there may be a loss or di-minishment of personal agency that is not only psychologically debilitating but morally troubling as well. In these cases, self-forgiveness enables achievement of inner peace, allow-ing one to go forward with one's life.

Third, self-forgiveness helps to *restore self-respect.* The issue of self-forgiveness typi-cally arises when one's actions have injured self-respect, though diminishment of one's sense of self-worth is not the wrong for which one needs to forgive oneself. Such diminishment is the result of actions that are properly the focus of concern, but the person who can forgive himself or herself is able to "recover enough self-respect to recognize that [he or] she is a valuable human being in spite of what [he or] she has done."[40] Self-forgiveness allows this person to absorb the full impact of the wrong he or she has done without losing sight of his or her humanity. Moreover, in repairing the damage to self-respect, the individual gains an important good because without self-respect, or with a diminished sense of self-worth, en-joyment of other goods diminishes. No matter how much wealth and power or how many opportunities one has, enjoyment of these goods is likely to be diminished if one lacks self-respect. A person who lacks self-respect is also unlikely to see much point in striving to rectify character flaws or habits that have caused injury to self or others in the past.

Thus, self-forgiveness serves crucial interests of the self-forgiver: It confers various psychological benefits, aids in the recovery of agency, and helps repair damage to self-re-spect. The realization that there is, after all, nothing for which to forgive oneself because one did nothing wrong can produce the same benefits. The *good* of self-forgiveness is only part of the story about the virtue of self-forgiveness, however. The virtue of self-forgiveness also requires that these benefits are secured as a result of examining oneself realistically and honestly, taking responsibility for what one has done, confessing one's flaws, and resolving to prevent repetition. The person who evades, explains away, or denies the harm he or she has done others, for example, does not respect his or her victims and does not exhibit the virtue of self-forgiveness, even if he or she thereby manages to free himself or herself of self-loathing and guilt.

Finally, I do not want to leave the impression that the virtue of self-forgiveness serves only the good of the one who possesses it. Indeed, in various ways it can also serve the interests of others even for minor missteps. For instance, a person who has unreasonably high expecta-tions of himself or herself and so cannot forgive himself or herself when he or she errs might also be unforgiving of others. The offender might beg for forgiveness and be deeply repen-tant, but the victim—expecting nothing less than perfection of herself and of others—is un-moved, thereby denying the offender the reconciliation he seeks. Even if the unself-forgiving person does not hold others to the same impossibly high standard to which she holds herself, she might withdraw from her victims because their presence is a painful reminder of her misdeeds, and this withdrawal might compound the initial injury. Moreover, there are certain role relationships in which the virtue of self-forgiveness has special other-regarding significance. One of these is the physician-patient relationship—to which I now return.

SELF-FORGIVENESS IN THE PHYSICIAN-PATIENT RELATIONSHIP

In the introductory section of this essay, I claimed that physicians who are not self-forgiving are less likely to perform well *as physicians* than those who are. I will now try to support this claim by proposing that the physician's refusal or inability to forgive himself or herself is an impediment to the physician's performance with respect to caring for seriously ill patients who are beyond cure or near death and disclosing medical errors to patients or their families. Physicians need the virtue of self-forgiveness to maximize their prospects of doing well in the job of looking after sick people. Though there are deficiencies and excesses of self-forgiveness among physicians, this discussion focuses only on avoiding the extreme of being unreasonably hard on oneself.

Caring for the Incurable

"There is a specific form of abandonment that is particularly common among patients near death from cancer," writes Sherwin Nuland: "abandonment by doctors."[41] Emotionally, and sometimes physically as well, doctors (and not only oncologists) tend to disappear when their efforts to cure—or to significantly prolong life—fail. Many reasons have been offered for this disturbing tendency of physicians to turn away from patients in their time of great need. Nuland mentions two reasons. One is a heightened degree of personal anxiety about dying: "We become doctors because our ability to cure gives us power over the death of which we are so afraid, and loss of that power poses such a significant threat that we must turn away from it, and therefore from the patient who personifies our weakness."[42] On this view, the feeling of invulnerability that is reinforced by working among the sick while being healthy is a defense against the physician's fear of illness and death, and the illusion of invulnerability is maintained by staying at a distance from the patient whose death the physician cannot prevent.

Another reason is the intense need to exert control over nature: "When control is lost, he who requires it is also a bit lost and so deals badly with the consequences of his impotence."[43] Physicians are trained to try to control disease processes and naturally are frustrated when that cannot be achieved. Not infrequently, however, physicians regard their failure to prevent death not just as a failure of medicine but as a personal defeat. Rather than accept that even the most competent physician cannot indefinitely extend life, they persist in viewing death as the "enemy" that must be vanquished, and they are likely to deal with their sense of defeat by putting emotional distance between themselves and the painful reminders of their impotence.

In addition to patient abandonment, the physician's sense of impotence to control nature, which physicians experience most acutely in relation to patients who are near death, may have other detrimental consequences. Nuland notes that "having lost the major battle, the doctor may maintain a bit of authority by exerting his influence over the dying process"[44] by unilaterally determining the manner and timing of the patient's death. The physician who is powerless to prevent death can maintain the illusion of omnipotence by controlling how and when the patient dies. In this way, "he deprives the patient and the family of the control that is rightfully theirs."[45] This disempowerment of patients and families is facilitated by the physician's lack of candor—resulting from the physician's sense of therapeutic impotence—about the efficacy of treatments and the patient's prognosis. When the physician's efforts to cure are frustrated, he or she can maintain some semblance of control over the information he or she gives to patients and families.[46] The physician thereby influences the patient's decision making in self-serving ways—although in most cases the physician is probably unaware that he or she is doing so and acts from the very best motives.

I suggest a further possible explanation of these phenomena—an explanation that is linked to those Nuland presents (but is not mentioned by him) and that I believe contributes to a more complete picture of the psychological dynamics at work. This explanation has to do with an aspect of the virtue of self-forgiveness—namely, accurate assessment of personal limitations and wrongdoing: The physician blames himself or herself unreasonably for not doing something that he or she is powerless to do. There is also a kind of grandiosity in supposing that one ought to be able to control nature and extend life indefinitely and holding oneself responsible for failing to do so. If part of the virtue of self-forgiveness is the ability to discern whether there is any need to forgive oneself, physicians who are prone to this sort of thinking and the emotions that accompany it are deficient with respect to the virtue. Strictly speaking, they do not need to forgive themselves; rather, they need to learn that there is nothing for which to forgive themselves.

An analogy might help explain why I include this sort of case in a discussion of self-forgiveness. Someone who possesses the virtue of courage not only knows how to act well in the face of danger—and so acts—but also has true or reasonable beliefs about what is dangerous. A paranoid person may run from danger, but it is not chiefly for this reason that we would say he or she lacks the virtue of courage. The paranoid person lacks the virtue because his or her perceptions of danger are regularly distorted by paranoid delusions. Similarly, the physician who reproaches himself or herself because he or she has exaggerated expectations of competence is lacking in the virtue of self-forgiveness. This physician lacks the virtue of self-forgiveness not because he or she does not let go of feelings of self-reproach—people might properly continue to reproach themselves for their wrongdoing even if they possess the virtue—but because the physician's self-conception or self-ideal distorts his or her assessment of blameworthiness. Among other things, the virtue of self-forgiveness functions as a corrective to erroneous or unreasonable beliefs about one's fault and hence to unreasonable self-blame.

Disclosing Medical Errors

Adverse outcomes in medicine may be neither preventable nor predictable; they may be unpreventable but may occur with predictable frequency even when the standard of care is practiced; or they may be preventable, either because they result from remediable deficiencies in the delivery system (i.e., systemic errors) or from carelessness or ineptitude (i.e., human errors). Human errors are more idiosyncratic and less predictable than system errors; they include errors of commission (for example, prescription errors) and errors of omission, such as "failure or delay in making a diagnosis or instituting treatment, and failure to use indicated tests or take precautions to prevent injury."[47]

Even when treatment does not fall below the standard of care and the physician has done everything that could reasonably be expected, there is no guarantee of a positive outcome. The nature of medicine and medical practice is such that adverse events are always possible and not uncommon. Although adverse outcomes are never welcome, it is especially difficult for physicians to acknowledge human error on their part because the "processes that motivate the physician to maintain excellent standards of practice do not incorporate the notion of fallibility."[48] If physicians do admit that a mistake was made, they may attribute it to some failure in the system of delivering care or to uncertainty inherent in the current state of knowledge in medicine rather than to a personal fault, thereby evading acknowledgment of responsibility.

There are several possible grounds for the physician's ethical duty to disclose medical errors to the patient or the patient's family and several explanations of physicians' reluctance to do so. Among the former is the risk of further physical harm if the victim is not notified: Failure to disclose mistakes can deny patients the opportunity to seek further treatment to mitigate harm, leading to continued illness and even death. The principle of respect for patient autonomy—which underlies the doctrine of informed consent—supports a duty to disclose as well, and "respect for patient autonomy is required to achieve the ends of medicine."[49] Among the barriers to disclosure are fear of medical malpractice litigation, strong professional pressures to conceal error, concerns about destroying the relationship of trust with the patient, and the belief in physician infallibility.[50]

Belief in physician infallibility may be responsible for the nondisclosure of medical error in part because of the physician's inability to confront and accept his or her failings and to forgive himself or herself for having committed errors. Before the physician can approach those he or she has harmed and disclose his or her mistakes in a true confessional spirit, the physician must first acknowledge them to himself or herself and take responsibility for them. The physician must also be humble and courageous enough to expose himself or herself to the judgment and anger of others and be ready to make amends for what he or she has done. The physician who cannot face himself or herself honestly and come to terms with his or her failings is unlikely to step forward and disclose his or her mistakes—least of all to those he or she has harmed. Indeed, the physician who does not disclose his or her mistakes may by that very fact show that he or she has not forgiven himself or herself because disclosure is itself part of the process of self-forgiveness.[51]

Psychological resistance to disclosure is only part of the problem, however. It is also necessary to change the legal and professional environment within which the physician is socialized and practices medicine. Several features of this environment make it difficult and costly for physicians to disclose error to the patient or the patient's family, even if they are so disposed.

Atul Gawande claims that "virtually everyone who cares for hospital patients will make serious mistakes, and even commit acts of negligence, every year."[52] Moreover, with the advent of managed health care, errors—especially errors of omission—are likely to occur more often because physicians are under intense pressure to increase their productivity and control costs. Some of these errors will result in harm to the patient; some will not.

Even if most physicians seldom make serious mistakes, however, my argument for why the good physician needs the virtue of self-forgiveness is not predicated on the assumption that the individual physician will frequently commit serious mistakes. Self-forgiveness is an essential medical virtue because without it the physician is unlikely to disclose mistakes to those he or she has harmed—although the physician has an ethical duty to do so—and because serious mistakes are always *possible*. We expect that the virtuous physician will exhibit the virtue of self-forgiveness when it is required and will be so habitually disposed to do so that those in the physician's care can depend on the physician to own up to and disclose mistakes when they occur.

NOTES

1. Self-forgiveness is a topic of interest to religious (especially Christian) writers, of course, but I am concerned here only with the philosophical literature. Exceptions are Nancy E. Snow, "Self-forgiveness," *Journal of Value Inquiry* 27 (1993): 75–80; Margaret R. Holmgren, "Self-forgiveness and Responsible Moral Agency," *Journal of Value Inquiry* 32 (1998): 75–91.
2. For example, Robert S. Downie, "Forgiveness," *Philosophical Quarterly* 15 (1965): 128–34; Howard J. N. Horsbrugh, "Forgiveness," *Canadian Journal of Philosophy* 4 (1974): 269–82.
3. Edmund Pellegrino and David Thomasma, *The Virtues in Medical Practice* (New York: Oxford University Press, 1993); see also Edmund Pellegrino, "The Virtuous Physician and the Ethics of Medicine," in *Virtue and Medicine,* ed. Earl Shelp (Dordrecht, The Netherlands: Reidel, 1985), 237–55.
4. Alasdair MacIntyre, *After Virtue* (Notre Dame, Ind.: University of Notre Dame Press, 1981).
5. Ezekiel Emanuel, *The Ends of Human Life* (Cambridge, Mass.: Harvard University Press, 1991), 16.
6. Pellegrino and Thomasma, *The Virtues in Medical Practice,* 52–53, 194.
7. See Lucian L. Leape, "Error in Medicine," *Journal of the American Medical Association* 272 (1994): 1851–57.
8. See Charles Bosk, *Forgive and Remember: Managing Medical Failure* (Chicago: University of Chicago Press, 1979).
9. For a moving account of the emotional toll that the expectation of perfection can take on physicians, see David Hilfiker, "Facing Our Mistakes," *New England Journal of Medicine* 310 (1984): 118–22.
10. I discuss patient non-abandonment, disclosure of medical mistakes, and their connection to self-forgiveness in Section IV of this essay.
11. Joram Haber, *Forgiveness* (Savage, Md.: Rowman and Littlefield, 1991), 40.
12. Downie, "Forgiveness," 130.
13. Jean Hampton argues that "the central difference between them [condonation and forgiveness] is that condonation involves accepting the moral wrong whereas forgiveness does not" (Jeffrie Murphy and Jean Hampton, *Forgiveness and Mercy* [Cambridge, England: Cambridge University Press, 1988], 40).

14. Norman Care, *Living with One's Past* (Lanham, Md.: Rowman and Littlefield, 1996), 11.
15. Michael Stocker, *Plural and Conflicting Values* (Oxford: Clarendon Press, 1990), 28.
16. Horsbrugh, "Forgiveness," 276.
17. Ibid., 278.
18. Thomas E. Hill, Jr., "Servility and Self-Respect," in *Autonomy and Self-Respect* (Cambridge, England: Cambridge University Press, 1991), 4–18.
19. Gabriele Taylor, *Pride, Shame and Guilt* (Oxford: Clarendon Press, 1985), 77–78.
20. Pauline Chazan, *The Moral Self* (London: Routledge, 1998), 147, 149.
21. Stephen Darwall, *Impartial Reason* (Ithaca;, N.Y.: Cornell University Press, 1983), 154.
22. Beverly Flanigan, *Forgiving Yourself* (New York: Macmillan, 1996), 58. I highly recommend Flanigan's book for its sensitive and insightful discussion of the process of self-forgiveness.
23. Robert C. Roberts, "Forgiveness," *American Philosophical Quarterly* 32 (1995): 290.
24. Ibid., 293.
25. Ibid., 303.
26. I say more about reconciliation in section III of this essay.
27. Taylor, *Pride, Shame and Guilt,* 81.
28. Richard Swinburne, *Responsibility and Atonement* (Oxford: Clarendon Press, 1989), 87.
29. On self-forgiveness as a second-best alternative to interpersonal forgiveness, see Snow, "Self-forgiveness."
30. Quoted in John Gartner, "The Capacity to Forgive: An Object Relations Perspective," in *Object Relations Theory and Religion: Clinical Applications,* ed. M. Finn and J. Gartner (Westport, Conn.: Praeger, 1992) 21–33.
31. Taylor, *Pride, Shame and Guilt,* 106.
32. Phillipa Foot, "Virtues and Vices," in *Virtues and Vices and Other Essays in Moral Philosophy* (Berkeley: University of California Press, 1978), 8.
33. I owe this point to William Ruddick.
34. This description of the process of addressing our wrongs echoes Holmgren, "Self-forgiveness and Responsible Moral Agency," and Flanigan, *Forgiving Yourself.*
35. As to whether certain acts are in principle unforgivable, see Berel Lang, "Forgiveness," *American Philosophical Quarterly* 31 (1994): 111–12.
36. Flanigan, *Forgiving Yourself,* 57–58.
37. Roberts, "Forgiveness," 294, 299.
38. See Gartner, "The Capacity to Forgive."
39. Care, *Living With One's Past,* 131.
40. Holmgren, "Self-forgiveness and Responsible Moral Agency," 76.
41. Sherwin B. Nuland, *How We Die* (New York: Vintage, 1995), 257.
42. Ibid., 258.
43. Ibid.
44. Ibid., 259.
45. Ibid.
46. See Robert Buckman, "Breaking bad news: why is it still so difficult?" *British Medical Journal* 288 (1984): 1597–99.
47. Lucian Leape, et al., "The Nature of Adverse Events in Hospitalized Patients," *New England Journal of Medicine* 324 (1991): 381.
48. John Christensen, Wendy Levinson, and Patrick Dunn, "The Heart of Darkness: The Impact of Perceived Mistakes on Physicians," *Journal of General Internal Medicine* 7 (1992): 430. The authors go on to suggest that "the absence of fallibility as a category in physicians' concepts of their profession may be a product of the lack of serious discus-

sion of mistakes in medical training, in the medical literature, and in the conferences, grand rounds, and symposia through which physicians are continuously socialized into the way that medicine works."

49. Pellegrino and Thomasma, *The Virtues in Medical Practice,* 53.
50. See Francoise Baylis, "Errors in Medicine: Nurturing Truthfulness," *Journal of Clinical Ethics* 8 (1997): 336–40; Daniel Finkelstein et al., "When a Physician Harms a Patient by a Medical Error: Ethical, Legal, and Risk-Management Considerations," *Journal of Clinical Ethics* 8 (1997): 330–35; Peter H. Rehm and Denise R. Beatty, "Legal Consequences of Apologizing," *Journal of Dispute Resolution* 115 (1996): 115–30; Joan Vogel and Richard Delgado, "To Tell the Truth: Physicians' Duty to Disclose Medical Mistakes," *UCLA Law Review* 28 (1980): 52–94.
51. I thank Bart Collopy for this point.
52. Atul Gawande, "When Doctors Make Mistakes," *The New Yorker,* 1 February 1999, 48.

Moral Courage: Unsung Resource for Health Professional as Healer and Friend

Ruth B. Purtillo

Humanism encompasses a spirit of sincere concern for the centrality of human values in every aspect of professional activity. This concern focuses on respect for the freedom, dignity, worth and belief systems of the individual person. . . .[1]

Edmund Pellegrino's work on medical humanism stands out among contemporary writings devoted to a deep understanding of the health professional as healer and friend. Time and again I have turned to Pellegrino's work to regain my moral equilibrium as a health professional and bioethicist. His examination is instructive for many scholars in their search for resources available to health professionals: What will assist professionals in their desire to walk the walk of respect for patients? What can educators do to nurture "the spirit of sincere concern" that initially motivated many professionals to enter their chosen field? As important, how can they sustain that motivation, and the behaviors reflecting it, over the course of a professional lifetime? In Pellegrino's work, virtues that help fix the professional's gaze on the "freedom, dignity, worth and belief systems of the individual person" are basic instruments for building a morally good professional life that encompasses the roles of healer and friend. The virtue of moral courage serves as one vital resource.

Most ethicists acknowledge the importance of virtues in morality, and I am no exception. Moral courage crept onto my horizon as a compelling topic of exploration from the identity crises that face one in the lifelong challenge of trying to do the right thing over time, especially in one's relationships—as health professional, faculty member, spouse, friend, and citizen. Like many people, I presume, I had entered into those relationships with optimism and in good faith, but with little preparation for the wide variety of situations that would present practical obstacles to Pellegrino's ideal of exercising respect. It would take courage— whatever that is—to persevere in my resolve and act in accord with values I hold dear.

Discussions with colleagues in the health professions about this desire to endure well as healer and friend led me to conclude that they, too, face situations in which moral fiber is required if they are to act consistent with "a spirit of sincere concern for the centrality of human values. . . . "[2] I concluded that we do not work often enough to recognize, nurture (in ourselves and others), and applaud a readiness to do the right thing—or even seek the basic dispositional resources to do so. The purpose of this essay is to help the reader more readily recognize the powerful resource that moral courage can be within one important relationship—the relationship between the health professional and the patient—when the professional's desire to be healer and friend is threatened.

WHAT IS MORAL COURAGE?

From the earliest discussions of the term *courage* within Western philosophy, *moral* courage has been the focus, the core notion—a special type of strength that individuals can call upon to support the moral life. A detailed historical development of this important idea is beyond the scope of this essay, but insights from Plato's writings are especially relevant for a working definition that elucidates the role of moral courage in maintaining moral values that are constitutive of a healer or friend in the health professions.

Plato focused his attempt to offer a coherent treatment of the nature of morality on an understanding of four cardinal virtues: courage, temperance, wisdom, and justice.[3] Early in his writings he situated each somewhere on the continuum between the sensual and intellectual aspects of human functioning.[4] The highest virtue was knowledge (i.e., wisdom)—a function of the intellect. Although courage (called *thymus*) was accorded relatively high standing, all other virtues ultimately were secondary to wisdom. (At one point in *Laches*—the dialogue most thoroughly devoted to courage—Plato temporarily equates courage with wisdom itself, attributing to it an overarching status among the virtues.[5])

Philosopher David Carr chronicles how the proper place of courage among the other cardinal virtues courses through several Platonic writings, creating a record of Plato's own evolving thinking about the virtues and his understanding of moral psychology. In the *Republic*, a distinct role for all four virtues emerges. Each relates to different dimensions of psychological experience ("human elements"), with courage belonging to the will.[6] Later, in the *Laws*, a new and important distinction is made. To that point in Plato's moral psychology, all the appetites, emotions, passions, and feelings are lumped together in the "lower" sensual or bodily realm of the person. In the *Laws,* Carr observes, Plato separates passion from pleasure and allows that courage governs passion whereas temperance governs pleasure. A person who can exercise his or her will to control sensual appetites may still be prone to disintegrate in that resolve under stress. Courage is useful not so much when prospectively making a choice but when acting for the good within a stressful situation that has been handed to one.[7] Although the virtue of moral courage does not guarantee wisdom, temperance, or a tendency to seek justice, it is a basic resource that provides a resolve to act in situations that have the potential to seriously compromise basic human values.

Plato viewed the virtues as traits and dispositions of character that assured that people would act in morally praiseworthy ways. When basic human values were threatened, the virtuous person could count on the morally courageous act to flow from a courageous disposition.

Plato's classical understanding of the centrality of virtue is the subject of debate to this day. Yet he set a course of inquiry that modern moral psychology generally affirms—namely, that humans are capable of grabbing hold of and developing dispositions that help prepare them for morally purposive action. This line of reasoning makes good sense as a resource for the health professional's moral task of maintaining focus in the face of forces that deter from the role as healer or friend. Commitment to the basic values may be sustained by a readiness to "screw up the courage" to act rightly.

In light of Plato's contributions to our understanding of moral courage as a virtue, what would a courageous act look like? It would be a voluntary act of will undertaken in the face of a realistic threat to protect something of moral value. Of course, a positive outcome is not necessarily assured.[8] At most, the actor can engage in what Catholic theologian Karl Rahner calls "hoping faith."[9]

Within the health professions context, the agent (one who has the capacity to act voluntarily) is the health professional. The moral value is an environment in which the health professional can serve as healer and friend—or, in Pellegrino's terms, an environment in which "the freedom, dignity, worth and belief systems" of the patient and others can be respected.[10] The threat is anything that generates fear or other types of stress in the health professional when he or she prepares to act in defense of those values.

SOME PRACTICAL BARRIERS

Under what conditions would an agent who is disposed to act according to the virtue of moral courage fail? Examples from the health professions environment highlight three types of barriers.

First, the person may not feel capable of acting voluntarily. Highly constrictive policies or institutional arrangements may stymie the courageous agent. One example is the gag clause physicians have been forced to sign in some employment agreements. This clause coerces physicians to refrain from disclosing that there are serious constraints on what they can offer a patient, even though those physicians believe the patient is being seriously shortchanged. Fear of losing one's job, fear of being sued by one's employer, or even altruistically believing that patients will be worse off if one is not there at all (i.e., in rural or other underserved settings) are realistic barriers that can create a coercive situation.

A second type of failure could result if the agent loses sight of the core values to be protected in the face of competing, but compelling, values. This failure does not require a moral lapse on the part of the agent. For example, in a recent editorial on managed care, Jerome Kassirer poses the following questions to his physician colleagues:

> . . . how can physicians provide optimal care for each of their patients and for the entire group at the same time? In agreeing to a distributive ethics, are physicians tacitly becoming agents of the plan instead of agents for their patients? How sturdy are our traditional medical ethics?[11]

Nowhere does Kassirer suggest that a disposition toward justice required for sensitivity to distributive issues is wrong. Instead, the situation calls for physicians, in their unique role, not to lose sight of the patient care-oriented values to which their own priority must be directed. Again, the disposition to act courageously is a resource, but in this case the many claims to which health professionals feel pulled to respond may dissipate the focus required for them to keep sight of appropriate moral priorities.

A third type of failure could result when the agent's disposition to do the right thing is thwarted by the newness and complexity of a clinical situation. The agent is free from coercion, is aware that core values are threatened, and has identified a source of the threat—*but is uncertain about what to do to curb the harm.* This type of stress is illustrated in the modern practice of employing life-sustaining technologies. A centerpiece of the art of healing always has been to identify the limits of what medicine can accomplish. The appropriate response is to withdraw from aggressive intervention when there seems little hope of further benefit.[12] In comparison with former times, it is more difficult today to strike a humane balance between trying another curative intervention and allowing the patient's illness to take its course while the health professional offers comfort measures. The process of ascertaining appropriate moral limits is confounded in part by the uniquely modern dilemma of so many possible technologies and the prodigious rate at which new ones are being made available. Pellegrino comments that whereas the introduction of new technology historically has been spaced so that humans have the time to make conscious choices about its dangers,[13] the situation has changed:

> In these times . . . our ability to make such choices has been overwhelmed by the endless capacity of our techniques and the awesome rate at which they are produced. We suffer acutely the twin fears of reverting to a barbarous existence either by using them too much or using them not enough. . . .[14]

The temptation to allay our anxiety by dumping new technologies for an earlier, "purer," hands-on medicine crumbles, however, beneath ample evidence of the remarkable ability of technology to save and improve the quality of peoples' lives.

Moreover, another stumbling block is that the mere availability of technology can be perceived by clinicians as a *moral* claim, urging them in the direction of interventions. During a conversation about percutaneous endoscopic gastrostomy (PEG)—when PEG was a relatively new type of intervention—a young internist lamented that the ease of the procedure itself "felt like a claim." She was experiencing what clinicians Heaney and Barger-Lux termed the "technological imperative" in medicine[15] and what philosophers often have termed the fallacy that "is implies ought": Because of the technology's very existence, it ought to be used.

In short, the health professional's third barrier to realizing the fruits of courageous action is the sheer number and complexity of the care-artist's materials with which modern health care is crafted. The courage to undertake a complex treatment regimen carries the hope that it may provide relief for the patient's suffering, but it also carries the worry that it may result in mere "spot-welding." The clinician relies on the fact that each individual intervention may fall within usual and customary medical practice and is based on widely acknowledged, scientifically substantiated findings. The problem is that the larger framework from which the contours of the patient's life and well-being took shape simply cannot hold up under the assault. This uncertainty and its potential for regret can be paralyzing.[16]

EXERCISING MORAL COURAGE IN HEALTH PROFESSIONS PRACTICE

The foregoing discussion spells out sobering barriers to the exercise of moral courage in the health professions environment. Yet each type of situation can be interpreted as an occasion for the exercise of courage.

For example, the barrier of coercive policies and employment arrangements should mobilize health professionals to purposive individual and group action designed to change such structures eventually. Courage also may account for an individual's willingness to seek positions on policy development or review committees with the express purpose of speaking out against arrangements that thwart professionals' ability to show respect for the freedom, dignity, and worth of patients. Several celebrated cases in which health professionals openly challenged "gag rules" in their health plans illustrate this type of courage. Some of these courageous individuals were "rewarded" with firings or other negative sanctions—an extreme price to pay, to be sure. Strikingly, however, federal and state legislation has now prohibited the use of gag rules. The courageous acts of some individuals in this situation of serious threat are resulting in dramatic change for the good.

The barrier of competing moral values that distracts a professional from keeping his or her primary focus on appropriate moral priorities as a healer also can become an occasion for courage. A health professional can conscript others through written communication, participation in policy making and review bodies, and other means, urging them to pay attention to important priorities to which they themselves cannot give their full attention. Such professionals often are not especially well liked. It takes a certain type of courage to be pigeon-holed as a "do-gooder" who "tries to solve the world's problems" or "badgers" others—but perseveres.

The barrier of complex, newly emerging technologies that create uncertainty about how to serve patients' best interests is an opportunity for courage as well. In the modern, knowledge-intensive health professions ethos, certainty is viewed as a value in itself; *not knowing* is perceived as a weakness. The student soon learns that not having "all the facts" is a sure sign of failure. This socialization has been exposed as failing to prepare students well for situations of uncertainty and how to respond to honest mistakes.[17] Courage requires admitting one's limits in the face of this threat to one's professional self image. It takes courage to admit that one does not exactly know the best clinical course to take and to seek help about what to do from colleagues, the patient, and, often, the patient's family.[18]

Modern society recognizes this shortcoming among professionals and acknowledges at patients' input is of great significance in such situations. Although a patient may not know the technical aspects of medical care, she or he usually does know first-hand what matters in his or her own life. Usually a clinician's dilemma reaches its zenith when more technology is available but the patient seems to be "losing ground" overall.[19] Although every stone must be turned to try to learn the patient's informed preferences, even the most arduous and thorough attempts may not always lead to certainty about the best course of action.

Great courage is required to act in the face of irreducible uncertainty. In this situation, the possibility of being negligent or wrongfully informed is combined with the threat of doing harm, which may, in fact, ensue. Such moments of reckoning with having to take full responsibility in the face of serious limitations as a fellow human being requires the courage to be humble and to seek forgiveness when necessary. In such a situation, the patient may recognize a friend when the health professional is least successful as a healer in the usual sense of the term.

LOOKING AHEAD

I hope that as these reflections have unfolded, the reader has seen more clearly why today's health professionals need moral courage to continue to practice as healer and friend. They are faced with coercive policies; competing, but legitimate, values; and the necessity of looking the limits of the art in the eye.

Excellence of character serves us well in many ways. The stakes are too high for traditional ideals of a humanistic type of health care to be compromised. Given these considerations, the opportunity to cultivate and exercise moral courage among today's health professionals is reason for rejoicing.

NOTES

1. Edmund D. Pellegrino, *Humanism and The Physician* (Knoxville: University of Tennessee Press, 1979), 118.
2. Ibid.
3. Plato, *The Collected Dialogues,* ed. E. Hamilton and C. Huntington (Princeton, N.J.: Princeton University Press, 1961).
4. Plato, "The Republic," in *The Collected Dialogues*, ed. E. Hamilton and C. Huntington (Princeton, N.J.: Princeton University Press, 1961), 575–844.
5. Plato, "Laches," in *The Collected Dialogues*, ed. E. Hamilton and C. Huntington (Princeton, N.J.: Princeton University Press, 1961), 123–44.
6. David Carr, "The Cardinal Virtues and Plato's Moral Psychology," *The Philosophical Quarterly* 38: 151, 186–200.
7. Ibid.
8. Earle Shelp, "Courage and Tragedy in Clinical Medicine," *Journal of Medicine and Society* 8 (1983): 417–29.
9. Karl Rahner, "Faith as Courage," in *Meditations on Freedom and the Spirit* (New York: Seeburg Press, 1978), 12–29.
10. Pellegrino, *Humanism and the Physician,* 118.
11. Jerome Kassirer, "Managing Care—Should We Adopt a New Ethic?" *New England Journal of Medicine* 339, no. 6 (1998): 397–98.
12. Hippocrates, *The Art VIII,* trans. W. H. S. Jones (Cambridge, Mass.: Harvard University Press, 1923), II, 203.
13. Pellegrino, *Humanism and the Physician*, 10.
14. Ibid., 10–11.
15. M. J. Barger-Lux and R. P. Hearney, "For Better and Worse: The Technological Imperative in Health Care," *Social Science and Medicine* 22, no. 12 (1986): 1313–20.
16. R. B. Purtillo, "Life Support: The Doctor's Dilemma," *Annals Academy of Medicine* 24, no. 2 (Singapore, 1995): 263–67.
17. David Hilfiker, "Making Medical Mistakes," in *Healing the Wounds*, revised ed. (Omaha, Neb.: Creighton University Press, 1998).

18. E. N. Forman and R. E. Ladd, "Telling the Truth in the Face of Medical Uncertainty and Disagreement," *American Journal of Pediatric Hematology and Oncology* 11, no. 4 (1989): 463–66.

19. A. O. Baumann, R. B. Deber, and G. G. Thompson, GG, "Overconfidence Among Physicians and Nurses: The 'micro-certainty, macro-certainty' Phenomenon," *Social Science and Medicine* 32, no. 2 (1991): 167–74.

The Six Transformations of
American Health Care

John Collins Harvey

The many chapters in the history of American medicine and American medical ethics tell a rich and interesting story. This story includes the history of medical education and the provision of health care to the population as they were affected by European influences to produce the ideal or "good" American physician.

Originally, American medical practice was British medicine transported to the colonies and incorporated into the life of the new nation. This incorporation was modified, to be sure, to fit the needs of pioneering people living in a vastly different environment and culture than that which prevailed in the home country.[1]

In Great Britain, hospitals and institutions of medical learning had been well established for centuries. In 1476, William Gregory, lord mayor of London, described the good works done in five of the major hospitals of London, all of which still exist—the Papey; St. Bartholomew; St. Mary of Bethlehem; St. Mary's, Bishopgate; and St. Thomas, Southwark.[2] The first medical college at Oxford University was established in 1486. Henry VIII granted charters to practice medicine and surgery to the Barber-Surgeons Guild in 1512 and to the Royal College of Physicians of London in 1518.[3] England had a tradition of social customs, a defined class structure, and recognized obligations of the upper classes with accepted and practiced social ethics.

In America, the institutions and customs were still evolving and not yet established. No health care facility like a hospital existed before 1760. There was no institution for medical education until 1765. There was no overall governmental licensure for the practice of medicine—though some colonies, and later states, did license physicians.[4] Social organization reflected the immigrants' desire for freedom from the Old World's customs and social fabric. Thus, the patterns, social ethics, and particularly the medical practice that developed in the colonies and eventually in the new country did not mirror those of the home country.[5]

As immigration into the new country increased in the nineteenth century from other European cultures, non-British ideas, concepts, and principles were introduced into American medical practice and health care.[6] Newly arrived immigrant physicians and other health care workers (primarily religious women) from Ireland, "Catholic Germany" (Bavaria), Spain, and Italy brought their philosophies and customs with them. These new ideas affected medical practice and modified the previously pure British influence. This foreign infusion enriched and improved American medicine in many ways. The result is the current American medical enterprise, which—though now beset by many problems—is recognized the world over as the most advanced and finest in the world.

Three transformations in the health care field that occurred in the nineteenth century and three in the twentieth century altered American medicine profoundly and permanently. These transformations, all of which occurred in medical education, have given American medical and health care practices their distinctive character. They have influenced in a profound way the production of the ideal or "real" American physician—scientist, humanist, and ethicist.

PHYSICIAN EDUCATION

In the colonial days and the early period of the new republic, physicians were educated as apprentices. Their teachers were either educated divines who knew some law, medicine, and theology or one of the rare English or Scottish-trained physicians in the colonies. For the most part, these physicians were to be found in the larger cities such as Boston, New York, Philadelphia, Annapolis, Williamsburg, Charleston, or Savannah. A French-trained physician might be found in Bards Town (Kentucky), Louisville, or St. Louis. Only rarely would a physician trained in Europe be found on the "backwoods" frontier.

The physicians who served the primitive "backwoods" areas all came from the apprentice system. Thus, west of the Alleghenies, American medicine took on a distinctly insular character—though this too was good medicine. Some very fine physicians developed from this educational system. William Beaumont (1785–1853), an Army surgeon who made brilliant physiological studies of digestion, trained entirely in the apprentice system.[7] Ephraim McDowell, a pioneering backwoods surgeon in Kentucky who performed the first successful ovariotomy in the world, was another apprentice-trained physician.

In early colonial days, study for a young colonist at an English or Scottish university medical school was rare though not unknown. Such study was limited, however, to young men from more affluent families—most often, sons of immigrant physicians who previously had received university medical training in the home country or training in one of the London teaching hospitals. In the later years of the colonial period and the early years of the republic, an increasing number of Americans studied medicine in Britain. Most colonial students studied at the University of Edinburgh, whose medical school had been established in 1726. Returning home, they tended to settle in the larger cities, rarely going to the less-populated areas of the colonies.

In the later colonial period, several medical schools were established in America, usually by physicians trained in Britain. At this time, there were almost no care institutions that could be called hospitals. Thus emerged the distinctly American pattern of *university* education for physicians, distinguished from the British system based on training in a health care institution (i.e., a hospital or infirmary). These university medical departments began to do an excellent job of training physicians on this side of the Atlantic.

The medical school of the University of Pennsylvania was founded in 1765 by the intellectual leaders of Philadelphia, among whom were Benjamin Franklin and Benjamin Rush (both of whom were signers of the Declaration of Independence). Samuel Bard, a distinguished American-born physician who was trained in Edinburgh, established a medical school at King's College (later Columbia University) in New York in 1768. The Harvard Medical School started in Boston in 1783. Shortly thereafter followed medical schools at Dartmouth College in 1798, at Baltimore in 1812 (the forerunner to the medical school of the University of Maryland), and at Yale College in 1813.

Thus, the training of physicians in America was university-based—in contrast to the British system, which originated in teaching hospitals and infirmaries. As in Britain, however, medical practice in the colonies and early republic was based on the developing sciences of anatomy, botany, chemistry, and physiology of the Age of Reason in Europe.

During the colonial period and the early years of the republic, women proficient in nurturing skills provided primitive care with herbal remedies and various home-made potions in areas where there were few physicians, particularly on the western frontier; women also practiced midwifery. There were also a number of itinerant "healers" (poorly trained apprentices; ship's surgeons who had jumped ship; immigrant physicians from somewhere in Europe, perhaps suffering from chronic alcoholism or escaping from the law or an unhappy and burdensome marriage; as well as charlatans or con artists with only rudimentary knowledge of medicine) who passed themselves off as physicians in the less-populated areas of the country. These practitioners provided some rudimentary care but introduced a great deal of quackery into medical practice.

In the first half of the nineteenth century, many trained physicians began joining together to teach apprentices. Income from this practice was excellent. These physician-teachers frequently organized primitive "medical schools," and such schools proliferated before 1850. A few of these medical schools were very successful, producing excellent physicians. For example, William Worral Mayo—the immigrant English tailor who apprenticed himself to Elizur Deming of Lafayette, Indiana—subsequently studied for one year at the Indiana Medical College at La Porte and received his M.D. degree from that institution in 1850.[8]

Most of these proprietary schools, however, did not do an effective job. The doctors they turned out were generally poorly trained and poorly motivated for service to the population; they regarded the profession of medicine as a lucrative employment enterprise. As new knowledge about electricity and chemistry was developed by the European scientists of the Enlightenment, medical charlatans invented electrical or chemical "cure" gadgets. They pawned off these spurious devices and treatments on the unsuspecting and ignorant public as miraculous medical nostrums or even cures.

THE FIRST TRANSFORMATION

In colonial America, British medical ethics—such as they were—prevailed. The physician was a "learned gentleman" who exhibited all the "virtues of a gentleman" in his practice. The "ethics" that guided the medical practice at this time was based on the Hippocratic oath that had directed Western medical practice for more than 2,000 years.[9] Therefore, paternalism was the order of the day. This ethics was also cognizant of the physician's proper living out of the "virtues" to be found in Aristotle's *Nicomachean Ethics*[10]—influenced, to be sure, by the empiricists of the Scottish Enlightenment (Locke, Mill, and Hume).

Quackery became a growing concern of legitimate physicians in the United States—particularly in the eastern states, and most notably in New York City. The concerned physicians endeavored to do something about this situation. At the annual meeting of the New York State Medical Society in February 1844, Nathan Smith Davis, a young physician from the Broome County Medical Society (later professor of medicine and dean at Northwestern University Medical School in Chicago), proposed that a national convention be called in May 1846 to discuss the need for uniform national standards for medical education and licensure.[11] Although these attempts to reform medical education and eliminate quackery would lead nowhere at the time, the physicians involved in the effort would have been surprised at the onset of their meeting to know that their efforts would instead lead to the development of a code of medical ethics to govern the practice of medicine in the United States and to the organization of a national medical association.

On May 5, 1846, 122 delegates assembled in the medical department of the University of the City of New York.[12] They represented medical societies in fourteen states, twelve medical colleges, two hospitals, and one asylum. This group was not representative in any way of the nations' physicians, medical colleges, or health care institutions. Upon a resolution by Isaac Hays of Philadelphia, the delegates undertook to organize a national medical association that could act not only regarding physicians' medical education and licensure but "for the protection of physicians' interest, for the maintenance of their honor and respectability, for the advancement of their knowledge, and the extension of their usefulness." A committee was to draw up a plan of such an organization and present it at a meeting in Philadelphia in the following year. Another committee invited delegates from all regularly organized medical societies and chartered medical schools in the United States to the organizing convention. Somewhat as an afterthought, Hays moved to appoint a committee to report a code of ethics. Although these actions gave short shrift to the problems of haphazard medical education and quackery, they lent legitimacy to the meeting and set the stage for the foundation of the American Medical Association (AMA).[13]

The model for the ethics proposed at the national meeting in Philadelphia in 1847 was Hays' revision of Thomas Percival's work.[14] Percival, a well-respected physician of the Royal Infirmary of Manchester, had in 1800 developed a "code of ethics" to which the Governors of the Royal Infirmary could hold all physicians and surgeons appointed to the Infirmary. This request was occasioned by an ongoing and increasingly bitter struggle among the Infirmary's professional staff concerning matters related to medical practice, including individual physicians' rights over control of patients, splitting of fees, and ghost surgery. The physicians had split into bitter rival factions and were so divided that their fighting actually threatened the very continued existence of the Manchester hospital.

The Governors turned to Percival, a member of the Infirmary staff and the epitome of the "gentleman physician." His character was impeccable, and all factions respected him. The Governors asked him to establish a set of guidelines for physicians and surgeons to follow in their medical practice. The Governors felt that if each physician and surgeon followed these guidelines, there would be gentle but firm control of medical practice in the hospital and an end to the bitter disagreements and fighting that had taken such a toll within the Infirmary. Percival's work, *Medical Ethics,* was published in 1803.

The efforts of the Governors and Percival indeed brought peace and order back to the Infirmary. The hospital expanded its services, increased its size, and flourished mightily, setting a pattern that was followed in most other hospitals in Great Britain. In 1896, the British Medical Association accepted Percival's work as modified by Styrap.[15] Subsequently, the public accepted it also. Thus, a real recognized medical ethics came to exist in Britain.

Joseph Knight of New Haven, president, and John Bell of Philadelphia and Edward Delafield of New York, vice presidents, convened the meeting of the AMA in Philadelphia on May 5, 1847. Hays and John Bell, chairman, along with W. W. Morris of Delaware, T. C. Dunn of Rhode Island, A. Darius Clark of New York, and R. D. Arnold of Georgia formed the committee to report on medical ethics. All but Clark were graduates of the Medical School of the University of Pennsylvania. The delegates spent two days debating their concerns about the quackery and charlatans that had invaded American medical practice and the proliferation of "medical trade schools." Giving scant attention to the report of Bell's committee, they adopted the presentation summarily with no debate. It was published on June 5, 1847.

The committee insisted that a medical ethics to which all legitimate American physicians could subscribe was needed. Indeed, there had been some codes of ethics developed earlier by groups of physicians in different areas of the new country, such as that of the Association of Boston Physicians—who, in 1807 developed the "Boston Medical Police."[16] Such codes, however, were local and not authoritative. The convention thus established a Code of Ethics for medical practice that they felt strongly had authority nationwide.

Though this code was based on the English Code, it was actually a radical reformation. In contrast to Percival's code—which said that physicians and other gentlemen of high station have a duty to society that is automatically incurred by their station in life—this new American Code (consisting of three chapters containing eleven articles and requiring thirteen printed pages)[17] has been described as "a brilliant tripartite social contract between physicians, patient, and society, in which each of the three parties has reciprocal obligations and rights, fitting well into the spirit of the new nation."[18] It recognized patients' and communities' rights to medical care—a radical concept that suggested that patients have an inalienable right to health care even if they are unable to pay. The code dealt with many of the societal and commercial aspects of the practice of medicine and less with the technical aspects. Above all, it protected patients. Over the years, many modifications have been made to this code, some of which have diluted the original basic guiding principles concerning patients' rights.

This document transformed American medicine in the nineteenth century by introducing into the practice of medicine a concern for ethics. With the subsequent development of the Judicial Council of the AMA, this concern of physicians has persisted and flourished. Even the great blossoming of bioethics that developed among philosophers in the United States in the 1970s was really only an expansion of this earlier conviction—and a mere incremental change compared to that transformation of 1853.

THE SECOND TRANSFORMATION

The practice of medicine in the nineteenth century was based on the sciences that had been developed primarily in France during the Age of Reason. There was fairly good knowledge of anatomy and some knowledge of physiology and chemistry as it applied to medical practice. Viner has reported "while American physicians in the early nineteenth century looked to the empirical clinical and pathological studies of the Paris school as the scientific basis for orthodox medicine, American therapeutic practice valued personal experience and heuristically proven remedies over the claims of experimental science."[19] American physicians in the late eighteenth century and the first three-quarters of the nineteenth century carried out little scientific investigation. There were some prominent exceptions, however. Benjamin Rush, for example, studied vaccination in 1790. William Beaumont, an Army physician on the western frontier, studied gastric physiology on his famous patient, Alexis St. Martin, a Native American who survived an abdominal injury that left him with a traumatic gastrostomy. Beaumont recognized this opportunity to study the digestive process and over a ten-year period did extensive and brilliant experiments on gastric physiology.

In Europe, by contrast, a medical research enterprise of the highest caliber was being developed in various universities' medical school laboratories, particularly in Prussia and the other German states. In these same universities, there was much political activity in the first part of the nineteenth century that attempted to bring ideas about democratic reform from the French revolution to the German states. Faculty members in the medical schools eagerly joined in this political activity. They wished to free medicine from strict state control and Schelling's *Naturphilosophie*.[20] Liberal physicians such as Johannes Muller, Emil DuBois-Reymond, Herman Helmholtz, and famed pathologist Rudolf Virchow felt that if medicine were reformed on material and chemical grounds, its role in the modern democratic state would be secure. Some of these physicians—particularly Virchow—claimed that medicine and politics were the same undertaking and that the reform of medicine would bring about the reconstruction of society along scientific, physiological lines.[21]

Natural science had become the new model for public and political life just as the reformers embraced democratic government to bring about German unity. Marx had issued his *Communist Manifesto* in 1848. Engels published the first part of his seminal work *Anti-Duehring: Socialism, Utopian & Scientific*, in 1850.[22] The result of all this activity, however, was the failed revolution of 1848.

Many of the revolutionaries sought asylum in England or in the New World. A large group of German-speaking liberal political refugees ended up in New York City. Among them were numerous young physicians of liberal political views who had been trained in the scientific methodologies of the German medical schools, many of whom had embraced the revolutionary ideals with great enthusiasm. Among these doctors was a young physician who had studied medicine under Virchow and had been a leading figure in revolutionary activities in Frankfurt. After the coup failed, this young physician had been tried and served some time in prison, after which he went to England. When he could not establish a medical practice in England, he came to Boston and finally settled in New York City. His name was Abraham Jacobi.

Most of these political refugees were poor and unable to speak English, and they were able to find only sporadic work of the most menial kind. They were crowded into tenements on the Lower East Side of New York in an area called *Kleindeutschland*. Living conditions were far from ideal. Sanitary conditions were primitive. Medical care was almost nonexistent because the refugees could not afford to pay the fees then charged by doctors in the city. Epidemics of acute contagious diseases were common. Morbidity and mortality rates were high.

The members of the New York medical establishment, particularly physicians who had been German immigrants of an earlier time, did not accept the young radical physicians. The more recent immigrant physicians who banded together for mutual support and to arrange some kind of care for the poor German refugees formed the German Medical and Surgical Society.[23] They established the German Dispensary[24] for the care of the sick poor, modeling it after the universities' polyclinics in which they had studied. The polyclinic combined charity care with medical research and physician education.[25] Structuring the Dispensary as a university teaching service enabled these physicians to combine their radical agenda for poverty relief with efforts to improve their own medical knowledge. This structure also allowed them to carry out basic physiological and biochemical investigations, as well as clinical investigations on the diseases that they encountered.[26] Among the most active of these radical and idealistic physician-refugees in this medical and scientific enterprise was the young Dr. Jacobi.

Under Jacobi's leadership, monthly scientific meetings were organized for the mutual education of the physicians of the Dispensary. Jacobi and fellow radical-socialist physicians Karl Heinzen and Frederic Knapp organized public lectures on health, medical science, popular science, politics, and culture.[27] A library of European medical journals was established. Jacobi became scientific editor of the New York German socialist publication, *Die Reform,* and he wrote pieces for the popular New York German literary magazine, *Belletristiches Journal.*

Jacobi worked diligently in the Dispensary and established its Children's Department— the forerunner of a modern medical school's department of pediatrics. Jacobi studied epidemics among the children in *Kleindeutschland* and reported on them in the New York State medical journal.[28] He studied and reported on various medications used as expectorants in respiratory diseases in children, and he studied the actions of various antipyretics in children using the methods of German physiological research. His studies on diphtheria were classics, as were his studies on the intestinal diseases of infants and children.[29]

Soon the science reported in these papers on studies done in the German Dispensary began to attract notice in wider medical circles in New York City. The New York Academy of Medicine, the New York Pathological Society, and the *New York Medical Journal* recognized favorably the work of these young, scientifically trained, and socially enlightened "refugee" physicians. The work of the radicals of the German Dispensary introduced into American medicine the concept that experimental physiology could guide therapeutic practice. Young, influential American medical reformers such as Stephen Smith, the editor of the *New York Medical Journal,* and Elisha Harris, the great sanitary reformer, recognized and adopted the Dispensary radicals and their scientific approach to medical care. Smith and Harris gave wide publicity to the Germans' work, thereby helping to build the radicals' reputation for scientific medicine in the wider American medical enterprise. The most sympathetic forum for the radical refugee physicians and their scientific approach to medicine was the New York Pathological Society.[30]

Jacobi was invited to a professorial chair at the New York Medical College in 1860. Since its founding in 1850, the College had been a center for medical educational reform, attempting to implement the recently formed AMA's agenda to improve the standards of medical qualification. During the course of his long career, Jacobi developed the specialty of pediatrics, through which he pursued his political agenda.[31] In this latter activity, he involved himself with housing reform, infant public health, the anti-tuberculosis movement, milk stations, settlement houses, and the development of highly scientific infant-feeding practices. Jacobi subsequently abandoned his radical political activities, focusing his reform efforts instead on the application of German science to American children.

William Henry Welch, the first faculty appointee to the Johns Hopkins Medical School and its leader in developing a new type of institution based on the German university model, worked for Jacobi when he was an intern and subsequently was a staff member in pathology at the Bellevue Hospital Medical College. Jacobi's interest in experimental physiology and the overall scientific approach to medicine obviously influenced the young Welch, who wrote many years later,

> When I came to Bellevue as an interne [*sic*] I first got to know Abraham Jacobi and he was the one who first directed my attention especially to the great position of German medical science in the world. He used to invite me occasionally to come to his own house, where we would talk over the cases that had interested us in the hospital. . . . It was an inspiration to me.[32]

Turning out properly educated physicians had been the objective of the physicians who had called for the first national medical congress. They wished to curtail the wholesale and quick production of physicians by the proprietary medical schools. They wanted physicians to have correct and proper medical knowledge. The concept of "proper medical knowledge" to replace quackery was very high on their agenda. The "scientific medicine" that the immigrant German refugee physicians advocated was not the Americans' idea of proper medical knowledge, however. For them, proper medical knowledge was related to the quick recognition of signs and symptoms of disease and knowledge of proper treatment for the diseases once recognized. This approach, of course, was a tradition in French medicine and the *Naturphilosophie* of European thought of the mid-nineteenth century. The introduction of the German tradition of scientific medicine into the medical curriculum had to wait for the revolution in medical education that began in 1910.

The closing of many proprietary medical schools and the introduction of experimental science into the curricula of the remaining medical schools occurred as a direct result of a study of medical education in the United States and Canada carried out by Abraham Flexner during the 1909/1910 academic year, under the auspices of the Carnegie Foundation for the Advancement of Teaching.[33] This report, the genesis of another transformation in American health care in the twentieth century, profoundly affected the concept of the real physician.

THE THIRD TRANSFORMATION

Hospitals were almost nonexistent in the United States until the middle of the nineteenth century. There were some, of course, which had been established in earlier times—such as the Pennsylvania Hospital in Philadelphia, founded by Benjamin Franklin in 1755, and the Massachusetts General Hospital, established in 1821 in Boston. Some of the big cities such as New York, Baltimore, Chicago, Cincinnati, Baltimore, New Orleans, Atlanta, and Savannah had public institutions for the care of the sick poor, homeless, and insane that were little more than almshouses or asylums, providing only primitive care. These institutions, however, could not be considered hospitals in the modern sense of the word.

Most individuals were cared for in their own homes. Surgery was performed on the kitchen table. People felt that care at home was safer, more secure, and less fraught with complications than going off to a hospital. Hospital nurses were ill-trained, coarse women with little compassion; very often they were alcoholics. Mortality rates were exceedingly high, so going to the hospital was considered almost a signed death warrant.

Immigration to America increased in the early years of the nineteenth century as successive waves of families and individuals arrived from Ireland, Scandinavia, the Rhineland, and other German states. Toward the middle of the century, immigrants from Italy and the Slavic states of Eastern Europe arrived. These immigrants were almost always followed shortly afterward by the arrival from the same area in Europe of ministers, religious workers, teachers, and other professionals, each more educated and skillful than the earlier groups. Such individuals—highly motivated, deeply concerned for the welfare of their compatriots, and driven by a sense of duty and beneficence—ministered to the religious, educational, and social needs of their "cousins."

Many religious women, such as Roman Catholic and Anglo-Catholic nuns and Lutheran deaconesses, realized that there were important missions for them in the New World. The immigrant children needed secular and religious education. Widows and orphans needed care. There was even a new mission in which the religious women could take part: The native "heathen" population of the West needed to be evangelized. Thus, there were many opportunities in the New World. These immigrants came to America and spread all over the new country, particularly westward to the frontier areas. There they set up their institutions: schools, orphanages, chapels, and missions—whatever seemed to be needed in that particular area.

These religious workers established—often by chance—the first hospitals of the Midwest, the far West, and the Pacific Northwest. Where an epidemic or a natural disaster such as a flood or tornado occurred, these women were often asked by the community to provide for the nursing care of the victims, though they were busy with their other occupations. Although the religious community's original mission was not nursing, these formally untrained women stepped into the breech and provided emergency care as best they could. These incidents frequently led to a transition from their original mission of teaching or evangelizing to health care. At times, fearing contagion when a deadly epidemic struck, people abandoned their sick and dying—and these women, eschewing danger to themselves and out of a sense of religious duty and love of God, stepped into the void and organized needed care. Such chance events were often the genesis of a hospital in a given community.

A good example is the story of the founding of St. Mary's Hospital in Rochester, Minnesota—the hospital associated with the world famous Mayo Clinic.[34] On August 21, 1883, a tornado struck Rochester at 6:33 P.M. Much damage to the town occurred; one section, North Rochester, was totally destroyed: In this section, only 1 or 2 of about 130 houses remained standing. Rescue efforts to search out the injured and dead were carried out by lantern light. The wounded were carried to hotels or doctors' offices in the town. Forty victims were put into the parlor of the motherhouse of the Sisters of St. Francis, a teaching congregation of sisters who had been in Rochester for ten years.

The next morning, the mayor held a meeting at the town hall. The need for a centralized area to treat the hundreds of wounded residents prompted a treatment center in a dance hall and in the nearby lodge of the German Library Association. To avoid favoring any one doctor in particular and to avoid any disagreements among doctors, the mayor appointed a veterinarian to be in charge of the temporary hospital, the supplies, and the nurses. After areas were curtained off and beds and other supplies were brought in by the town's women who had volunteered to nurse the patients, the wounded were gathered from the scattered quarters in which they had been placed on the previous evening, including the convent of the Sisters of St. Francis, and doctors treated the wounded.

Soon, however, dissension broke out. Several of the doctors tried to assume authority and issue orders for all of the patients. Other doctors disagreed over the appropriateness of these orders. Among these dissenters was William Mayo, a very well-respected and unusually competent physician and surgeon who had practiced in Rochester since January 1864. Mayo, by virtue of his astute diagnostic ability and great surgical skills, was considered the leading physician and surgeon by most—though not all—of the physicians and townspeople of Rochester. That afternoon, the city council appointed Mayo head of the hospital.

It soon became apparent to Mayo that the volunteer nurses needed better discipline and direction. He knew that 100 sister-teachers of the Sisters of St. Francis were in Rochester at the motherhouse for summer vacation. He spoke to the superior, Sister Alfred, suggesting that a sister or two should look after things. Sister Alfred agreed at once and sent to the hospital two sisters, who supervised the nursing until the hospital closed in the fall of that year.

Sister Alfred had been born Josephine Moes in Luxembourg in 1829 to a prosperous family. She was educated at a boarding school in Metz, in Alsace. Like all proper young ladies of that time, she learned German and French, painting, tapestry, embroidery, singing, and proper manners. The life of domestic tranquility as wife and mother was not for her, however. She was strong-willed and dreamed of entering a convent, going to America, and evangelizing Native Americans. She traveled to America and in 1854 made vows as a Sister of the Holy Cross at Notre Dame, Indiana.

Sister Alfred became dissatisfied with the Sisters of the Holy Cross, however, and transferred her allegiance to the Third Order of the Sisters of St. Francis—a teaching order located in nearby Turkey Creek, Indiana. Eventually she was made mother superior of a new Franciscan congregation in Joliet, Illinois. After successfully establishing a school there, she was sent to Minnesota to open a convent school in that state. She established the school in Owatonna in September 1877; with the financial help of the two Catholic parishes in nearby Rochester, she opened another in that city the following December.

The sisters in Minnesota officially separated from the motherhouse of the order in Chicago. Sister Alfred and twenty-four sisters formed a new congregation of Franciscan sisters, the Congregation of Our Lady of Lourdes. Though life for a sister on the frontier was difficult, recruits were numerous. By 1883, the congregation had more than 100 members and operated several boarding and day schools in various towns of Minnesota, as well as other missions in Missouri, Ohio, and Kentucky.

A year before the tornado, the Bishop of St. Paul had suggested to Sister Alfred that the congregation might build a hospital in Rochester. Sister Alfred was not enthusiastic about doing so, for she and her sisters were trained as teachers, not nurses. After the tornado, however, and the success with which the sisters guided the nursing in the temporary hospital of Rochester, Sister Alfred gave additional thought to the bishop's suggestion and consulted Mayo about the possibility. At first he was not enthusiastic: He felt the town was too small for a hospital, that it would be too costly an undertaking, and that it would probably not be a successful venture.

Mayo's opinion of hospitals was not high. When he had come to America in 1845, he had worked as a chemist-pharmacist at Bellevue Hospital in New York City—and the Bellevue Hospital he knew was not an inspiring place. Under its roof were housed the charity hospital for the sick poor, the municipal almshouse, the insane asylum, and the city prison. The city prisoners were part of the derelict nursing staff. The nursing care at Bellevue was rough, unsympathetic, and considered too menial for anyone but the lowest members of society.

Mayo's experience had taught him that with few trained nurses, the best nursing care was given at home by loving and nurturing family members under a physician's directions. The hospitals of his day were still little more than almshouses where the sick poor went to die, and they had not improved over his days at Bellevue. Mayo's opinion of hospitals was shared by the public and most physicians of his day. More affluent members of society never sought care in these dreary asylums for the sick poor.

There were few hospitals in Minnesota at the time. St. Paul had St. Joseph's Hospital, run by the Sisters of St. Joseph, as well as St. Luke's Hospital, which had recently separated from St. Luke's Orphanage and was operated by Anglo-Catholic sisters. Duluth had recently opened a hospital under the auspices of the Episcopal Church. There were no other hospitals in the vast expanse of southern or western Minnesota—nor in the Dakota Territory just west of Minnesota (although some Sisters of St. Benedict were beginning to offer care in rented rooms in a hotel in Bismarck).[35]

As Sister Alfred persisted in her discussions, Mayo softened his opposition, and she and the congregation gradually raised sufficient money to proceed. On July 26, 1887, the sisters of the Congregation of Our Lady of Lourdes voted to build the hospital. They completed the purchase of land four months later. Mayo was asked to plan the hospital, and his sons Charlie and Will helped their father with this task.

The townspeople showed a great deal of interest and support, although there was some opposition from the Rochester chapter of the anti-immigration and anti-Catholic American Protective Association. Despite the opposition; financial difficulties; and hardships in building, supplying, and staffing, the hospital prospered and gained an excellent reputation. The Mayos used it exclusively for hospitalization of their Rochester clinic patients. They also used its facilities to help teach the many young doctors who began coming to Rochester to observe and learn surgical techniques from the Doctors Mayo—whose fame as surgeons was spreading rapidly around the world.

Thus, St. Mary's Hospital, operated by the Sisters of St. Francis of the Congregation of Our Lady of Lourdes—and one of the most outstanding teaching hospitals in the world—came about by chance. A natural disaster in a small frontier town led some teaching sisters to help a community care for its injured. The result was a change in the mission of the order from teaching to nursing and the development and operation of a hospital.

THE FOURTH TRANSFORMATION

As a result of Abraham Flexner's study of medical education in the United States and Canada for the Carnegie Foundation for the Advancement of Teaching, the reform of medical education envisioned by the founders of the AMA sixty years earlier came to fruition—though in a different way than the AMA's founders had planned. Within an incredibly short period of time, this reform led to a sharp reduction in the number of medical schools in the United States by causing many of the poorer medical schools to close altogether or to join forces with stronger ones. All medical schools adopted higher entrance requirements for prospective students, including a baccalaureate degree; restructured their curriculum; and lengthened the course of study to four years. Many of the medical schools introduced instruction for all students in basic and applied medical sciences—a movement toward a genuine university medical education proposed in the 1850s not by the founders of the AMA but by the "radical" refugee medical reformers of the German Dispensary in *Kleindeutschland*, led by Abraham Jacobi. Medical schools also became much more selective in picking faculty members and, most important, changed the way faculty members were compensated.

The Johns Hopkins Medical School was the model that other schools followed. Flexner had called particular attention to Johns Hopkins for its innovations in medical education. He was especially impressed that the students did not pay the faculty members for each course attended; instead, faculty members were salaried by the university. He wrote, "All the laboratory teaching is conducted by instructors who give their entire time to teaching and research; the heads of the clinical departments are salaried teachers attached to the Johns Hopkins Hospital."

Although Johns Hopkins University paid members of the basic science faculty a salary, the clinical faculty members were practicing physicians and surgeons whose principal income came from patient fees. The Johns Hopkins Hospital did pay the clinical department heads a small stipend for their services, but even these faculty leaders derived their principal income from patient fees. Nevertheless, this arrangement was an improvement over the system in effect in most other schools, where clinical faculty received some income directly from students—thus, the more students, the greater the income. Anyone who could pay was accepted, with little attention paid to training the "real physician."

There were several early supporters of this reform. Franklin Mall, the first professor of anatomy at Hopkins, supported a salaried medical faculty (preclinical and clinical). He felt that no faculty member should depend for his livelihood either on student or patient fees. He came to appreciate the advantages of this remuneration system of the German universities—where all faculty members, including those who were physicians, were salaried. Thus, they were able to expend their full energies on their teaching and research and did not have to curry favor with patients or students. Mall had advocated this practice at the University of Chicago, and after his appointment to the faculty of the Johns Hopkins University, he urged its adoption there.

Welch was also very much in favor of the concept, though he was not a "clinical" faculty member. In an address at the University of Chicago on December 17, 1907, he said, "The heads of the principal clinical departments, particularly the medical and surgical, should devote their main energies and time to their hospital work and to teaching and investigation without the necessity of seeking their livelihood in a busy outside practice and without allowing such practice to become their chief professional occupation."[36] William Howell, professor of physiology (a basic, not clinical, department) and dean of the Medical School at Johns Hopkins, spoke in favor of this practice in a public address in 1909 at Yale University.[37]

The concept of a full-time, salaried clinical faculty came to realization at Johns Hopkins Medical School in 1913 when the system was introduced into the departments of medicine, surgery, and pediatrics at Hopkins. This action was the fruition of intense, cooperative work carried out by, among others, Welch; Frederick T. Gates, the confidential advisor to John D. Rockefeller, Sr., and chairman of the General Education Board; Rockefeller himself; and Flexner. Ultimately, Rockefeller gave more than $50 million for medical educational projects.[38]

The story of their work is very interesting. Welch had discussed the concept of a "full-time" system with Gates at a private meeting in January 1911. Immediately after this meeting, Gates requested an estimate of funds to secure the best possible teaching in the various departments—teaching uncomplicated with the professional work outside, the model being the very best of the European schools and the best European practice and spirit.[39] Welch's initial estimate dismayed Gates, who did nothing further on the subject until much later in 1911.

When Gates read Flexner's report on medical education in 1911, he was greatly impressed. Subsequently he invited Flexner to lunch at his home. (Whether this meeting took place before or after Welch's visit with Gates, no one knows, though Chesney surmises that the Gates-Flexner meeting took place after the Welch-Gates meeting.[40]) During the course of the meal, Gates asked Flexner what he would do " . . . if you had a million dollars with which to make a start in the work of reorganizing medical education?"[41] Flexner replied without hesitation that he would give the sum to Welch. Flexner argued that Welch had created the ideal medical school and that this work had had such a great effect in reorganizing medical schools elsewhere that Welch certainly would do much more good with such a sum.

Two years later, the General Education Board made final arrangements to give an endowment to enable Johns Hopkins University to place its three major clinical departments (medicine, surgery, and pediatrics) on a salaried full-time system—setting a pattern that was subsequently adopted by most other medical schools in the country. From this time onward, teaching and research in the clinical departments of America's medical schools were wholly for the benefit of medical students. Clinical faculties no longer had divided loyalties; faculty members were freed from dependence on patient fees for their livelihood and could devote all of their energies to their academic duties.

The Hopkins Medical School became the glittering symbol of the reformers' desire for a genuine university medical education—a transformation in American medicine not in the pattern advocated by the original AMA reformers but in the pattern advocated some fifty years earlier by the radical German refugee physician reformers of New York's *Kleindeutschland*, led so ably by Jacobi.

The Hopkins Medical School had been developed on the German university model of a graduate school by the great American educator, Daniel Coit Gilman (the first president of Johns Hopkins University),[42] and William Welch, the brilliant young pathologist who was the first professor in the medical faculty. Gilman had organized and directed Yale's

Sheffield Scientific School from 1866 to 1874; later he was president of the University of California at Berkeley. Welch had spent the years 1876–78 in Germany, studying first microscopic anatomy and pathology in the laboratory of the distinguished pathologist Ernst Wagner in Leipzig and afterward physiology with Carl Ludwig in the same city. Later, in Breslau, he studied experimental pathology under renowned medical scientist Julius Cohnheim. Welch also spent some time in Vienna studying under Von Recklinghausen.[43]

The radical refugee reformers led by Jacobi had brought with them to America the idea of the German university, devoted to scientific study and research. After the Civil War, these ideas had penetrated, to a limited degree, into the American medical education system, particularly in New York. Certainly Jacobi would have had great opportunity to influence Welch while they worked together at Bellevue Hospital.[44] New York's proximity of New Haven—where Gilman was organizing the Sheffield Scientific School of Yale University[45]—would have enabled Gilman to be aware of Jacobi and his associates and their ideas.

Jacobi's ideas also penetrated into New England and reached Boston, the "Athens of America." Under president Charles Elliot, Harvard introduced a graded curriculum into its medical school in 1871 and at the same time lengthened the course of instruction to three years. The school also introduced a written examination for the completion of any medical course. After 1877, all students entering Harvard Medical School had to possess a collegiate degree or be able to pass a qualifying examination in a foreign language (Latin, French, or German) and physics.[46]

Influenced by the ideas of Jacobi and by their personal experiences in the universities of Germany and Austria, Gilman and Welch emphasized basic and applied research undertakings in medicine and surgery by faculty and students.[47]

THE FIFTH AND SIXTH TRANSFORMATIONS

The fifth transforming change in the American health care enterprise occurred during the Great Depression of the 1930s. A group of schoolteachers in Houston, Texas, realized that they could not pay high *per diem* fees[48] for inpatient hospital care, so they decided to create a pool of money that each could draw on whenever they were in need of hospital care. The teachers each contributed about fifty cents a week to this fund. This insurance program would pay members' bills for any needed hospitalization and for attending physicians' services. This transformation—indeed, revolutionary change—introduced a payer system for physician and hospital care that interposed a third party between the physician or hospital and the patient. This action by the Houston schoolteachers was the beginning of what is now known as the Blue Cross/Blue Shield Hospital and Medical Insurance program. The success of this program led many life insurance companies to enter the health insurance field. Labor unions succeeded in obtaining health insurance for themselves and their families that was written into union contracts with employers. This development ultimately led to health care insurance coverage for approximately 60 percent of the population in this country.

Several factors, including remarkable advances in health care brought about by high technology, resulted in an exponential rise in health care and premium costs between 1970 and 1990. Employers were forced to purchase contracted health insurance at the lowest possible rates. Some employers even altered their personnel practices, hiring only part-time employees (for whom they do not need to provide health insurance). Others renegotiated their union contracts to enable them to reduce some of the benefits that the health care insurance provided for employees and their families. If an employee lost his or her job, he or she lost health insurance. As premiums and copayments rose, some employees simply dropped the coverage for their families. A total of 40 million individuals (a large proportion of whom are children) in the United States now have no health care insurance.

Many incremental changes have affected this health insurance transformation since 1933. One important change took place when the federal government undertook in 1965 to provide Medicare and, in conjunction with the several states who elected to join, the cooperative Medicaid system to provide health care for the poor.

The sixth transformation in the American health care delivery system occurred in 1994, when Congress failed to enact the national health system recommended by the Clinton administration. Following this failure, the private health insurance sector was driven by market forces to capture more Americans into managed care plans. More than 40 percent of the total population of the United States enrolled in various managed care plans in less than a year.

Managed care not only imposes a third-party payer between the physician and the patient but adds to this imposition a second reviewer, a "case manager"—another truly revolutionary change. This employee of the health insurance company is a trained nurse or social worker who monitors the advice, actions, suggested tests, treatments, and prescriptions of the physician to ensure that the health care insurance plan provides for payment for these requested items. If the plan does not cover these services, payment is denied. If the patient does not forego the physician's instructions, or if the physician does not change his or her instructions to comply with the directives of the case manager, the patient will have to pay "out of pocket" for treatment that is denied by the program's health care manager.

In essence, this case manager becomes the authority who decides what the physician may do—what the physician may prescribe, when the physician may test, and when the physician may hospitalize a patient—if the insurance program is to pay. The final authority for health care has passed from the physician to the case manager. A less well-trained individual than the physician has become the decision maker in the physician-patient relationship. This concept is, indeed, revolutionary.

EFFECTS OF THE FIRST FOUR TRANSFORMATIONS

The first four transformations in health care in the United States occurred because the need for changes in medical education was uppermost in the minds of the reformers. The educational changes that the reformers wished for were not always accomplished. Indeed, sometimes the change did not affect medical education at all. Those that did occur, however, brought momentous change to one or another aspect of health care—many totally unexpected by the initiating reformers. Witness the organization of the AMA and the development of its Code of Ethics or the introduction of German scientific medicine into American medical practice in the nineteenth century.

The fifth transformation—the development of insurance for medical and hospital expenses—greatly enhanced medical education even though the reformers had no idea that it would do so. Health insurance stabilized hospitals' operations. No longer did hospitals depend primarily on bequests and endowment income to sustain patient care. Now (for the most part), payment for all hospital services was realized. The cost of charity care and of residents and interns could even be included in a hospital's *per diem* costs: The insurance plans paid *per diem* costs or charges, whichever was less. This bonanza for teaching hospitals had an enormous effect on the clinical education of medical students and the training of interns and residents in the specialties of medicine.

As a result of this development, the number of total hospital beds in the country devoted to the education of health care personnel greatly increased. The length of stay for a patient who exhibited the classical course of a disease process could be extended for the benefit of students' observation and education. The patient was not paying directly for the hospital costs engendered for this educational activity; the insurance plan was. A group of beds in a hospital could be set aside for a teaching service to be directed by the resident staff, who were wholly responsible for patient care under the oversight of the clinical faculty. Such teaching services greatly enhanced the medical students' education and contributed immeasurably to the development of many specialists in all fields of medicine and surgery, primarily after World War II.

Payment for the care given to patients directly by residents or secondarily through their supervision was easily recovered from the third-party payers. These monies provided for a better salary structure and augmentation of the numbers of full-time clinical faculty. Clinical research could be carried on in a more convenient way by the faculty investigators. In one sense, the period from 1960 to 1980 was a golden age for medical education. Costs didn't seem to be a contentious arena between the patient and the physician or hospital.

Beginning in the 1980s, however, the situation began to change. The development of synthetic drugs and antibiotics by the pharmaceutical industry added greatly to health care costs. The development of high technologies that could be applied in health care also contributed to rising prices. Moreover, health care is labor intensive. Prior to 1955, hospital workers were poorly paid, and negotiations for just wages during the late 1950s and 1960s were a third source of added costs. The appearance of the AIDS epidemic increased tremendously the costs of direct patient care in hospitals in the inner areas of large cities where AIDS was nearly epidemic. Finally, the growing practice of defensive medicine by physicians frightened of malpractice law suits from a litigious public added to expenses.

By 1990, about 15 percent of the United States' gross domestic product (GDP) was being spent on health care. Because health economists had preached that if a country spends more than 10 percent of its GDP on health care it will eventually go bankrupt,[49] such rapidly rising costs became alarming. The Clinton administration tried to address the situation, but the attempt was defeated in Congress. Thus, managed care became the order of the day.

Medical educators have tried to adjust to managed care by altering medical pedagogy. To date, however, they have not been successful in overcoming the deleterious effects managed care has had upon medical education. The number of patients in teaching hospitals has decreased so drastically that there is not enough clinical material to allow hospitals to carry on adequate clinical teaching. The length of stay of patients has been reduced so that the average is now close to 3.5 days. Such a short period is not adequate to observe the natural history of an acute disease process completely; students cannot get to know patients in any meaningful way, so they are deprived of the opportunity to learn how to participate in proper and adequate patient-doctor interactions.

With the advent of outpatient surgery advocated by managed care plans, students do not have the opportunity to take an adequate history from a patient who arrives at the hospital on the morning of an operation; thus, students do not learn adequately the signs and symptoms of various surgical conditions that require planned or emergency interventions. When the surgical patient leaves six or eight hours later, the student has no opportunity to learn post-operative care. The attempt to shift clinical training to outpatient settings such as clinics or doctor's private offices, where managed care insurance companies require that a physician see six patients an hour, has been a failure. Students' encounters with patients in such settings are antithetical to good educational practice and violate all canons of medical ethics.

Managed care plans will not reimburse hospitals for the cost of residents and students or charity care. Thus, teaching hospitals across the country that have been forced to downsize by managed care practices are rapidly running into monumental debt. Full-time clinical faculty members are being forced to do direct patient care to earn money to contribute to the financial stability of the medical school and its teaching hospital. Their clinical investigations, research efforts, and teaching are being curtailed by the necessity to earn money. Thus, the many positive effects of the fourth transformation in American health care—the establishment of the system for a full time salaried clinical faculty—have been totally vitiated.

CONCLUSION

The medical educational enterprise in this country will undoubtedly attempt to modify its pedagogical methods to adjust to the managed care health system, which has now captured about 80 percent of the population. If managed care survives, these adjustments will have to be drastic. Will we ever again see the likes of "good" physicians such as Francis Peabody of the Harvard Medical School and Boston City Hospital, Louis Hamman of the Johns Hopkins University School of Medicine and Johns Hopkins Hospital, or Connie Guion of Cornell Medical College and New York Hospital (all now deceased)? Will there still be among us, as there are now, "good" physicians and surgeons such as Edmund Pellegrino of the Georgetown University Medical School and its University Hospital, or David C. Sabiston of the Duke University Medical School and its University Hospital, or Carol Johnson Johns of the Johns Hopkins University School of Medicine and Johns Hopkins Hospital? These are but a few of the many thousands of "good" physicians who were trained in the glorious American medical educational system described above.

That system was surprisingly and unexpectedly affected by transformations (whose origins were European) that occurred in the American health care system prior to 1990. Consideration of these sweeping transformation raises a compelling question. Will the sixth transformation—namely, the coming of managed care in 1992—prevent or permit the American medical educational enterprise to continue to produce "good" physicians: those who are at once scientists, humanists, and ethicists? Only time will answer this question. The development of medicine in the early years of the republic caused great concern among well-trained and legitimate physicians of the great cities of the eastern seaboard. They wanted to ensure that physicians were well educated so that the medicine they practiced would be excellent and legitimate, and they wanted to get rid of the charlatans who were swindling the public by passing themselves off as trained physicians. Consequently, a group in the New York State Medical Society in 1844 called for a national conference of physicians to reform medical education and establish national standards for the education and licensing of physicians.[50]

Indeed, problems related to the education of physicians and quackery will remain. Every time organized medicine attempted to correct problems in the education of physicians and eliminate fraudulent practice, it failed. Surprisingly enough, however, these attempts inevitably brought about unexpected changes in medical education that transformed American health care. These changes molded the ideal of the real physician.

NOTES

1. James S. Goodwin, "Culture and Medicine: The Influence of Puritanism on American Medical Practice," *Perspectives on Biology and Medicine* 40 (1996): 977–82; Michel Foucault, *The Birth of the Clinic: An Archeology of Medical Perception,* trans. A. M. Sheridan Smith (New York: Pantheon Books, 1973).
2. Nicholas Orme and Margaret Webster, *The English Hospital 1070–1570* (New Haven, Conn.: Yale University Press, 1995), 2.
3. Gordon Wolstenholme, ed., *The Royal College of Physicians of London, Portraits* (London: Churchill Ltd., 1964), 7.
4. Rosemary Stevens, *American Medicine and the Public Interest* (New Haven, Conn.: Yale University Press, 1971), 22–23, 58–63.
5. Stevens, *American Medicine and the Public Interest,* 11–20.
6. Russell Viner, "Abraham Jacobi and German Medical Radicalism in Antebellum New York," *Bulletin of the History of Medicine* 72 (1998): 434–63.
7. William Osler, "William Beaumont: Backwood Physiologist," *Journal of the American Medical Association* 39 (1902): 1223–31.
8. Helen Clapesattle, *The Doctors Mayo* (Minneapolis: University of Minnesota Press, 1941), 24.
9. William Henry Samuel Jones, *The Doctor's Oath: An Essay in the History of Medicine* (Cambridge: Cambridge University Press, 1924).
10. Aristotle, *Nicomachean Ethics,* trans. Terence Irwin (Indianapolis: Hackett Publishing Company, 1985).
11. Nathan S. Davis, *History of Medicine with the Code of Medical Ethics* (Chicago: Cleveland Press, 1903), 36–45.
12. American Medical Association, *Minutes of the Proceedings of the National Medical Convention held in the City of New York, 1846* (New York: H. Ludwig, 1846).
13. Robert Baker, "The Historical Context of the American Medical Association's 1847 Code of Ethics: The Codification of Medical Morality," in *The Codification of Medical Morality,* ed. Robert Baker, Dorothy Porter, and Roy Porter (Dordrecht, The Netherlands, and Boston: Kluwer Academic Publishers, 1995), 47–63.
14. Thomas Percival, *Medical Ethics: Or, A Code of Institutes and Precepts. Adapted to the Professional Conduct of Physicians and Surgeons* (London: J. Johnson, 1803).
15. Peter Bartrip, "An Introduction to Jukes Styrap's *A Code of Medical Ethics,*" in *The Codification of Medical Morality,* ed. Robert Baker, Dorothy Porter, and Roy Porter, 145.
16. Baker, "The Historical Context," 41.

17. American Medical Association, "Code of Ethics," *Minutes of the Proceedings of the National Medical Conference held in the City of Philadelphia, in May 1847* (Philadelphia: T. K. & P. G. Collins Printers, 1847).
18. Baker, "The Historical Context," 58.
19. Viner, "Abraham Jacobi and German Medical Radicalism," 452.
20. Rhoda Truax, *The Doctors Jacobi* (Boston: Little Brown, 1952) 149.
21. Timothy Lenoir, "Laboratories, Medicine, and Public Life in Germany, 1830–1849: Ideological Roots of the Institutional Revolution," in *The Laboratory Revolution in Medicine,* ed. Andrew Cunningham and Perry Williams (Cambridge: Cambridge University Press, 1992), 14–71.
22. Gustav Mayer, *Friedrich Engels, a Biography,* trans. Gilbert and Helen Highet (New York: H. Fertig, 1969).
23. "A New German Medical Society," *New York Journal of Medicine* 15 (1855): 158.
24. Later this became the Lenox Hill Hospital.
25. Rudolf Virchow, *Collected Essays on Public Health and Epidemiology,* ed. L .J. Rather (Canton, Mass.: Science History Publications, 1985).
26. Charles E. Rosenberg, "Social Class and Medical Care in Nineteenth-Century America: The Rise and Fall of the Dispensary," in *Explaining Epidemics and Other Studies in the History of Medicine,* ed. C. R. Rosenberg (Cambridge: Cambridge University Press, 1992), 154–77.
27. "On Lectures given in New York by Various German Physicians," *Neu-Yorker Belletristiches Journal und Criminal Zeitung (BJCZ),* 12 December 1856; Carl F. Wittke, *Against the Current: The Life of Karl Heinzen* (Chicago: University of Chicago Press, 1945), 140.
28. Abraham Jacobi, *Report on the Clinic for Diseases of Children, Held in the New York Medical College, Session 1860-61* (New York, Balliere, 1861); also in *American Medical Monthly* 15 (1861): 401–26; 16 (1861): 9–23, 97–107, 146–50, 263–70.
29. *Proceedings and Addresses at the Complimentary Dinner Tendered to Dr. A. Jacobi on the Occasion of the Seventieth Anniversary of His Birthday, May Five, Nineteen Hundred* (New York: Knickerbocker Press, 1900), v–x.
30. Viner, "Abraham Jacobi and German Medical Radicalism," 454.
31. Truax, *The Doctors Jacobi,* 152; Victor Robinson, "The Life of A. Jacobi," *Medical Life* 35 (1928), 213–306.
32. Simon Flexner and James T. Flexner, *William Henry Welch and the Heroic Age of American Medicine* (New York: Viking Press, 1941), 69–70.
33. Carnegie Foundation for the Advancement of Teaching, *Bulletin Number Four: Medical Education in the United States and Canada* (New York: Carnegie Foundation for the Advancement of Teaching, 1910).
34. Clapesattle, *The Doctors Mayo,* 242–67.
35. Ibid., 248.
36. William Henry Welch, *Papers and Addresses by William Henry Welch,* Vol. III (Baltimore, Md.: Johns Hopkins Press, 1920), 89–103.
37. William Howell, "The Medical School as Part of the University," *Science* 30 (1909): 129–40.
38. Abraham Flexner, *I Remember* (New York: Simon & Schuster, 1940), 147.
39. Alan Mason Chesney, *The Johns Hopkins Hospital and the Johns Hopkins University School of Medicine: A Chronicle,* Vol. III (Baltimore, Md.:Johns Hopkins Press, 1945), 131–32.
40. Ibid., 136.
41. Abraham Flexner, *I Remember,* 178.

42. H. Harlan, *Johns Hopkins University Circular* XXVII (10) (December 1908), 11–16.

43. Simon Flexner and James T. Flexner, *William Henry Welch and the Heroic Age of American Medicine,* 88–110.

44. It is interesting to note that Bellevue Hospital's Training School for Nurses, organized in 1877, was headed by an Anglican nun from London who had come to the "New World" to give service to immigrants: Sister Helen of the Anglican All Saints Sisterhood. See Mary Adelaide Nutting and Levinia L. Dock, *A History of Nursing, Vol. II* (New York: G. Putnam & Sons, 1935).

45. F. Franklin, *The Life of Daniel Coit Gilman* (New York: Dodd, Mead and Co., 1910), 82–109.

46. F. Brown, *The Medical Register for New England, 1877* (Cambridge, Mass.: Riverside Press, 1877), 109–18.

47. Chesney, *The Johns Hopkins Hospital,* Vol. I, 74–97.

48. The per diem cost of a day in a Houston hospital at that time was $2.00.

49. Dr. Murray Feshbach, personal communication.

50. Davis, *History of Medicine,* 35.

The Principle of Dominion

David C. Thomasma

You have made us a little less than the angels;
You have crowned us with dignity and honor;
You have set us over the works of Your Hands.

—Psalm 8:5

Nothing is rich but the inexhaustible wealth of nature.
She shows us only surfaces, but she is a million fathoms deep.

—Ralph Waldo Emerson[1]

. . . what Sinatra evokes is not strictly urban. It is a very particular American loneliness—that of the self adrift in its pursuit in the destiny of "me," and thrown back onto the solitude of its own restless heart.

—John Lahr on Frank Sinatra[2]

This essay examines a principle proposed as fundamental to health care ethics and environmental ethics. The principle of dominion establishes responsibility for every act of intervention into natural processes. This principle may be stated simply as follows: *For every act of intervention into natural processes there is a corresponding requirement to manage and respect the vulnerabilities that occur from the intervention, now and in the foreseeable future.* As we shall see, this initial formulation will need further refinement as additional considerations and objections are met.

The principle arises in medical ethics because of the vast array of interventions available to the modern physician and patient. Indeed, in our age—at what is actually only the beginning of the scientific age[3]—not only are we able to intervene in natural processes, we are able to alter them to such a degree that we may appropriately wonder if a state of "pure" nature exists any longer. This process of improving nature through activities as diverse as medicine and husbandry demonstrates the endless search for the underlying structures of existence and the restless energy of the human race.

The powers of dominion reclassify the bond between doctor and patient because in the past, this bond arose in a context of working with nature, in and through the body, to bring about healing. Indeed, this is how Edmund Pellegrino and I defined the goal of medicine.[4] Having a new power over nature that can not only work in and through the body but also redesign the natural world means that we require an exploration of its deeper implica-

133

tions. In this essay, I explore the impact that the control of nature has on our moral reasoning in medical ethics and the philosophy of medicine.

BACKGROUND

As the quotations above show, Western civilization has had a long relationship with the natural world. By comparison to the Buddhist or Native American view, the Western perspective on nature is more complex. Buddhists and Native Americans are much more reverential and accepting of nature than Western culture has been. The West has long thought that humans, by divine command, are rulers of the world, with the power to dominate nature—and by controlling it, to transform it. The Book of *Genesis* includes a command to increase, multiply, fill the earth, and "name" (i.e., control) all the life forms—especially the animals. Medical ethics and the philosophy of medicine are only two of the contemporary responses to the challenge this heritage brings to human concourse: How are we to direct our technologies and interventions to good human ends?[5]

The unbridled endpoint of this controlling attitude, we now see, is a strange isolation from nature that pushes us back onto the solitude of the autonomous self. Thus, despite incredible scientific advances, Western civilization also has introduced a tragic flaw into the thinking and conduct of those of us who share this civilization.[6] To dominate—in contrast to exercising dominion—is somehow to destroy. Furthermore, to objectify and control nature is to miss its inexhaustible riches and simultaneously to alienate ourselves from our environment. We create the urban loneliness of which Sinatra sang. Alienated from nature, alone with all our cityscape designs and projects, the task for the coming century will be to reconstitute nature in an ethical way.

I cited the Old Testament with regard to the divine command to take dominion over life. Note that taking dominion—at least for the purposes of this essay—is different that dominating. The Psalm implies something quite less than the freedom to dominate the world: Not only are human beings "set over the works of God's hands," they are custodians and caretakers, not dominators. A great deal of contemporary cultural analysis rubs up against the enormous stretch from the custodial care of nature to its transformation and betterment.[7]

THE ETHICAL PROBLEM

Whatever creature it is that lies sleeping along the twists and turns of your nerves is awakened. . . . Your dragon calls to the dragon of the natural world and receives a gorgeous reply.

—Stephen Wright[8]

In bioethics and environmental ethics, an enormous number of issues arise from intervention into natural processes. These interventions draw us further and further into the natural world, as Wright describes. Consider, in bioethics, concerns we have about germ line therapy. Germ line therapy introduces changes in the genes that affect not only the current participant but every succeeding generation. This alteration changes things "down the line" long after the original researchers or interveners are dead. Of course, when and if we can introduce an alteration in the present, there is no reason we cannot change it later should it prove disastrous in some unforeseen way.

Nonetheless, any change we contemplate—even a change so obviously good that everyone considers it an improvement in human, animal, or plant makeup—requires caution about the consequences. This concern for consequences is particularly cogent because Western civilization tends to introduce changes for efficiency and control under the guise of progress and human betterment. Domination is not very reflective about subsequent effects, which leads to moral "catch-up"—a posture that medical ethics often must take in trying to deal with the consequences of innovative technologies. Who can forget the way nuclear development was portrayed in the 1950s as providing safe and cheap fuel? The later "oopsie" resulting from this dominion over nature is too little, too late. Caution, therefore, must be a moral *a priori* of our culture. This experiential prudence is the basis of the principle of dominion.

Human beings have long intervened and refined the processes of nature, from plant and animal husbandry to today's technological reshaping of the world around us. We have diverted rivers, rearranged mountains (strip-mining), and genetically engineered square tomatoes that can be shipped without damage; in health care, we have overseen the creation of life, determined its sex, challenged traditional family relationships, installed lifelong burdens on parents by saving their damaged newborns, prolonged dying, ended pain, mastered the direction of death.

If intervening in nature is not new in human history, what makes current ethical issues so challenging that we find the use of past wisdom and ethical principles difficult, even inadequate to the current task? One reason is that we now have the power not just to change nature and our environment but also to alter its very makeup for the future. This new relationship represents an apogee of the Enlightenment goal of refining nature. A walk in the Versailles gardens shows how regular and controlled is the imposition of reason on nature; outside the walls, the forest looks exuberantly wild by comparison.

A similar change has occurred in medical theory. Aristotle argued, for example, that the art of healing was a kind of partnership between the healer and nature itself. Today, the art of healing seems to entail redesigning nature, improving it, entering into evolution and aiming it in directions not found in its history. Only outside this "garden of Eden" is the uncontrolled world left to its own devices. Is it not interesting in this regard that only when we have exhausted all our abilities in caring for the dying that we appeal to the morality of "letting nature take its course"?

Without over-emphasizing this new influence (we also continue merely to reshape nature without redirecting it), we could claim that the primary ethical issue of the twentieth and of the twenty-first centuries has been and will continue to be the responsibility that attends this remarkable power. Most often this responsibility or duty is developed in terms of the rights of the vulnerable: the frozen embryo, the fetus, the defective newborn, the retarded, the poor, animals, unaltered nature where the air always smells cleaner. Does it make sense to speak of the rights of nature and of regulating our intercourse with it? At the very least, our double take on nature—altering it and redesigning it—requires double duty to care for and oversee the consequences of these actions. The principle of dominion expresses this requirement. Is it enough? On what basis could the world community find its moral compass regarding so great an effort?

American culture, with its emphasis on autonomy, does not appear to offer much help for a foundation of caution because of its unbridled and individualistic enthusiasms. As the quote about Sinatra shows, the push for individual achievement as the source of an ethics is particularly lonely. The only source for redesign of nature would be individual perceptions of the good, and our ethics could not transcend the obvious problems of pluralism presented by post-modernism today.[9]

Instead, a more common basis for the new relation to nature is created by a triad:

- nature as it has evolved to the present;
- interventions by humans in the evolution of nature—producing that which may never have appeared if left alone (e.g., the square tomatoes that conform to shipping cartons, animal clones and possible human ones, mining environments on the moon or on asteroids);
- the effect of redesigned nature on future generations—especially unforeseen developments—even when the greatest care is taken to divine the future to bring about good and minimize harm.

COMMON EXPERIENCES

What common experiences of modern life could lead to ideas for moral monitoring of this kind of power? A good example of the role of person, dominion, and the context of life is provided by one of the United States' greatest novelists, Thomas Pynchon, who set three anti-heroes in immediate, post World-War II Germany in his novel *Gravity's Rainbow*.[10] In that novel, all three anti-heroes—one German, one Russian, and one American—are sent into the "zone," a euphemism for the area of life that is controlled by forces that are anti-human and anti-nature. These nihilistic forces, known as "The Cartel," promote the dominance of things in place of the lush, green life that existed before humankind appeared on earth.[11] All three individuals discover that, in the words of Mr. Information:

> The truth about the War is keeping things alive. *Things.* . . . The German-and-Jap[anese] story was only one, rather surrealistic version of the real War. The real War is always there. The dying tapers off now and then, but the War is still killing lots and lots of people. Only right now it is killing them in more subtle ways. . . .[12]

The virtuous right people—those the Cartel finds to be in its way, in the way of progress—keep getting killed.

The American, Slothrop, is plucked and denuded; with his growing awareness of the truth about human control of nature, he falls apart spiritually. In the novel, the prehuman world was, in Slothrop's words, an "overspeaking of life so clangorous and mad, such a green corona about Earth's body that some spoiler *had* to be brought in before it blew the Creation apart."[13] This spoiler was the human being, who promotes death by considering nature to be dead, "transputrified into oil or coal."[14] What a powerful image: nature, the unimaginable green force, in genetic disarray, producing human beings who subdue it by considering it a dead object, "transputrified."

Our struggle then—with environmental as well as biomedical ethics—is linked through the problem of objectification of subjective life, the deadening into categories of what is rich and abundant without them. This trans-historical and cross-cultural problem explains how we are able to meet in communities of common concern about our pressing international problems.

Dominion emerges from the West's emphasis on autonomy and domination—the notion that we can subject all things to the human will with little or no consideration of the consequences. The challenge of dominion is and will be the greatest moral task of Western civilization.

AUTONOMY AND DOMINION

Medical technology gives us enormous power at all levels of life, especially at the end of life. Euthanasia and physician-assisted suicide are the most obvious examples of how conflict between autonomy and dominion arises. The temptation to employ technology rather than to give oneself as a person in the process of healing is really a "technological fix." The technological fix is much easier to conceptualize and implement than the more difficult engagement required by the principle of dominion. The training and skills of modern health professionals overwhelmingly foster the use of technological fixes. By instinct and proclivity, all persons in a modern civilization are tempted by technical rather than personal solutions to problems: If we cannot solve problems, at least we can control them.

Daily life is full of interactions with "things"—including some things that are fundamentally incomprehensible to persons who are not technologically proficient or expert. At other times, we become so accustomed to technological processes that we substitute them for human and compassionate care. Eating is replaced by tubes; participating in the spiritual and material values is replaced by "merely surviving." As Illich observes:

> Medical civilization is planned and organized to kill pain, to eliminate sickness, and to abolish the need for acts of suffering and dying. . . .[15]
>
> The new experience that has replaced dignified suffering is artificially prolonged, opaque, depersonalized maintenance.[16]

These concerns relate not only to the impersonalization of dependency on a specific technology but also to the goals of technology. Although such technology seems to give us more autonomy as it increases our choices, it may dangerously compress our personal dignity in the process. Dominion over life and death is a two-edged sword. It can offer relief of suffering, prolongation of life, and increased quality of life. Yet these good features can be accompanied by alienation, environmental assaults, and impersonalized dying.

Thus, from a deeper analysis of autonomy versus dominion, concerns about euthanasia should not be confined to the notion of dispatching persons without meeting their physical and social needs. Far from belittling these concerns, the control over death that we seek through euthanasia parallels our efforts to control and prolong life. As a result of life-control, another form of the "technofix" society is the ability to prolong suffering in conditions of hopeless injury to life. "Hopeless injury," as Braithwaite and I once defined it, is:

> . . . a condition in which there is no potential for growth or repair; no observable pleasure or happiness from living . . . and a total absence of one or more of the following attributes of quality of life: cognition or recognition, motor activity, memory or awareness of time, consciousness, and language or other intelligent means of communicating thoughts or wishes.[17]

Examples such as these show that the dominion we have taken over life and death is accompanied by legitimate concerns that we not overstep our bounds by prolonging life too long or by creating new, chronically dependent forms of living. In both cases, the goals of medicine are subverted because both entail a kind of suffering from dependence on machines and technology, products of our own creativity. Part of taking responsibility for our technology is to avoid this subjugation of human life to machinery in the first place, through more thorough discussion of possible outcomes and patient values. Normally, the way out is by restraining the use of that technology—especially through the use of advance directives.

Concern still exists that doctors and institutions ignore advance directives, especially if the patient becomes incompetent yet stable (e.g., after a stroke). When advance directives include foregoing fluids and nutrition or the respirator, health care professionals worry about "standing by and letting someone die" when that person is not considered to be terminally ill. Because many patients and families have heard such stories or seen the conflict of autonomy and paternalism displayed through movies such as *Whose Life is It Anyway?* or on talk shows or soap operas, pressure exists for a final "way out"—a right to die.

For some medical ethicists—such as former Surgeon General C. Everett Koop—withholding treatment from incompetent patients violates the patient's constitutional right to life. Few physicians would employ this vitalist position at the bedside.[18] Alternatively, the late Joseph Fletcher continuously and strongly proposed a right to die: "Death control . . . is a matter of human dignity. Without it persons become puppets. To perceive this is to grasp the error lurking in the notion that life, as such, is the highest good."[19]

THE ROLE OF PHYSICIANS

Armed with powerful technology, then, physicians can increase their power or dominion over life and death. Fascination with that power can cause even extraordinary mortals to overstep their boundaries and intervene when, as it turns out, they probably should not have. The use of the qualifier "probably" is well-considered because it is not always clear initially that the intervention will fail to accomplish the desired goals of treatment. Many physicians, however, will not let go of that power even when the patient is visibly declining and most family members, colleagues, and co-workers acknowledge that it is time to stop.

Based on this scenario, today's physicians understand their role as trying to achieve a balance between relief of suffering and non-harm.[20] With the rise of the autonomy ethic, a counterbalance to the Hippocratic view has arisen. The emphasis on autonomy and the pluralism of today's society has raised questions about the internal morality of the profession that used to place beneficence over all other values.

Consider a meeting between Jack Kevorkian, who has assisted at the suicides of many patients, and the Michigan State Medical Society. Kevorkian argued that because certain procedures for assisting in dying are clearly medical and have been performed for centuries, they can be considered ethical and should be legalized. This view received little credence. Yet Howard Brody, who chaired the committee that Kevorkian met with, said that Kevorkian "impressed many people in the room by his presentation."[21]

If patient autonomy and control of nature prevail over the value of the medical profession to preserve life, what is the moral difference between Kevorkian and anyone else who responds to patient requests? Only procedural differences distinguish between them. The tension between supporters and objectors of physician-assisted suicide lies in the doctor-patient relationship itself and in the limits and powers of that relationship. In other words, the principle of dominion reveals that the autonomy/beneficence conflict is actually an argument about control over natural processes: Who should possess that control, and what should limit it, if it is to be limited?

Leon Kass argues that the internal morality of the profession requires that doctors "give no deadly drug" and that rather than press for physician-assisted suicide, we should accept the limits of the medicalization of life and death and instead learn to live with mortality. In other words, we must respect the limits of dominion over life. The residual human wholeness in dying persons, however precarious, demands that they should be cared for even in the face of incurable illness. In opposition to Kevorkian and Quill and others who support them, Kass claims that, should doctors abandon their posts during the dying process in favor of the "technical dispensing of death," they will set the worst example for the community at large.[22]

Serious concern about dominion arises when physicians are involved in voluntary active euthanasia.[23] Kass presents a thoughtful articulation of what the physician owes a dying patient. He argues that humanity is owed humanity, not just "humaneness" (i.e., being merciful by killing the patient). Kass argues that the very reason we are compelled to put animals out of their misery is that they are *not* human and thus demand from us some measure of humaneness. By contrast, human beings demand from us our humanity itself—for the relationship "between the healer and the ill" is constituted essentially, "even if only tacitly, around the desire of both to promote the wholeness of the one who is ailing."[24]

THE NAZI EXAMPLE OF SOCIAL DOMINION

The greatest danger is to ignore lessons about dominion from world history and to misconstrue similar terms from totally different cultural contexts. Factors shaping today's debate about controlling life and death resemble those in Nazi Germany that led to social programs to eliminate the vulnerable and weak.[25] No examination of the principle of dominion would be complete without some exploration of the misuse of medical technology by the Nazi state.

The euthanasia movement was widely discussed in Nazi Germany, as it is in the United States and the world community today. Considerations of mercy allowed Adolph

Hitler to sign into law (in his first official act as Chancellor) permission (*Gnadentod*) for designated physicians to kill patients judged "incurably sick by medical examination."[26] This order seems to be parallelled in Kevorkian's suggestion that only certain trained physicians, called obitiarists, would be allowed to carry out euthanasia for those who request it.[27]

Hitler's orders soon focused on the retarded and mentally ill, however. By 1941, 70,000 patients in mental institutions had been euthanized, paralleling similar mercy killing in other countries.[28] For the Nazis, this action was just another step toward greater social hygiene: the elimination of gypsies, Jews, and socialists. It takes a powerful state to unleash these destructive forces within the medical community—and the power of the state, rather than the empowerment of individuals, formed the cultural background. What is becoming more and more obvious as research on this era continues is that the Nazi party did not initiate these ideas; they came from medicine itself.

Germany after World War I exemplified social control and a type of dominion.[29] Weimar Germany was the first modern state to control the health of its populace and the first to have a national health plan; German medical care was the envy of the world. Within the context of this plan, efforts were made to reduce costs through the prevention of serious diseases. Some attention focused on altering behaviors that led to ill-health, such as smoking. Dresden, for example, was the first city to issue a citywide ban on smoking in public places (in 1939).[30] Other research and activities focused on sociobiology and crime, the ill-effects of exposure to X-rays and asbestos, support for midwifery, high-fiber and low-fat diets, and laws requiring every German bakery to produce whole-grain bread. Nazi physicians restricted the use of DDT and rationed tobacco for pregnant women because it would harm the fetus. Most attention, however, was paid to prevention through eliminating the sources of genetic "impurities." All of these good interventions in society and nature lacked the very care or caution I have emphasized as essential to the principle of dominion.

The emphasis on social hygiene and the incorporation of many of the newest scientific ideas about human behavior, social health, and technological innovations made the Nazi party very popular. The Nazis were not "foisted" on an unwilling populace; they rose to power on wings of popularity. By 1942, more than half of Germany's physicians had joined the Nazi party. Even more startling, 8 percent had joined early on, before the party ever came to power.[31] Hence, physicians not only cooperated in varying degrees with the party and its goals, they helped shape them. Most physicians joined from self-interest, realizing that by embracing Nazi views they would be wresting power from the socialists and communists. More than half of the physicians in Berlin were Jewish, many holding prominent positions in the profession, so racism also was involved.

The moral problem lay in the conflict between traditional medical duties and virtues that promoted the best interests of patients and the goals of social hygiene embraced by a powerful state. Although some physicians surely had qualms of conscience, most did not think that promoting hygiene and the other goals of civil society was evil. In fact, no one forced them to participate in the euthanasia project; it seemed to be their duty as citizens and as professionals to encourage social hygiene.

Among the most dramatic discoveries at the turn of the twentieth century was the role of genetics in producing poor health and retardation. The world's medical journals were filled with insights about this major cause of disease. The literature contained not only scientific discoveries but also proposals for reducing genetically based disease. Removing the "polluters" of the genetic purity of the human race was the first and foremost interest of persons promoting social hygiene.[32]

The Nazis were not the only ones to think about this problem. Sterilization of the retarded—as a major step toward cleaning up the genes of the human race—was practiced in the United States as well. Foster Kennedy, in the *American Journal of Psychiatry* in 1942, advocated killing retarded children, whom he described as "nature's mistakes."[33] In fact, German physicians worried constantly about how far ahead of them the United States was—in attitude and in willingness to improve eugenics. By the late 1920s, 15,000 individuals had been sterilized in the United States:

> . . . most while incarcerated in prisons or homes for the mentally ill. German racial hygienists throughout the Weimar period expressed their envy of American achievements in this area, warning that unless the Germans made progress in this field, America would become the world's racial leader.[34]

The power of eugenics as a scientific discipline was coupled with an intolerance for other races in the United States as well as in Nazi Germany. The American Medical Association refused to admit black physicians, for instance. As Proctor points out, this attitude permitted the Nazis to argue that they were not the only ones to protect racial purity in the profession and in society as a whole.[35] The goals of social hygiene and eugenics rapidly destroyed individual autonomy and tolerance for pluralism.

Perhaps the least-understood feature of Nazi Germany's euthanasia effort was the explicit use of wartime triage as a reason for eliminating "valueless life." If times were different, Nazi physicians argued, economics would not be a factor in the problem of social hygiene. The high inflation rate and the need for beds for soldiers and others needed for the war effort demanded the elimination of "unnecessary eaters," a major burden on the state.

Proctor, for example, says that "the fundamental argument for forcible euthanasia was economic."[36] This argument involved a preemptive triage to free up beds for the coming war. Hitler's first directive authorizing euthanasia for special cases occurred in 1939, coinciding almost exactly with the invasion of Poland—making euthanasia more easily justifiable. Quickly, however, euthanasia turned into mercy killing. Proctor notes that the first mental patients were gassed in Posen, Poland, on October 15, 1939—just 45 days after Germany's invasion.[37] By 1941, euthanasia was part of the normal hospital routine in Germany. At one point, psychiatrists worried that they would have no more patients and the field would become too small.[38]

The application of "mercy" to this population had a history, moreover. During World War I, half of all German mental patients starved to death, according to one estimate—including 45,000 in Prussia alone. These "useless eaters" were simply too far down on the ration list to obtain food. This practice, coupled with the long campaign to stigmatize the handicapped and the mentally ill as having lives not worth living, led to the inauguration of the liquidation program. The idea that certain human lives are expendable entails a judgment regarding the value of life of vulnerable individuals and the needs and wants of society itself. From a purely utilitarian standpoint, those who contribute nothing to society and drain its resources are expendable.

DOMINION OVER LIFE

The story of the Nazi physicians exemplifies dominion as a *non*-moral concept. Drs. Binding and Hoche, Nazi party euthanasia theorists, called the lives of vulnerable persons "ballast existence." In their view, when economic times are prosperous, society does not ask questions about caring for expendable individuals. When times get difficult, then such "ballast existence" must be eliminated:

> The question of whether the expense of maintaining these categories of ballast existence is in every aspect justifiable was not an urgent one in former times of prosperity. Today conditions are different and we have to consider it.[39]

Note how easily the wartime triage justification conflates with the economic justification for mercy killing. Similar reasoning in our day leads to the marginalization of individuals who are cut off from power and recourse. At first blush, explicit downgrading of the intrinsic value of human life seems foreign to our way of thinking. Most people today would react with dismay, even anger, at a statement like Binding's and Hoche's. We also have the advantage of hindsight about the horrible, devastating consequences of such thinking: The stench of the death camps is a pall that still hangs over Western civilization.

Yet attitudes of superiority and the disvaluing of individual lives creep into our own thinking as well. They creep in while we construct what we consider to be rational allocation plans for health care. Although we intend to minimize suffering and maximize the common good, individual persons in high numbers face neglect of their needs.

Perhaps the biggest concern about euthanasia today is the forthcoming crisis in health care that will be created by an increasingly elderly population. In the next fifty years, the number of Americans who are more than 85 years of age will increase fivefold, from 3 million to 15 million citizens. Most of these elderly persons will be graduates of our technological interventions; many will be dependent on long-term nursing home care—the most expensive medical cost for the elderly. In all state budgets, Medicaid is the second largest budget item after education. Persons over the age of 85 expend four times as much money for hospitalization as those under 85. There will be fewer individuals "in the middle," able to bear the burden of caring for the young and the elderly. Already the phenomenon of the elderly (70–85 years of age) caring for the "old old" (those over 85) has begun. How soon would we turn our attention to the high cost of caring for extremely elderly and debilitated persons? The discussion of euthanasizing the demented elderly has begun again in the United States.[40]

Recall that the fundamental argument for forcible euthanasia is economic. Once active voluntary euthanasia is in place, habits of finding other areas for "mercy," coupled with hard economic times, could easily lead to involuntary euthanasia. This scenario is another form of the traditional slippery slope argument. It is based on fears about the violence in American society and the natural human propensity to find "technofix" solutions to difficult problems we can only imagine for the future but that our children must face soon enough. If we set the wrong precedents in the present, why should we believe that the sort of thinking and policy that occurred in Nazi Germany would not arise again?

Proponents of direct euthanasia usually argue that fences can be built on the slope—legal requirements that would eschew even the most remote possibility of a society turning mercy into murder once more. What the Nazis did was not euthanasia but murder, purely and simply for the good of the state. If quality-of-life judgments and social utility judgments are constantly held in check by our cultural and historical memory of the Holocaust, we will be well on the way toward providing a humane solution to the problem of suffering not only at the end of life but throughout it as well. Academic and public policy debate must include an awareness of the social violence in American society today—where individuals are killed simply because someone wants their sports jacket, small children are killed in projects on their way to school, and, increasingly, children themselves kill students and teachers in schools. This violence does not manifest itself only in the inner city; it is a pandemic of our society. It infects us even when we are wary of it; it barrages us in the "previews of coming attractions" in the movie theaters. President Clinton has called for more research on the relation of media and film violence and its imitation in youth culture.[41]

If a broadly adopted principle of dominion were in place, depictions of violence would be regarded as artificial interventions into the generally orderly life of society. The depiction itself would be regarded more explicitly as an effort to take control over others. Responsibility for the outcome of this "intervention" would be readily acknowledged as a moral responsibility—something that has not been forthcoming from the National Rifle Association or the film and television industry: Instead of accepting what can be foreseen as a consequence of portrayals of violence, they make excuses and appeal to constitutional rights and privileges.

THE PRINCIPLE OF DOMINION

All future generations potentially exist, just as frozen embryos potentially would grow to human stature as persons if not impeded by technological intervention. In this respect, there is a connection between future bioethics and environmental ethics. Both must employ a concern about natural development unimpeded by technology. As a consequence, a general principle can be constructed that domination of the environment and human beings through technological intervention brings an intensification of duties to protect that which is in custody. This attitude is the proper understanding of the principle of dominion that should result from responsible use of our autonomy.

In other words, development of individual freedom is inherently bound with moral responsibility because that freedom is circumscribed by duties to self, family, society, and environment. Autonomy is not rule-less or norm-less; instead, the concept of autonomy recognizes the need for boundaries and setting up one's own moral rules (e.g., not harming others or the environment). To that growing freedom of humans is now added in the Principle of Dominion: the explicit duty to care especially well for the foreseeable consequences of interventions into natural processes.

For this reason, dominion is a major ethical and philosophical concern in bioethics. At most we ask rhetorical questions about doctors "playing God" in the lives and deaths of patients; physicians and researchers developing new forms of life that are the subject of patents;[42] vast, contemplated interventions into the genetic makeup of the human race after the map of the genome is completed—or even before it is completed;[43] concerns created by cloning Dolly;[44] and current concerns about genetic implants in the ovum.[45]

The image of playing God usually is aimed exclusively in the direction of public policy; it could be redirected at the deeper question of the duties that emerge from (or arise with) dominion.

Dominion is a primary concern in issues of unduly prolonging life, when physicians might ignore the wishes of patients and families about stopping treatment. It also is the central problem in the use of animals in research: Are they here for human beings to control and manipulate for our own purposes, or are they subject only to our custodial care?[46]

As with the environment, then, all of our technological capacities require greater responsibility than we have displayed in the past. In this respect, bioethics is just a footnote to the larger problem of directing our technology to good human ends.[47]

CONCLUSION

Rousseau's "smile of reason," depicted in a statue of him from the Enlightenment, is today an anachronism. Humanism does not take sufficient account of the power of evil in human society and in human hearts.[48] To take this evil into account, I began this essay with the challenge of dominion and its consequences, the struggle of ordinary people to adapt to new circumstances, the pointed neglect and elimination of most of the world's most vulnerable people, the wholesale destruction of the environment. A modern, international bioethics concerning dominion over the environment and over human lives is our challenge.

The challenge of the future in international bioethics will concentrate on the question of development. Should economic interests in development take precedence over other human values in health care? As we have seen, too much power concentrated in the state over the health care needs of its citizens can lead to a belligerent overriding of individual autonomy, inappropriate quality-of-life judgments about the value of vulnerable populations to the social system, and subsequent acts of destruction and violence. A tolerance for pluralism and a respect for fundamental disagreements about social policy must check these tendencies.

On the other hand, too much concentration on individual autonomy abandons persons in need, ignores the common good and the need for social health care policy, and damages majority interests while respecting the few.

Some refinements of the principle of dominion would be the following:

- A properly "environmentally respectful" bioethics would not move too quickly toward easy "technical" solutions to difficult moral and personal problems.
- A presumption against the taking of human life is embedded in the foundational moral traditions of society.[49] Losing sight of this foundational ethic turns control of human life over to society's judgments of quality of life and to technical solutions to profound human problems.
- Invoking a technical solution also invokes realms of control over individual lives that accompany technology.[50] With that control comes the power of the state. It is always a dangerous move to empower the state over individuals; this is even more true today than it was fifty years ago, when technology itself had not developed to the extent it that it has today.

- We should cultivate a healthy respect for the role of evil in the human heart and human affairs. Such a respect is often missing in humanistic and autonomy-based writings, yet it is, as we have seen, germane to the bioethics issues I have raised in this essay.

The chief Nazi physician and medical ethicist, Rudolph Ramm, wrote, "Only a good person can be a good physician."[51] No one could disagree with this sentiment. Yet because of the evils perpetrated by the Nazis, these words echo a warning through time. They demonstrate how closely linked our sense of moral duty is with social goals presented by our government and our culture. If we accept the latter uncritically, our moral duty is in jeopardy. Not only is unexamined life not worth living, as Socrates said long ago; it is also dangerous. How could intelligent and well-educated persons have participated in programs that wrested dominion over individual, vulnerable human lives? How might we be doing the same?

NOTES

1. As cited in Carl Sagan, *Broca's Brain: Reflections on the Romance of Science* (New York: Random House, 1979).
2. John Lahr, "Sinatra's Song," *The New Yorker*, 3 November 1997, 88.
3. For example, more than three-quarters of all scientists that ever lived are alive today.
4. Edmund D. Pellegrino and David C. Thomasma, *A Philosophical Basis of Medical Practice* (New York: Oxford University Press, 1981).
5. Bertrand Russell, as quoted in "Medicine's Technical Feats Forcing New Emphasis on Study of Ethics," *American Medical News*, 2 December 1974, 17.
6. Edmund Husserl, *Krisis der Europäischen Wissenschaften und die transzendentale Phanomenologie*, trans. David Carr (Evanston, Ill.: Northwestern University Press, 1970).
7. See, for example, Lewis Mumford, *Pentagon of Power: The Myth of the Machine, Vol. 2* (New York: Harcourt Brace Jovanovich, 1974).
8. As quoted in Craig Seligman, "A Touch of Evil," review of *Going Native*, by Stephen Wright (New York: Farrar, Straus, and Giroux, 1994), *The New Yorker*, 17 January 1994, 90.
9. H. Tristram Engelhardt, Jr., *The Foundations of Bioethics*, 2nd ed. (New York: Oxford University Press, 1997).
10. Thomas Pynchon, *Gravity's Rainbow* (New York: Viking, 1973).
11. Dwight Eddins, *The Gnostic Pynchon* (Bloomington: Indiana University Press, 1990).
12. Pynchon, *Gravity's Rainbow*, 645.
13. Ibid., 720.
14. Ibid.
15. Ivan Illich, *Medical Nemesis: The Expropriation of Health* (New York: Pantheon Books, 1976), 106.
16. Ibid., 154.
17. S. Braithwaite and D. C. Thomasma, "New Guidelines on Foregoing Life-Sustaining Treatment in Incompetent Patients: An Anti-Cruelty Policy," *Annals of Internal Medicine* 104 (1986): 711–15.

18. Erich Loewy, "Treatment Decisions in the Mentally Impaired: Limiting But Not Abandoning Treatment," *New England Journal of Medicine* 317 (1987): 1465–69.
19. Joseph Fletcher, "Four Indicators of Humanhood—The Enquiry Matures," *Hastings Center Report* 4 (1974): 7.
20. Eric Cassell, "The Relief of Suffering," *Archives of Internal Medicine* 143 (March 1993): 522–23.
21. "Missouri and Kevorkian Continue to Provoke Controversy," *Hospital Ethics* 8, no. 6 (November/December 1992): 9.
22. Leon R. Kass, "'I Will Give No Deadly Drug': Why Doctors Must Not Kill," *American College of Surgeons Bulletin* 77, no. 3 (March 1992): 7–17.
23. W. Gaylin, L. Kass, E. D. Pellegrino, and M. Seigler, "Commentaries: Doctors Must Not Kill," *Journal of the American Medical Association* 259, no. 14 (8 April 1988): 2139–40.
24. Leon Kass, "Arguments Against Active Euthanasia by Doctors Found at Medicine's Core," *Kennedy Institute of Ethics Newsletter* 3 (January 1989): 1–3, 6.
25. David C. Thomasma, "The Ethics of Caring for Vulnerable Individuals," in *Reflections on Ethics* (Washington, D.C.: American Speech-Language-Hearing Association, 1990), 39–45; Edmund D. Pellegrino and David C. Thomasma, "Dubious Premises—Evil Conclusions: Moral Reasoning and the Nuremberg Trials," *Cambridge Quarterly of Healthcare Ethics* 9, no. 2 (winter 2000): 261–74.
26. R. N. Proctor, "Nazi Doctors, Racial Medicine, and Human Experimentation," in *The Nazi Doctors and the Nuremberg Code,* ed. George Annas and Michael A. Grodin (New York: Oxford University Press, 1992), 23.
27. Jack Kevorkian, *Prescription—Medicide: The Goodness of Planned Death* (Buffalo, N.Y.: Prometheus Books, 1991).
28. Proctor, "Nazi Doctors," 23–27; R. N. Proctor, *Racial Hygiene: Medicine under the Nazis* (Cambridge, Mass.: Harvard University Press, 1988), 179–89.
29. Robert J. Lifton, *The Nazi Doctors: Medical Killing and the Psychology of Genocide* (New York: Basic Books, 1986); Karl H. Roth, ed., *Erfassung zur Vernichtung, von der Socialhygiene zum "Gesetz ueber Sterbehilfe"* (Berlin: Verlagsgesellschft Gesundheit, 1984).
30. Proctor, "Nazi Doctors," 28, footnote 23.
31. Ibid., 26.
32. Proctor, *Racial Hygiene*.
33. Foster Kennedy, "The Problem of Social Control and the Congenitally Defective: Education, Sterilization, Euthanasia," *American Journal of Psychiatry* 99 (1942): 13–16.
34. Proctor, "Nazi Doctors," 21.
35. Ibid.; "Keine Negeraerzte in der amerikanischen Standesorganisation," *Archiv fuer Rassen-und Gesellschaftsbiologie* 33 (1939): 276.
36. Proctor, "Nazi Doctors," 24.
37. Ibid.
38. Benno Mueller-Hill, *Murderous Science: Elimination by Scientific Selection of Jews, Gypsies, and Others, Germany 1933–1945* (New York: Oxford University Press, 1988), 42.
39. K. Binding and A. Hoche, *Die Freigabe der Vernichtung des Lebensunwertens Lebens, 1920,* as quoted in H. Lauter and J. E. Meyer, "Active Euthanasia without Consent: Historical Comments on a Current Debate," *Death Education* 8 (1984): 89–98.
40. Stephen Post, "Severely Demented Elderly People: A Case Against Senicide," *Journal of the American Geriatrics Society* 38, no. 6 (June 1990): 715–18; David C. Thomasma, "Mercy Killing of Elderly People with Dementia: A Counterproposal," in *Dementia and Aging: Ethics, Values, and Policy Choices,* ed. Robert Binstock, Stephen Post, and Peter Whitehouse (Baltimore, Md.: Johns Hopkins University Press, 1992), 101–17.

41. Gary Dretzka, "Clinton Orders Study of Kid Violence, Films," *Chicago Tribune*, 2 June 1999, sec. 1, p. 4.
42. "U.S. OKs Patents for Strains of Mice," *Chicago Tribune*, 30 December 1992, sec. 1, p. 12.
43. "U.S. Clears Gene Therapy for Woman's Brain Tumor," *Chicago Tribune*, 30 December 1992, sec. 1, p. 10.
44. Arlene Judith Klotzko, ed., *Cambridge Quarterly of Healthcare Ethics* 7 (spring 1988).
45. Donald S. Rubenstein, David C. Thomasma, Eric A. Schon, and Michael J. Zinaman, "Germ-Line Therapy to Cure Mitochondrial Disease: Protocol and Ethics of *In Vitro* Ovum," *Cambridge Quarterly of Healthcare Ethics* 4 (summer 1995): 316–39.
46. Baruch A. Brody, ed., *The Ethics of Biomedical Research: An International Perspective* (New York: Oxford University Press, 1988).
47. Jeremy Rifkin, *Biosphere Politics: A New Consciousness for a New Century* (New York: Crown, 1991); J. Ronald Engel and Joan Gibb Engel, *Ethics of Environment & Development* (Tucson: University of Arizona Press, 1990).
48. David C. Thomasma and Erich Loewy, "Exploring the Role of Religion in Medical Ethics," *Cambridge Quarterly of Healthcare Ethics* 5 (spring 1996): 257–68.
49. Courtney S. Campbell, "'Aid-in-Dying' and the Taking of Human Life," *Journal of Medical Ethics* 18 (1992): 128–34.
50. David C. Thomasma, *Human Life in the Balance* (Louisville, Ky.: Westminster Press, 1990).
51. Proctor, "Nazi Doctors," 17; R. Ramm, *Ärtzliche Rechts- und Standeskunde* (Berlin: Akademie Verlag; Stuttgart, Druckenmüller, 1942), 88–89.

Organizational Ethics and the Medical Professional: Reappraising Roles and Responsibilities

George Khushf

The idea of an individual who serves as healer and friend has a strong hold on our psyche. It responds to a basic need we all have. When we are confronted with illness, we need a person who has the knowledge and skills required to effectively intervene (the healer). Yet we also require a person who appreciates our personal experience and responds in a personal way (the friend). Although our need calls for an intimate link between these two roles, in practice there has been tension between them. The challenge for the physician-humanist has been to integrate the roles: simultaneously advancing the scientific ideal and establishing a practice that is fully responsive to the needs of the individual patient as a person.

Edmund Pellegrino has been one of the most prominent advocates of this integrated ideal. Pellegrino was at the forefront of the developing field of bioethics and has served as a leader in medical education; he has championed scientifically based, individual-oriented care that takes seriously the fiduciary character of the physician-patient relationship and the ideals of medical professionalism. Today Pellegrino is also one of the most outspoken opponents of current transformations in health care associated with the rise of managed care. Pellegrino's current crusade is not separate from the positive ideal of the physician humanist. He believes that managed care establishes an institutional context that undermines the classic scientific and ethical ideals of medicine and thus works against the possibility that physicians can be friends and effective healers.

In this essay, I suggest that there is another, more positive side to managed care. I also suggest that there are tensions in Pellegrino's own thought—and that some of his best insights lead to an alternative assessment of the prominent role now being played by organizations. Medicine is in the midst of a paradigm shift. We are moving from individually practiced, individual-oriented medicine toward an institutionally practiced, community-oriented health care. This shift requires a reconfiguration of the older ideal, so that one focuses on an organization that fosters humane personal interaction and simultaneously realizes a scientific ideal. Previously the challenge was to integrate personal and scientific ideals, and challenge remains. Now, however, the focus is on organizations rather than on individual physicians. Thus, I seek to affirm Pellegrino's general ideals but show that one must move to an organizational perspective for their further development.

My argument proceeds in two steps. First, I identify three elements of what I call the "classical paradigm of medicine." These elements are scientific foundationalism, an individual patient orientation, and an assumed complementarity of medical and social interests. Within this classical paradigm, however, there were competing schools of thought. Pellegrino sought to develop a balanced approach between a reductionistic, scientific positivism, on one side, and an overly simplistic emphasis on art and subjectivity, on the other. In pursuing his ideal, he saw that normative ethical reflection could not come in as a second step; instead, a foundational, critical reflection on medicine was needed to articulate ethical ideals together with the scientific ideals of practice. In this philosophical project, tensions emerge in Pellegrino's thought that are never fully resolved. These tensions reflect the depth and richness of Pellegrino's focus and manifest deep tensions in medicine itself.

In the second section of this essay, I highlight the tensions between art and science, between individual and society, and between the perspectives of physician and patient. I suggest that these tensions cannot be resolved within the classical paradigm of medicine. At the heart of the classical paradigm is a focus on the physician-patient relationship as the central context for health care practice. Pellegrino bases his whole philosophy on an intuition about the centrality of this relationship and fights against anything that undermines it. This intuition is a premise of his project, however, not a conclusion. By highlighting the way medicine has been transformed, I suggest that the central focus is now on the institution-patient relationship. Pellegrino's own discussion of institutions supports this conclusion.

My intent in this essay is to show how roles and responsibilities need to be reassessed and to show how recent developments hold the promise for addressing ethical issues that remained unresolvable in the older paradigm. The longing for a physician who is healer and friend has its counterpart in the longing for a community that is simultaneously responsive to personal values and scientifically grounded in its structure and practice, so that it can effectively respond to the health needs of the community. The two ideals—that of the healer/friend and that of community—must work together; one cannot have the former without the latter. A true healer and friend is responsive not simply to the individual but to that individual as a member of the community.

SCIENCE, ETHICS, AND THE SOCIAL GOOD: CORE ELEMENTS OF THE CLASSICAL PARADIGM OF MEDICINE

There have always been significant differences of opinion in medicine, not only regarding ethical issues but also in the way medicine is conceptualized as a science. Despite these differences, however, there are common background assumptions that are simply taken for granted by nearly everyone and rarely made explicit. These background commitments constitute a "thought collective"[1] or "paradigm."[2]

I focus on three core commitments that jointly characterize the traditional paradigm of modern medicine. These core commitments have characterized medicine since it emerged in its clinico-pathological form with the Paris School in the early nineteenth century. The three core commitments are scientific foundationalism, an individual patient orientation, and an assumption about the accord of medicine and social interest. Within the classical paradigm, these elements are hierarchically ordered in a way that will be specified later in this section.

Modern medicine understands itself as scientifically foundational. As David Thomasma makes clear, the meaning of *foundationalism* is complex.[3] The term need not imply a Cartesian method, in which complex ideas are built stepwise from simple, "clear and distinct" points of departure. Nor need it imply the alternative, empiricist version (perhaps seen best in the ideals of logical positivism, which suggests that knowledge arises from increasing levels of generalization from pure sense data, and all empirical knowledge is reducible to logical and observational terms). Although both of these more reductionistic foundationalisms are found in medicine,[4] I use the term in a broader sense. To claim that the modern medical paradigm assumes scientific foundationalism implies that medical theory and practice are built on "basic sciences"—which, as science, involve knowledge that is (relatively) independent of place and time and thus applicable to all humans. Although particular clinical interventions may not be independent of individual values and sociocultural context, the basic sciences that inform those interventions should be. The sciences—also known as the "laboratory sciences"—provide a basic knowledge of normal and pathological anatomy and thus the language for configuring biomedical disease. Thus, scientific foundationalism is intimately intertwined with the clinic-laboratory dialectic that constitutes modern medicine.[5]

Differences within the traditional paradigm emerge in interpreting this scientific foundationalism. Although there are many variants of interpretation, the most important distinction concerns how the basic sciences are related to clinical medicine. The dominant strand of interpretation can be aligned with the tradition of logical positivism. Science is sharply divided from the humanities, and priority is given to science in configuring clinical practice. On this model, clinical medicine seeks to emulate the laboratory sciences and, to this extent, can be regarded as a simple extension of theoretical science into the realm of practice. Clinical judgment is modeled in Bayesian terms, and decision theory is used to provide the basis for interventions. To the degree that irreducibly aesthetic or otherwise subjective considerations play a role, clinical decision making is regarded as falling short of its ideal. Ethical and culturally relative values are to enter only as a second step—concerned with the use and abuse of the independently formulated, scientifically configured practice.[6]

The viewpoint of what may be called the "medical humanist" stands in opposition to the logical positivist interpretation. From the medical humanist perspective, the scientific foundationalism of modern medicine signifies its dependence on basic or laboratory sciences, but clinical medicine is not simply a science or even primarily a science. Instead, medicine is a practice that uses science to address the needs of an individual patient and thus involves a mode of practical reasoning that bridges science and the humanities. Clinical reasoning can never be reduced to an algorithm or decision tree: It is a form of prudence, a practical wisdom.

Pellegrino is one of the most prominent advocates of medical humanism. He does argue that medicine is scientifically based.[7] He claims that one "must reject the suggestion that the 'scientific paradigm' should be replaced by a paradigm drawn from the humanities."[8] To offer just one example, Pellegrino's scientific foundationalism is apparent in his account of the importance of the autopsy:

[T]he properly performed autopsy remains the gold standard of clinical practice. . . . It is as close to a 'final' court as one can devise to detect serious errors in diagnosis or treatment, to ground the accuracy of the newer invasive and noninvasive techniques, and to provide that integrated view of a disease entity subsumed under its natural history.[9]

Clearly, Pellegrino's thought is wed to the clinico-pathological dialectic that emerged with the Paris School of medicine, in which "disease" is specified in terms of pathoanatomy (and later pathophysiology). To appreciate the importance of the autopsy, one must situate the discussion in the context of the distinction between "basic sciences" and "clinical experience" and the attempt to configure clinical phenomena in terms of a disease concept that is specified by the knowledge found in the basic sciences.[10]

Yet Pellegrino also insists that this description is not enough. Clinical medicine works with two kinds of data. One kind of data is associated with the activity and knowledge base of the scientist; the other is derived from the individual patient's illness experience. Thus, in addition to the patient's biomedical disease, one should also consider the patient's dis-ease. For Pellegrino, these two approaches must be integrated in clinical judgment.[11] The focus on the patient's values and experience cannot enter as a second step, after a scientific clinical judgment has taken place. This emphasis on the patient's values distinguishes Pellegrino from the medical positivist.

The second element of the modern medical paradigm is its focus on the individual patient. Medicine is not primarily socially or population oriented.[12] This element of the paradigm has scientific and ethical dimensions. Scientifically, there is a challenge associated with applying generalized knowledge to a particular case. Each case is unique, and one must develop the skills for discerning where special adaptation or individualized methods of care are required. Often, the term "the art of medicine" is used to describe the ability of a physician to be responsive to the unique and particular.[13] Ethically, the individual patient focus means that the physician must act as the patient's agent, promoting the patient's best interest. This obligation characterizes the physician-patient relationship as a fiduciary relation.

Traditionally, these fiduciary obligations were grounded in the vulnerability of the patient and the trust that the patient places in the physician. The physician's appraisal of the patient's needs and best interests directed the healing activities—thus placing the physician in a paternalistic role. More recently, however, there has been a shift away from paternalism and the assumption that patient vulnerability implies an inability to be an active participant and agent in the physician-patient relationship. Patients are now regarded as autonomous, capable of determining their own best interests and articulating those interests. The physician-patient relationship is redescribed as a more symmetrical and collaborative interaction in which patients articulate their needs and the physician works with the patient to address them.[14]

Pellegrino strongly affirms the individual patient focus and attempts to integrate the older emphasis on the patient's vulnerability with more recent criticisms of paternalism.[15] Yet there is a tension between these two approaches because the emphasis on patient vulnerability assumes an asymmetry of power and knowledge, whereas the emphasis on autonomy assumes a symmetry. Pellegrino resolves this tension by developing an essential linkage between the two elements of the paradigm; namely, scientific foundationalism and individual patient orientation. This linkage is worked out in clinical judgment. Here one finds the ethical motivation for the account of practical wisdom that was evident in Pellegrino's response to the positivist bifurcation of the scientific and humanistic sides of medicine.

In clinical judgment, the physician applies scientific knowledge, with its biomedical disease concept, to a particular patient. Through a philosophy of the lived body, Pellegrino distinguishes between the "organic dysfunction" associated with the object body and the disrupted life-world associated with the patient's illness experience. For Pellegrino, the primary goal of medicine is to address the lived body disruption; it achieves this goal by curing the organic dysfunction, which is "a necessary but not a sufficient step toward this goal."[16] Pellegrino also recognizes that the activities of other people—such as pastoral care workers, psychologists, and family—play an important role in addressing the life-world disruption. Thus, medicine's cure orientation is only one component of the broader activity of care; and medicine must coordinate this curing activity with those of other healers if it is to rightly address its ultimate goal.[17]

This relatively modest appraisal of medicine enables Pellegrino to integrate the traditional, vulnerability-based approach with more recent autonomy-based approaches to patient care. With regard to organic dysfunction, there is a clear asymmetry between the knowledge and power of the physician and the patient. In this cure orientation, the physician draws on science. The ultimate goal, however, is to address the patient's life-world disruption, which depends not just on the organic dysfunction but also on the patient's culture and individual narrative—including particular valuings of the organic dysfunction and its import. The broader perspective of the patient determines which medical interventions are appropriate and how they should be coordinated with other healing activities (such as those of priest, nurse, psychologist, and family). In the case of organic dysfunction, the physician knows best what is at issue and what should be done, but the patient knows best how the illness affects the patient's own life and what notion of "best interests" should determine care.

The contrast between the medical positivist and the medical humanist can be summarized by stating that for the former, "medically indicated" is a function of science; values enter as a second step, to address whether the patient's goals support that which is so indicated. For the medical humanist, however, medical indication is a function of a prudential integration of science and the humanities. Clinical judgment is a form of practical wisdom in which generalized knowledge (the science), with its organic notion of disease, is applied to an individual patient whose life is potentially or actually disrupted. Thus, clinical judgment is an activity in which scientific foundationalism is integrated with an individual patient focus, and the core clinical relationship is specified as a fiduciary one between physician and patient.

Although medicine focuses on the individual patient, nearly all physicians are confident that medicine advances the social good; for this reason, social and economic structures should be established to protect and foster good medicine. Yet according to the traditional paradigm, social and economic factors are *not* supposed to play a role in configuring *how* medicine is practiced.[18] That would be a violation of its scientific foundationalism and compromise the individual patient orientation that is central to its ethic. Yet physicians recognize that medicine depends on economic and social factors. To avoid distortion of medicine, a second foundationalism is introduced: Social and economic structures are to be developed so that they foster rather than interfere with the scientifically grounded, individually oriented practice of medicine. This approach to social and economic conditions is most apparent in Pellegrino's thought in his criticisms of managed care and his call for a universal health system.[19]

The three elements of the classical paradigm are constructed with a lexical priority. First, the paradigm assumes that the foundational science is developed independent of historically or culturally conditioned values and that it is therefore valid for all cultures. To the degree that contingent factors are part of the science, they are eventually to be excluded as the science is further developed. Second, clinical medicine has a focus on the individual patient. Although there are different approaches to relating these two elements, all physicians agree that medicine must integrate the universal, general knowledge of science and the unique characteristics of the patient. The physician-patient encounter is regarded as the condition for this integration, and this relationship is given priority in health care. Finally, as a third element, the classical paradigm assumes that society benefits from medicine and that social and economic structures should be established in a way that fosters and protects the configurations of medical reality that arise from the first two core elements of the paradigm. This lexical interrelation of the three elements, not just the individual elements taken singly, constitutes the classical medical paradigm.

INTER-ETHICS AND MANAGED CARE: NORMS FOR A NEW PARADIGM OF HEALTH CARE

In Pellegrino's philosophy of medicine, nearly all of the important strands of modern medicine are integrated. He has attempted to incorporate the science and the art, the imaginative/intuitive and the algorithmic, the biomedical disease and the patient's illness experience, the values and perspectives of physician and patient. He has come as close as anyone to accomplishing this integration. Important tensions remain, however—tensions that disclose an insufficiency in the paradigm itself. As a next step, we must move away from the individually oriented, individually practiced understanding of medicine toward an institutionally practiced, community-oriented form. Only in such a communal form of health care can Pellegrino's humanist ideal be realized.

The tensions in Pellegrino's thought become apparent when we consider his criticisms of managed care. Although Pellegrino does not provide a definition of managed care organizations (MCOs), we can identify their characteristics by considering the features that he finds problematic. First, MCOs are oriented toward patient populations; thus, they configure health care in a community-oriented, rather than individually oriented manner.[20] Second, MCOs transfer authority away from physicians and use that authority to place limits on clinical discretion and influence how medicine is practiced.[21] Third, MCOs directly employ physicians, thus generating an obligation on the part of physicians to the organization—which can be in tension with a physician's obligation to patients.[22] Fourth, MCOs pursue profits and allow economic considerations to influence how care is practiced. Thus, MCOs transform medicine into a commodity and distort its character as a profession and public good.[23]

Pellegrino clearly is most troubled when all four of these characteristics are combined, although he speaks of each of these four elements as individually problematic. At the same time, he suggests that managed care is not inherently unethical—although he says this in contexts in which he seems to equate managed care with an organization that is "properly organized around providing quality and a more equitable distribution of care."[24] It is not clear whether Pellegrino thinks the four characteristics listed above are necessary for accomplishing this quality and access. In places, however, he implies that they are not necessary and that the socially oriented goals are directly advanced by pursuing the ideals of a scientifically based, individually oriented medicine. Although he recognizes that the "everything for every patient" mentality is no longer appropriate, he still insists that "[t]he physician's prime obligation is as his patient's advocate. . . . A distant threat to the economic well-being of society cannot compete morally with the immediate and urgent need of the patient."[25] The individual patient focus is the basis for his rejection of MCOs.

Pellegrino distinguishes between a macro-ethic that focuses on broader social and economic concerns and a micro-ethic that focuses on the physician-patient relationship.[26] He points to possible areas of equilibrium between the two, arguing that many things that make for good medicine simultaneously advance the social good. For example, there is a need for good clinical trials and the development of clinical skills such as history taking, which will lead to lower utilization rates and thus save costs.[27]

Ultimately, however, Pellegrino clearly sides with the priority of the physician-patient relationship; in the discussion of managed care, he uses the classical micro-ethic to argue against the introduction of social concerns that would be advanced by a particular organization. He insists that if such social concerns are to be advanced, they must be addressed at a truly macro level—by democratic, social deliberation leading to just health policy. Until that process is carried out and other useful means are exhausted (good clinical trials, history taking, etc.), the types of rationing and physician double-agency found in MCOs should be rejected.[28]

Thus, Pellegrino's solution to the problems raised by managed care involves a reaffirmation of the elements of the classical paradigm, with its lexical ordering of scientific foundationalism, individual patient orientation, and presumed harmony of medical and social good. The problems with that paradigm become apparent when we further consider the elements of MCOs that Pellegrino considers problematic.

MCOs focus on patient populations rather than on individuals.[29] Consider, for example, a network of hospitals and physician group practices that accepts financial responsibility for a large population in a metropolitan area. The functions of insurer and provider are combined, and the network's annual funding consists of the sum of individual insurance premiums. To remain financially viable, the MCO must provide services to the population within the total dollar amount available. (Let us assume that this network is a nonprofit MCO.)

There will be cases in which this population-oriented system comes into conflict with the traditional, individually oriented approach of physicians. Such conflicts will occur when there is a high-cost, low-yield intervention that falls into a gray area regarding its indication (for example, certain uses of bone marrow transplantation).[30] Generally, discussions of such conflicts frame them as a choice between the economic interests of society and the health care need of the individual. The premise is that one clearly knows that a certain procedure is "medically indicated," and now the question is whether that treatment should be provided or rationed. When the key tradeoff is between "a distant threat to the economic well-being of society" and "the immediate and urgent need of the patient," it seems to be most appropriate to address the immediate and urgent need.

This approach to characterizing the conflict is inappropriate, however. The medical humanist should reject this analysis because it requires positivist assumptions about the way medical indication is determined. For the medical positivist, science alone provides a basis for determining what is medically indicated; values enter as a second step, providing a basis for determining whether the medically indicated action is also morally indicated. Further, this analysis assumes that decisions about medical indication can be isolated in an atomistic way from other individual and communal decisions. In Pellegrino's philosophy of medicine, however, clinical judgment is a function of science *and* the needs and values of the patient. One must weigh the values and needs of patients in the determination of medical indication. When this weighing is carried out, a different way of framing the tension between individually oriented and community-based approaches comes into view.

In *Clinical Decision Making*, David Eddy notes that the "public health or societal perspective" and the "patient perspective" can be framed as two different kinds of individual perspectives:

> The two perspectives roughly correspond to the two positions each of us can be in with respect to health care service. We are in one position (the "first position") when we do not yet have a health problem that would need the service and are deciding whether to buy coverage for the service. We are in another position (the "second position") when we have a disease, we know much more about what services we want, and this year's bills have been paid. With admitted simplification, society is people when they are in the first position, whereas patients are people when they are in the second position. The conflict arises because what is best for us when we are in one position is not necessarily best for us when we are in the other position.[31]

For Pellegrino, it is self-evident that the physician must consider the second position alone in health care decision making and that any patient who binds himself or herself to the first position is simply unwise. Thus, the callousness of the MCO is evident in the attitude that "if a patient at a young age opts unwisely for a cheaper plan with fewer or inappropriate benefits, that's just too bad."[32]

There are reasons, however, why an older, wise person may also want to opt into a plan that covers only what a person regards as indicated from the first position.[33] Moreover, there are prudential and moral reasons for saying that a person should opt into such a plan. Although I do not elaborate on these reasons here, it is worthwhile to note that if an individual has values that support a benefits package that is tied to the first position, the clinical determination of what is medically indicated should take these values into account. MCOs can be viewed simply as an organizational embodiment of such values regarding the determination of medical indication.

From this perspective, the deeper tension between community-oriented and individually oriented systems is not *whether* medically indicated services are provided. The issue is *how* medical indication is determined. Critics of MCOs tend to view individual patients in terms of their needs while ill—severing their values from the broader framework of their lives and alleviating them of any responsibility to the community. This criticism severs patient autonomy (with the individually relative specification of values) from responsibility (with accountability for previous choices and accepted constraints).[34] That atomistic approach to patients actually is a form of disrespect because it fails to treat them as moral agents.

Even if one focuses only on the patient's perspective when ill (the second position), there are still good reasons why a patient may opt into a system that allows for constraints on physician authority and involves organizational incentives that lead to alternative configurations of medical indication. Because patient need is broader than the cure of organic dysfunction, and there are many other professionals that contribute to addressing the patient's disrupted life-world, there may be times when physician activities and interests need to be subordinated to those of other professionals (e.g., when nursing takes priority, and physicians should be subordinate). Physicians are accustomed to being the "captain of the ship," however, and they may not be willing to take a subordinate position. Problems can emerge when physicians use their authority to resist reasonable limits on their role. Although such an imposition of medical values at the expense of patient's own values is hard to identify in particular cases, it is not rare. The comprehensive disregard within medicine for patient values and preferences is well documented by the SUPPORT study.[35] It may thus be reasonable to have administrative and organizational incentives that respond to the medical propensity to aggressively intervene.

Bioethicists have proposed informed consent and advance directives as means of navigating plural values and protecting patient choice. Such mechanisms, however, have very limited influence. They are insufficient as a guard against physician paternalism and the legislation of medical reality. Physicians control the way information is provided, and patients often passively acquiesce to recommended treatments. Furthermore, because values go to the root of health care decisions, physicians' own values unavoidably play a role in the determination of medical decisions. A recognition of this fact has recently lead Robert Veatch to argue against informed consent as it is currently practiced and to claim that patients should opt into health care institutions that reflect their values.[36]

Thus, it may be quite reasonable for patients to opt into organizational systems that limit physician authority and use incentive structures and policies (including guidelines, profiling, clinical pathways, and so forth) to influence their practice. Such limits on medicine do not necessarily imply limits on care. Instead, they involve configurations of care that acknowledge nonmedical components that are responsive to patient well-being. Considerations of the incentives in MCOs should not focus solely on how they motivate limits. One should also evaluate how they alter care and weigh benefits and deficits in a realistic manner. In the aforementioned hypothetical MCO, with its combination of insurer and provider responsibilities, there are incentives to decrease the utilization of high-cost, low-yield medical services. When that MCO is compared to alternative fee-for-service arrangements, there are also incentives to increase certain services. For example, there are incentives to provide patient education, which empowers patients to manage their own care and keeps them out of the physician's office. There also are incentives to develop outcomes information; to integrate and coordinate care; and to advance services such as nursing and pastoral care, which are known to have a positive influence on patient satisfaction rates. Not coincidentally, there has been an explosion in research on these kinds of activities just as MCOs have begun to play a prominent role in health care.

When MCO incentives are considered in the medical literature, they are almost always assessed in terms of their potential influence on a particular decision at a given moment—for example, whether a physician has a disincentive to provide a marginally indicated test.[37] This analysis misses the whole point of MCOs because it evaluates them from the perspective of a fee-for-service system. To properly consider MCO incentive structures, one must evaluate them as a whole and consider how they shift care away from the intervention, acute care, atomistic approach. In MCOs, "medically indicated" is a function of a comprehensive, coordinated kind of medicine.

The aforementioned modifications in the determination of "medically indicated" were not called for merely by the social good. They were motivated by a more nuanced account of what it means to address individual patient values; those values have a social dimension, and they involve an account of "best interest" that is more comprehensive than the organic function addressed in medicine's cure orientation. As these implications have been developed, however, it becomes increasingly clear that the elements of the classical paradigm, with their lexical ordering, are problematic and that communal ends cannot be excluded. The classical paradigm can probably be sustained only under the conditions of medical positivism. By working out the implications of Pellegrino's philosophy of medicine, we have found that there must be an evolution of the framework of analysis such that the communal context increasingly comes into view. MCOs can be regarded as the material embodiment of this recognition.

When we look at the way health care is practiced today, we find additional warrant for a radical reassessment of the classical paradigm. Health care is no longer practiced by individual physicians situated within a dyadic physician-patient relation. It involves teams comprising many professions, it is practiced by institutions as well as individuals, and it is individually and population-oriented. This reality was not brought about by MCOs; it is the result of the scientific development of health care. MCOs simply make this altered reality of health care practice explicit. Thus, the question is not whether we will have MCOs but what form they will take and how they should be configured. These developments demand a shift from traditional clinical ethics to an organizational ethic that is responsive to the new roles and responsibilities of institutions and teams.

Organizational ethics has recently emerged as an important area in bioethics, largely motivated by concerns about the role of business and market influences on health care. The literature on this topic is heavily influenced by business ethics.[38] One often finds the assumption that an organizational ethic *qua* business ethic is separable from traditional clinical ethics because the former is concerned with administrative and bureaucratic matters, whereas the latter is concerned with patient care. Thus, these forms of ethics are aligned with macro- and micro-ethics, respectively. Although Pellegrino's criticisms of managed care and the market fit with this approach, his medical humanism and philosophy of organizations point toward a much richer basis for organizational ethics—one that has remained largely undeveloped in the literature.

Before the topic of organizational ethics exploded on the scene, Pellegrino anticipated the major issues,[39] edited a journal issue on the topic,[40] and (with David Thomasma) published an important essay that provides theoretical foundations for such an ethic.[41] In this work, Pellegrino notes that health care is no longer just practiced by individuals; it is now practiced by interdisciplinary teams and by institutions. There are multiple, complex interprofessional relations between physician generalists and specialists, nurses and pharmacists, administrators and the host of technicians and technology that are required for modern medicine's practice. In this context, difficult questions arise about conflicting roles, interprofessional obligations, and responsibility to the "team" as well as the broader community.

Pellegrino's criticisms of MCOs assume that dual obligations—for example, to the patient and to the organization—are self-evidently problematic.[42] In his discussion of the current reality of health care, however, he sees such "dual agency" (with its dual obligation) as an inevitable consequence of the way medicine is now practiced.[43] Pellegrino recognizes that health care is practiced by a team that is "held together by a common purpose"—a purpose that is not separable from the goal of the organization.[44] Furthermore, he sees that "today an increasing number of patients now enter the same relationships with a hospital which formerly was obtained solely with physicians."[45]

When Pellegrino describes the altered reality of health care, he appreciates the depth of the challenge to traditional ideals and the need for a complete, foundational reassessment of the classical paradigm. In accord with the broader criticism of medical positivism, he insists that such a rethinking must involve a critical philosophy of medicine in which normative issues are addressed, as well as an account of the conditions of health care practice itself. This approach provides an important alternative to the kind of separation of business and clinical ethics that informs current approaches to organizational ethics (and informs Pellegrino's criticisms of managed care)—a separation that can be regarded as the organizational form of the medical positivist's assumption regarding the separability of science and values. Already in 1981, Pellegrino set forth such a foundational reassessment as urgent:

> The era in which the ethics of all the health professions could be conceived only in terms of individual transactions with individual patients is over. Dyadic moral obligations are as important as ever, but now they take place within institutional and collective contexts. The attribution of responsibility, the resolution between conflicts of obligations to patients and obligations to the collectivity, and the exercise of moral agency are therefore subjects of urgent importance for society and the health professions.[46]

Unfortunately, when Pellegrino considers MCOs and discusses the relationship between medicine and economics, he simply assumes that physicians *and institutions* have as their primary focus the individual patient.[47] He reasserts the elements of the classical paradigm, with their lexical priority.

The challenge posed by Pellegrino and Thomasma in their work on institutional ethics is formidable. They bring us a good part of the way, but they hover between the old and new paradigms. This hesitation is understandable. Not only does the new health care context call for a thorough reassessment of the core elements of the medical paradigm, it also calls for a kind of social and ethical theory that moves beyond the traditional contrast between micro- and macro-ethics. Such a theory must provide an alternative to the oppositions between market and government and between liberal and communitarian approaches to the problem of pluralism.[48] A genuine organizational ethic cannot be formulated merely as a concatenation of the individual-individual relationships that are the focus of micro-ethics. Nor can it simply be nested in a social ethic that focuses on governmental policy. A genuine third way is needed: an inter-ethic for middle-level institutions.[49]

Ultimately, Pellegrino's use of the micro-ethical versus macro-ethical distinction—more than any other factor—probably motivated his negative appraisal of MCOs.[50] Pellegrino speaks of the balancing of individual and communal ends in MCOs as if they were merely a balance between the economic interests of society and individual patient need. He then states that the social balancing issues should be resolved at the policy level through democratic deliberation. By moving to the government level, Pellegrino missed the opportunity to develop an alternative to the contrast between micro and macro levels of analysis.

To appreciate the challenge and opportunity afforded by managed care, the link between the micro-ethical and macro-ethical forms of the problem of pluralism must be acknowledged. At the micro-ethical level, the problem of pluralism is manifest as a concern with negotiating different values of physician and patient. In the United States, a classically liberal solution has been advanced. Through informed consent, the patient is supposedly empowered to obtain only those forms of care that advance his or her account of best interest. In practice, however, this solution has been inadequate because it fails to appreciate how physicians and institutions configure the way patient decisions can be made—for example, how "medical indication" is unavoidably a function of the values of persons other than the patient. People are not isolated islands, and any realistic approach to health care decision making must address the communal context that conditions choice.

At the macro-ethical level, the problem of pluralism is manifest in several forms—for example, in the problem of determining the basic benefits package for health care. At this level, there has been significant tension between liberal and communitarian solutions. Pellegrino advances a universal health system with a democratically determined basic benefits package. In countries that have such systems (e.g., Canada or Great Britain), however, hospitals have incentives that are similar to those in our MCOs. In fact, if one were to compare the services in the worst MCO in the United States with those found in national systems with global budgeting, the MCO would have a more generous level of benefits. Why is the MCO inappropriate but the system of global budgeting legitimate?

One cannot simply point to access because one could address access issues independently of how the services are provided and regard the development of MCOs in the United States as a decentralized way of initiating the kinds of balancing needed in any system of universal access. The key question in comparing the two systems is: Would it be better to have a centralized or decentralized system of configuring health benefits?

The most significant problem with a universal system is that it configures benefits according to the values of the majority and takes undue regard for the values of the individuals in the system. In such a system, individuals are supposed to make values decisions in the context of the physician-patient relationship. This process depends on informed consent as a means for navigating differences, however; for reasons already discussed, such means are unrealistic. The problem is that one cannot neatly divide the health care world into individual and social components. Middle-level institutions configure the most important decisions.

MCOs offer an alternative to this classical impasse between individualist and socialist options. They configure an integration of individual and communal values that involves a particular determination of "medical indication." As patients come to be informed about the way MCOs offer services, however, they can opt into organizational structures that reflect their own values.[51] By fostering a pluralistic, decentralized approach to the way individual and community are integrated, MCOs allow for the full range of choices needed to respect cultural and religious differences in our society.

Interestingly, Pellegrino recognizes the need for this pluralism:

> Moral pluralism is a fixture in our society. . . . [W]e can expect that patients will choose physicians and health-care institutions on the basis of their moral commitments as much as their technical capabilities.[52]

Yet Pellegrino considers such decisions as if they primarily regard whether an institution offers services such as abortion or euthanasia. He does not sufficiently consider how such value decisions should go all the way to the root, addressing every aspect of medicine and health care.

MCOs provide a first step toward a genuine alternative to the individualism and fragmentation in our society. At this stage, of course, they are in a very immature form. The next phase in their development must involve sustained reflection and concrete practices that make explicit how organizational values configure care. This judgment must be disclosed to those who are insured within a given network, so that they have the knowledge and ability to select among available options and work toward establishing systems that reflect their own values.

We must develop an inter-ethic and philosophy of health care so that conceptual and normative guidance can be provided for the realization of this emergent opportunity. To do so, however, we must move beyond criticisms of MCOs that are rooted in the traditional paradigm of medicine and the long-standing impasse between macro- and micro-ethics. We must thoroughly reappraise the roles and responsibilities of everyone involved in health care. Pellegrino leads us to the threshold of that reappraisal. Now we must take the next step.

NOTES

1. Ludwik Fleck, *Genesis and Development of a Scientific Fact* (Chicago: University of Chicago Press, 1979).
2. Thomas Kuhn, *The Structure of Scientific Revolutions,* 3rd ed. (Chicago: University of Chicago Press, 1996).
3. David Thomasma, "Antifoundationalism and the Possibility of a Moral Philosophy of Medicine," in *The Influence of Edmund Pellegrino's Philosophy of Medicine* (Dordrecht, The Netherlands: Kluwer Academic Publishers, 1997), 127–43.
4. On the Cartesian influence, see Drew Leder, "A Tale of Two Bodies: The Cartesian Corpse and the Lived Body," in *The Body in Medical Thought and Practice* (Dordrecht, The Netherlands: Kluwer Academic Publishers, 1992), 17–35. The positivist influence is complex. Historically, medicine informed Auguste Compte's thought, which in turn informed prominent thinkers in the logical positivist tradition; see Georges Canguilhem, *The Normal and the Pathological* (New York: Zone Books, 1991) for the influence of medicine on Compte. Thus, medical positivism is in some ways prior to the

logical positivist movement and finds in that movement a conceptually refined account of the premises that were associated with the emergence of modern medicine.

5. The elements of scientific foundationalism may best be seen in Abraham Flexner, *Medical Education in the United States and Canada* (New York: Carnegie Foundation for the Advancement of Teaching, 1910).

6. On the "positivist bias" of medicine, see Edmund Pellegrino and David Thomasma, *A Philosophical Basis of Medical Practice* (Oxford: Oxford University Press, 1981), 17.

7. This theme is consistently re-emphasized in Pellegrino's writings. For an early example, see Edmund Pellegrino, "What Makes a Hospital Catholic?" *Hospital Progress* (1966): 67–70.

8. Edmund Pellegrino, "Clinical Judgment, Scientific Data, and Ethics: Antidepressant Therapy in Adolescents and Children," *Journal of Nervous and Mental Disease* 184, no. 2 (1996): 107.

9. Edmund Pellegrino, "The Autopsy: Some Ethical Reflections on the Obligations of Pathologists, Hospitals, Family and Society," *Archives of Pathology and Laboratory Medicine* 120 (August 1996): 730.

10. On the link between the organic notion of disease and the clinico-pathological dialectic of the Paris School, see George Khushf, "Why Bioethics Needs the Philosophy of Medicine: Some Implications of Reflection on Concepts of Health and Disease," *Theoretical Medicine* 18, nos. 1–2 (1997): 145–63.

11. Pellegrino and Thomasma, *A Philosophical Basis of Medical Practice*, chapter 6.

12. Jerome Kassirer, "Managing Care—Should We Adopt a New Ethic?" *New England Journal of Medicine* 339, no. 6 (1998): 397–98.

13. Pellegrino and Thomasma, *A Philosophical Basis of Medical Practice*, 110.

14. Stephen Wear, *Informed Consent* (Dordrecht, The Netherlands: Kluwer Academic Publishers, 1993).

15. These themes pervade nearly all of Pellegrino's writings. For a representative essay, see Edmund Pellegrino, "The Ethics of Medicine: The Challenges of Reconstruction," *Transactions and Studies of the College of Physicians of Philadelphia* ser. 5, vol. 9, no. 3 (1987): 179–91.

16. Pellegrino and Thomasma, *A Philosophical Basis of Medical Practice*, 76; see also pp. 49, 55.

17. Ibid., 73, 77–81; chapter 11.

18. For a more detailed discussion of this assumption, see George Khushf, "A Radical Rupture in the Paradigm of Modern Medicine," *Journal of Medicine and Philosophy* 23, no. 1 (1998): 98–122.

19. Edmund Pellegrino, "Managed Care: An Ethical Reflection," *Christian Century* (August 12–19, 1998): 748–51; Pellegrino and Thomasma, *A Philosophical Basis of Medical Practice*, chapters 10 and 12.

20. Edmund Pellegrino, "Medical Economics and Medical Ethics: Points of Conflict and Reconciliation," *Journal of the Medical Association of Georgia* 69 (March 1980): 174–83.

21. Pellegrino, "Managed Care: An Ethical Reflection," 749; Pellegrino and Thomasma, *A Philosophical Basis of Medical Practice*, chapter 7.

22. Pellegrino, "Managed Care: An Ethical Reflection," 748; Edmund Pellegrino, "Words Can Hurt You: Some Reflections on the Metaphors of Managed Care," *Journal of the American Board of Family Practice* 7, no. 6 (November-December 1994): 505–10.

23. Ibid.

24. Pellegrino, "Managed Care: An Ethical Reflection," 751.

25. Pellegrino, "Medical Economics and Medical Ethics," 176.

26. Ibid., 175.
27. Ibid., 180–83.
28. Ibid., 183.
29. Mark Hall and Robert Berenson, "Ethical Practice in Managed Care: A Dose of Realism," *Annals of Internal Medicine* 128 (1998): 395–402.
30. Norman Daniels and James Sabin, "Last Chance Therapies and Managed Care: Pluralism, Fair Procedures, and Legitimacy," *Hastings Center Report* (March-April 1998): 27–41.
31. David Eddy, *Clinical Decision Making: From Theory to Practice* (Sudbury, Mass.: Jones and Bartlett, 1996), 112.
32. Pellegrino, "Managed Care: An Ethical Reflection," 748.
33. Mark Hall, "Physician Rationing and Agency Cost Theory," in *Conflicts of Interest in Clinical Practice and Research,* ed. Roy Spece, David Shimm, and Allen Buchanan (Oxford: Oxford University Press, 1996), 228–50.
34. E. Haavi Morreim, *Balancing Act: The New Medical Ethics of Medicine's New Economics* (Washington, D.C.: Georgetown University Press, 1995).
35. "A Controlled Trial to Improve Care for Seriously Ill Hospitalized Patients," *Journal of the American Medical Association* 274, no. 20 (November 22–29, 1995): 1591–98.
36. Robert Veatch, "Abandoning Informed Consent," *Hastings Center Report* 25, no. 2 (1995): 5–12.
37. For a review of this medical literature, see George Khushf and Robert Gifford, "Understanding, Assessing, and Managing Conflicts of Interest," in *Surgical Ethics,* ed. Laurence McCullough, James Jones, and Baruch Brody (Oxford: Oxford University Press, 1998), 342–66.
38. George Khushf, "The Scope of Organizational Ethics," *HEC Forum* 10, no. 2 (June 1998): 127–35.
39. Pellegrino, "What Makes a Hospital Catholic?"
40. *Journal of Medicine and Philosophy* 7, no. 1 (1982), which was devoted to organizational ethics.
41. Pellegrino and Thomasma, *A Philosophical Basis of Medical Practice,* chapter 11.
42. Pellegrino, "Managed Care: An Ethical Reflection," 748.
43. Pellegrino, "The Ethics of Collective Judgments in Medicine and Health Care."
44. Pellegrino and Thomasma, *A Philosophical Basis of Medical Practice,* 256.
45. Ibid., 251, 252.
46. Pellegrino, "The Ethics of Collective Judgments in Medicine and Health Care," 8.
47. Pellegrino and Thomasma, *A Philosophical Basis of Medical Practice,* 269.
48. George Khushf, "Solidarity as a Moral and Political Concept: Beyond the Liberal/Communitarian Impasse," in *Solidarity,* ed. Kurt Bayertz (Dordrecht, The Netherlands: Kluwer Academic Publishers, 1999), 57–79.
49. Dennis Thompson, "Hospital Ethics," *Cambridge Quarterly of Healthcare Ethics* 3 (1992): 203–10; George Khushf, "Administrative and Organizational Ethics," *HEC Forum* 9, no. 4 (1997): 299–309.
50. Pellegrino uses this distinction in several contexts to set up his discussion of medicine and economics; see, e.g., Pellegrino, "Medical Economics and Medical Ethics," 175.
51. Veatch, "Abandoning Informed Consent."
52. Pellegrino, "The Ethics of Medicine: The Challenges of Reconstruction," 187.

PART III

Current Challenges

Reproductive Technologies: Where Are We Headed?

Richard A. McCormick, S.J.

The birth of Louise Brown on July 25, 1978, in Oldham, England, was greeted with enormous fanfare. She was the first baby born from *in vitro* fertilization (IVF) and embryo transfer (ET), the crowning work of the late Patrick Steptoe and Robert Edwards. The fanfare included questions, accusations, expressions of fears and doubts, warnings, hopes, and joyful congratulations (including that of Pope John Paul I)—in short, just about every human reaction that greets a medical breakthrough that touches human life. People wondered whether Louise would suffer the effects of being a medical freak. They expressed misgivings about the embryos lost in the procedure, the safety of IVF, the future use of the technology.

Since that time, tens of thousands of babies have been born by IVF, and many of the early Frankenstein-factor questions have dissolved into unconcern. Physicians entered further into the goals of families and societies. Not all ethical concerns have been put to rest, however. The contemporary overemphasis on autonomy tends to trump and absorb all other considerations and leaves the impression that the disappearance of a question is equivalent to its satisfactory resolution. Our moral health depends on our ability to resist such facile and deceptive moves.

The title of this essay—"Where Are We Headed?"—is misleading. I am a moral theologian, not a bioethical prognosticator. Clearly the thrust of this essay is "Where *Should* We—and Where Should We Not—Be Headed?" My interest is the underlying ethical and value considerations that are at play in our deliberations about how we should use the technologies we currently possess.

This interest is intensified by the fact that the reproductive technology industry is completely unregulated at present. True, we do have the American Society for Reproductive Medicine's (ASRM) *Ethical Considerations of Assisted Reproductive Technologies.*[1] These directives have no legal clout, however; compliance is voluntary.

We must continue to press the ethical questions that are inseparable from reproductive technologies. There are many ways of doing so. My reflections are organized under five headings that cover some (not all) of the major ethical concerns about reproductive technologies: anthropology; the status of the preembryo; heterologous procedures; homologous artificial insemination and IVF; and the role of law in regulating reproductive technologies.

165

These five categories are based on the Roman Catholic *Instruction on Respect for Human Life in its Origin and on the Dignity of Procreation* (hereafter *Donum Vitae*) of the Congregation for the Doctrine of the Faith.[2] *Donum Vitae* was dated February 22, 1987, but released somewhat later.

I do not use *Donum Vitae* as a reference point as an external, token bow to an official Catholic authority. The issues are broader than those posed by a particular religion. I consider *Donum Vitae* a guiding word, from a respected authority, on a runaway technology that touches basic human values. I also fully acknowledge the theologian's responsibility to disagree when disagreement is warranted. Indeed, I regard such disagreement as an expression of the *obsequium animi religiosum* expected of loyal Catholics.

With regard to the basic values at stake, columnist Charles Krauthammer refers to synthetic children, synthetic families, and synthetic sex. Krauthammer notes:

> Each has a different moral valence and should elicit a different moral response from the state. The first, fetal manipulation and experimentation, is a threat to human dignity. The second, third-party donation of gametes (egg or sperm), is a threat to the family. The third, artificial insemination or in vitro fertilization that enables marriage partners to have their own children, is a threat to sexuality.[3]

ANTHROPOLOGY

Donum Vitae begins by stating a general criterion for the use of science and technology: the integral good of the human person. This criterion is repeated in several different ways to contrast it with a merely technical criterion (efficiency) for the use of technology.

This criterion reflects the approach taken by the Second Vatican Council (Vatican II). The Council stated that the "moral aspect of any procedure . . . must be determined by objective standards which are based on the nature of the person and the person's acts."[4] The official commentary on this wording noted two aspects of the wording: This expression formulates a general principle that applies to all human actions, not just marriage and sexuality. Moreover, the choice of this expression means that "human activity must be judged insofar as it refers to the human person integrally and adequately considered" *(personam humanam integre et adequate considerandam)*.[5]

This criterion is extremely important for any moral methodology. I leave it to others how to flesh out this criterion.[6] I do want to underline, however, its difference from a criterion previously used: the finality of the faculty. For example, the purpose of speech was said to be the communication of true information. If one used speech to communicate false information, it was an abuse—that is, morally wrong. Similarly, human sexual expression was said to be ordained to procreation. Artificially impeding this purpose was judged morally wrong.

A good example of this "Roman approach" was the thinking of Franciscus Hürth. Hürth argued that "the intention of nature was inscribed in the organs and their function." He put strong emphasis on biological finality ("une téléologie presque incroyable"). Hürth wrote, "Man only has disposal of the use of his organs and his faculties with respect to the end which the Creator, in His formation of them, has intended. This end for man, then, is both the biological law and the moral law, such that the latter obliges him to live according to the biological law."[7]

Many contemporary theologians have moved away from this approach, regarding it as naturalistic fallacy. For example, Franz Scholz notes, "These natural ends are not the last word. They stand under the judgment of reason, as Thomas [Aquinas] clearly emphasized."[8] Similarly, Brendan Soane states, "Theologians seem to be generally agreed that the French hierarchy was right [in its commentary on *Humanae Vitae*] when it taught that the integrity of the marriage act is one value which can be balanced by others when couples decide what they should do."[9] John Wright rejected approaches that "suppose a kind of sacred structure to the physical act itself, a divine purpose in this particular activity that renders any attempt to control or interfere with it immoral." Wright rejected this approach because "immediate finality is always subordinate to the total finality of a reasonable human life."[10]

I emphasize the criterion "the person integrally and adequately considered" because in the clinical setting it is so easy to contract it into a narrower focus. I have heard clinicians say, "My responsibility is to give this couple a baby." Not so. Such a statement collapses every consideration into a single rubric—as does the finality approach. For this reason, I am happy to take responsibility for writing "The Basis for Evaluation of an Ethical Position" (chapter 1 of the ASRM's *Ethical Considerations of Assisted Reproductive Technologies*). A key section of this chapter reads as follows:

> Several things should be noted about this criterion. In principle, it calls for an inductive approach based on experience and reflection. In addition, there are some things that we have already learned and generally accepted from experience (e.g., that violence begets violence). Furthermore, there are other things that so offend an inner sense of what is held to be proper or sacred that no experience is necessary to expose their moral character (e.g., the Nazi medical experiments). These only underline the principle: that to judge the moral character behind many human actions, experience of their comprehensive impact on persons is essential. Still further, some actions remain ambiguous because they involve both beneficial and detrimental aspects, because their impact on persons is unknown, or because they are variously evaluated. For example, some persons will see benefit to a single person or couple as dominant; others will view potential risks to society as a whole as taking precedence over individual benefits. Such moral ambiguity and pluralism calls for openness, caution, and a willingness to revise evaluations. This attitude has proved especially important with medical technology, in general, and with novel patterns of reproduction, in particular. The personal criterion used here requires the basic willingness to say "no" where we have said "yes" and "yes" where we have said "no." Finally, in applying the personal criterion, one must take into account that the human person is both individual and social. Hence, what is promotive or detrimental to the person cannot be assessed solely in terms of individual impact but must take into account overall social impact as well. Because the assessment of what is promotive or detrimental to the person, integrally and adequately considered, is a broad one, it must be recognized that a moral "yes" or "no" is not always an absolute. Such a judgment may represent only a pause on a path toward a consensus that has not yet been clearly spelled out. In this report we seek to move toward such a consensus.[11]

THE STATUS OF THE PREEMBRYO

It is safe to say that this single consideration—the status of the preembryo—lies at the heart of nearly every protocol for reproductive technologies. It touches issues relating to surplus preembryos (their freezing and/or discarding); experimentation on the preembryo (and especially creation of preembryos for this purpose—whether the ultimate purpose is improved IVF or knowledge about the partitioning of pre-stem cells); and pre-implantation diagnosis for conditions such as Tay-Sachs disease, Huntington's disease, and others. The late Joyce Poole was certainly correct when she wrote that "the question that lies at the heart of all such ethical debate [about reproductive technology] concerns the moral status of any potential human being at any given point in its journey from unfertilized gametes to new-born child."[12]

The position of *Donum Vitae* is quite clear. From the moment the zygote has formed, it deserves "unconditional respect." The human being is to be "treated as a person from the moment of conception." Its "rights as a person must be recognized." *Donum Vitae* asks: "How could a human individual not be a human person?"[13]

Thus, the Congregation for the Doctrine of the Faith—without committing itself to an "affirmation of a philosophical nature"—for all practical purposes insists that germinating life at even the earliest stage must be treated as personal life, with all the rights accorded to persons. This position reflects the strong position of Pope John Paul II in his address to a meeting of the Pontifical Academy of Sciences: "I condemn, in the most explicit and formal way, experimental manipulations of the human embryo, since the human being, from conception to death, cannot be exploited for any purpose whatsoever."[14]

Three moral positions have emerged on the status of the preembryo. The first position is that the preembryo is for all practical purposes a person. The second is the polar opposite of the first—denying personhood to the preembryo and arguing that it may be used for scientific and therapeutic purposes across a range of protocols. We accord the preembryo the respect it deserves by recruiting it for human purposes. The third position insists that the preembryo deserves great respect, but not the same respect we give human persons. This third position remains open and flexible—some commentators would say *fuzzy*—about what constraints and safeguards this respect calls for.

This third position is the most widely held. The ASRM adopted this position in the 1994 edition of its *Ethical Considerations*:

> The preembryo is due greater respect than other human tissue because of its potential to become a person and because of its symbolic meaning for many people. Yet, it should not be treated as a person, because it has not yet developed the features of personhood, is not yet established as developmentally individual, and may never realize its biological potential.[15]

The status of the preembryo has been the subject of an ongoing contemporary debate.[16] I do not detail the issues here except to note that they center around *developmental individuality*. The phenomena that give rise to this concern are the totipotentiality of the preembryo, twinning, recombination, and the huge spontaneous loss of preembryonic life. Persons who are impressed by these phenomena believe that they point to a lack of developmental individuality at this state, a feature essential to personhood. (Here we must recall that personhood is an ascription—not, like ensoulment, a fact. Thus, it is legitimate to ask: When *should* we ascribe personhood to the developing organism, and in light of what considerations?)

I have favored the position that the preembryo is not yet a person but should be treated as one. This treatment of the embryo as a person should be a strong *prima facie* obligation, but it could admit of exceptions.[17] Not everyone will find this position satisfying. Those with research interests will find it too constraining; those who view the preembryo as a person will judge it too permissive.

Why not, with *Donum Vitae*, afford "unconditional respect" from the very beginning? Krauthammer answers: "Because most people reject the notion that personhood begins at conception. If drawing lines against fetal abuse is the object, drawing them at a place where they will not be accepted is not prudent."[18] I agree.

HETEROLOGOUS PROCEDURES

Under the rubric of "heterologous procedures," several different procedures are possible: donated sperm, donated ovum, donated embryo, donated uterus, or combinations of these activities. Most discussions have centered around the use of donated sperm (artificial insemination donor, or AID) because this procedure is by far the most common; therefore, I use it to review some of the issues involved in third-party participation in reproductive technologies.

The most thoughtful and stimulating study on AID is that of Paul Lauritzen.[19] Lauritzen examines some contemporary works on AID. One is by Lisa Sowle Cahill.[20] Cahill rejects third-party participation in reproductive technologies because they separate genetic and social parenthood. There are moral responsibilities that are directly contingent on genetic connection. These responsibilities are inalienable and cannot be completely transferred to others. In Lauritzen's words:

> Thus it could never be morally acceptable to create a child with the intention of separating genetic and social parenthood, for to do so would require an individual to create a set of moral obligations he or she had no intention of discharging.[21]

For Cahill, the responsibilities of parenthood do not root entirely in human choice. They root also in biological (genetic) connections. For this reason, "biological relationships can and should exercise some constraints upon freedom to choose (or not to choose) the parental relation." For Cahill, biological restraints restrict the freedom to choose AID and surrogate motherhood.

Lauritzen criticizes this view on the ground that it assumes that separating genetic and social parenthood abandons *all* constraints on reproductive choice:

> Yet in disagreeing with Cahill about the normative ideal, I am not abandoning all restraints on reproductive choice. Rather I am simply drawing the line of acceptable choice at a different place.[22]

Lauritzen's fine study does not clarify where he is drawing the line and, above all, why. The major ethical obstacles he sees to the responsibility of parenthood in AID are secrecy (deception at the heart of the parent-child relationship) and the problem of asymmetry. With regard to secrecy, Lauritzen cites the work of Baran and Pannor:

> For most of the men we interviewed, the choice of donor insemination had been an acute response to the pain they were experiencing. They never permitted themselves the time and opportunity to explore their feelings about the devastating ego blow. They prevented themselves from becoming comfortable with and accepting of their handicap. Instead, they cast the handicap in concrete, and their feelings of inadequacy were continuously reinforced by visual proof: their donor offspring.
>
> With this enormous deficit in place, the relationship between the husband and wife had to be realigned. The husband became weaker and more passive; the wife became stronger and more powerful. The wife was the real mother of the children, and this message, although never spoken, was clearly given to the husband in many ways. The husband could be devoted and caring toward the children, while, at the same time, recognizing the difference between his parental role and his wife's.[23]

Lauritzen seems to treat this scenario as a problem of secrecy; therefore, one could disperse the problem by candid revelation and discussion. Many people will see this situation, however, as an intrinsic problem that is inseparable from AID itself, regardless of whether secrecy obtains. Whatever the case, if secrecy and asymmetry are the two obstacles to responsible parenthood in using AID, and if both can be overcome, it is not clear where and why Lauritzen would "draw the line of acceptable choice."

This exchange between Cahill (emphasizing the basic importance of genetic connections) and Lauritzen (emphasizing the superior importance of the parenting function) is a kind of symbol of the way the ethical discussion is conducted. For instance, *Donum Vitae* regards the use of third-party gametes as "a violation of the reciprocal commitment of the spouses and a grave lack in regard to that essential property of marriage which is its unity."[24]

How is this unity to be understood? There are at least two possibilities. The first is nonconsequentialist at root. It appeals to the nature of marriage—at least, that is how I read *Donum Vitae's* presentation of the argument. After noting that the child must be the fruit and sign of the mutual self-giving of the spouses, of their love and fidelity, *Donum Vitae* states: "The fidelity of the spouses in the unity of marriage involves reciprocal respect of their right to become a father and a mother only through each other."[25] A certain notion of marriage as exclusive at all levels seems to undergird this statement, though I admit that if one pushes hard enough (e.g., "Why must unity be so understood?") one gets to consequentialist considerations.

The second possibility is posed by Lauritzen. AID introduces life experiences that cannot be fully shared, and "this lack of mutuality may interfere with the couple's ability to care for and to love the child that is created." Is this disunity an overwhelming obstacle? Lauritzen thinks not.

There is an additional consideration that is rarely discussed. *Donum Vitae* rejected any reproductive technology that is a substitute for sexual intercourse. My own experience with couples who have undergone IVF and ET is that they do not regard these procedures as a *substitute* for sexual intimacy but as a kind of technological continuation or extension of it. If that is indeed the case, then we must ask: Is it appropriate for third parties to be involved in such continuation?

In summary, there are two key issues on which strong disagreement is likely to continue: Does third-party involvement (via gametic donation or surrogate gestation) infringe on conjugal exclusivity? Does having a jointly raised child justify such infringement? My own answer is yes to the first, no to the second. I hold these positions because I believe that the notion of conjugal exclusivity should include the genetic, gestational, and rearing dimensions of parenthood. Separating these dimensions (except through rescue, as in adoption) too easily contains a subtle diminishment of some aspect of the human person.

One can argue that marital exclusivity ought to include the genetic, gestational, and rearing components in at least two different ways. First, one could argue that third-party involvement in itself violates the marriage covenant independent of any potential damaging effects or benefits. This argument is the thrust of Lisa Cahill's analysis, as well as that of Pope Pius XII. This view might be argued in purely ethical terms (Cahill) or in religious terms. Paul Ramsey supports the latter approach: "To put radically asunder what God joined together in parenthood when He made love procreative, to procreate from beyond the sphere of love . . . or to posit acts of sexual love beyond the sphere of responsible procreation (by definition, marriage) means a refusal of the image of God's creation in our own."[26]

There is a simpler way of making this point. As I noted, many couples regard IVF not as a *replacement* for their sexual intimacy but as a kind of *continuation* or *extension* of it. On that view, third-party presence (via egg or sperm) is presence of another in the intimacy itself—a presence that ought not be. One need not call this process adultery to make the point.

The second form of the argument is that any relaxation in marital exclusivity will be a source of harm to the marriage (and marriage in general) and to the prospective child. For instance, the use of donor semen means that there is a genetic asymmetry in the relationship of husband and wife to the child, with possible damaging psychological effects. If a surrogate mother is involved, conflicts could arise that damage the marriage and the surrogate.

William J. Winslade and Judith Wilson Ross raised some of the questions I have in mind:

> Is the child to know about the method of its birth? If so, how much information should the child have—only that which is deemed to be health-related data, or all of the other biological information about its heritage that most of us value? Whose interests, whose preferences, whose needs count here? Born into a society that is already fragmented by divorce and confused about alternative life styles, morals and sexual choices, the child may well have serious identity problems at a later time. Does such a possibility have to be seriously considered by those who want to undertake unusual reproductive methods? . . .
>
> The interests and well-being of the baby-to-be-made seem to be the last issues considered, and sometimes (when physicians promise anonymity to the donor or parents require it of the surrogate) seem not to be considered at all.[27]

Another form of the first argument is the assertion that third-party involvement separates procreation from marriage *in principle.* That separation opens the door, by human proclivity and by the logic of moral justification, to a litany of worrisome problems such as single-women insemination and insemination of a lesbian couple.

The second argument, which is built on possible harmful consequences, is subject to empirical verification. We must admit in all honesty that the data are thin at best, often even conjectural. Fears of what might happen once marital exclusivity is relaxed are legitimate, even if they do not always lead to clearly established absolute prohibitions. In the past I have argued that the risks and potential harms involved would support a "safe side" moral rule (procreation should be restricted to marriage at all levels—genetic, gestational, social) against the slide to abuse. This prudential calculus gives greater weight to institutional risk of harm than to individual benefit.[28]

In summary, then, I agree with *Donum Vitae* that third parties should be excluded from reproductive procedures for the good of the marriage partners, the prospective child, and marriage itself.

HOMOLOGOUS PROCEDURES

This category comprises all procedures that use the gametes of husband and wife, but without sexual intercourse. In particular, it includes artificial insemination by the husband (AIH), as well as IVF and ET.

Donum Vitae's exposition begins as follows:

The Church's teaching on marriage and human procreation affirms the "inseparable connection, willed by God and unable to be broken by man on his own initiative, between the two meanings of the conjugal act: the unitive meaning and the procreative meaning."[29]

The quotation within this passage is drawn from Pope Paul VI's encyclical letter *Humanae Vitae* regarding birth regulation. *Donum Vitae* refers to this "inseparable connection" as a "principle based on the nature of marriage and the intimate connection of the goods of marriage."[30]

Donum Vitae goes on to note that just as contraception separates the unitive and procreative dimensions, IVF and ET do so in an analogous way. Therefore, procreation by IVF and ET is "deprived of its proper perfection." The instruction sees in such procreation a procedure not "in conformity with the dignity of the person" because it fails to respect the unity (body-soul) of the human being.[31]

A few remarks are in order at this point. First, it is difficult to suppress the impression that on this matter, *Donum Vitae* is much more concerned about contraception than about reproductive technology. I mean, of course, that if the Holy See were to allow IVF and ET, it would be allowing a procedure that provides for a separation of the unitive and the procreative. Thus, it would implicitly be undermining the inseparability principle it appealed to in condemning contraception. Rather than clinching the rejection of IVF and ET, however, this concern only raises the question of the meaning and validity of the inseparability principle, at least as an absolute. In other words, just as the inseparability principle fails to persuade where the rejection of contraception was involved, so too with regard to reproductive technology.

Second, there is the issue of procreation "deprived of its proper perfection." We can admit that IVF procedures are a kind of "second best." They involve certain disvalues (what some contemporary theologians refer to as "premoral evils") that, absent sterility, we would not entertain. Yet a procedure "deprived of its proper perfection" is not necessarily morally wrong in all cases. There are many human actions that we judge morally acceptable even though they involve disvalues.

Third, although the "inseparability principle" embodies a legitimate esthetic or ecological concern, the Congregation has improperly elevated this principle into an absolute *moral* imperative. As I suggested above, this conclusion applies to contraception as well as IVF and ET.

Fourth, what is responsible for this elevation into an absolute moral imperative? In my judgment, it traces back to the early history of theological thought on human sexuality. For centuries, Catholic thought regarded procreation as the *only* legitimate meaning and purpose of sexual intercourse. The contemporary Catholic teaching that every act of intercourse must be open to procreation (thus, no artificial contraception) is a linear descendent from that earlier view—and from the inadequate biology on which it rested.

Fifth, the Congregation correctly notes that "the one conceived must be the fruit of his parents' love."[32] The movement from that general premise to the conclusion that the child must be conceived via sexual intercourse, however, involves a gap in logic that implies that sexual intercourse is the only loving act in marriage.

Sixth, this gap is underlined in the Congregation's attitude toward technology: "The one conceived must be the fruit of his parents' love. He cannot be desired or conceived as the product of an intervention of medical or biological techniques."[33] This is a false opposition. Being a product of a medical intervention is not opposed to being "the fruit of his parents' love." If experience is our guide—and it clearly is not in the Congregation's document—medical interventions to overcome sterility between husband and wife are *precisely* concrete manifestations of their love. Why is IVF not a help to sexual intercourse and *ergo* acceptable on Congregation terms?

In summary, then, I find the Congregation's analysis and reasoning unpersuasive on "the simple case." So do many other commentators. It is understandable, therefore, that several Catholic institutions (in France, Belgium, Holland) indicated that they intend to continue to provide IVF and ET. It is also understandable that individual couples and physicians might draw the same conclusion.

THE ROLE OF LAW IN REPRODUCTIVE TECHNOLOGIES

I can be brief on this subject. The relationship between morality and public policy is difficult and delicate. There are two extremes here. One is that morality and public policy should be identical, especially where basic rights are concerned. Thus, the move from moral conviction to public policy should be simple and smooth. This analysis, however, presupposes the ideal—a situation we do not have. The other extreme is that there is no relation between morality and public policy, as if what promotes the common good (or even, minimally, of public order) has no relation to what is helpful or harmful to persons—in short, to what is morally right or wrong.

Some Vatican documents tilt toward the first extreme. For example, *Evangelium Vitae* takes insufficient account of the complexity of public policy in a pluralistic democracy: "*Donum Vitae* correctly argues that the new technological possibilities . . . require the intervention of the political authorities and of the legislator, since an uncontrolled application of such techniques could lead to unforeseeable and damaging consequences for civil society."[34]

So far, so good. Great caution is required, however, in specifying which penal interventions are warranted. Specifically, *Donum Vitae* asserts that "the child has the right, as already mentioned, to be the fruit of the specific act of the conjugal love of his parents."[35] In short, the child has the right to be conceived *only* by sexual intercourse.

Later on, the instruction states that "the law must provide appropriate penal sanctions for every deliberate violation of the child's rights."[36] In other words, the prohibition of AIH, IVF, and ET (using gametes from husband and wife) should be on the penal code. This form of maximalization of policing power will make it too easy to put aside and disregard the many serious and legitimate moral concerns of *Donum Vitae*.[37]

Ultimately, therefore, I agree with Krauthammer in his appreciative but critical essay: "To avoid the horrors of the new reproductive science, our most important weapon may be nuance."[38]

NOTES

1. American Society of Reproductive Medicine (ASRM), Ethics Committee, *Ethical Considerations of Assisted Reproductive Medicine* (Birmingham, Ala.: American Fertility Society, 1994).
2. Congregation for the Doctrine of the Faith, *Instruction on Respect for Human Life in its Origin and on the Dignity of Procreation* (Vatican City: Vatican Polyglot Press, 1987).
3. Charles Krauthammer, "The Ethics of Human Manufacture," *New Republic*, 4 May 1987, 17–21.
4. "Pastoral Constitution on the Church in the Modern World," in *Documents of Vatican II* (New York: America Press, 1966), n. 51.
5. *Schema Constitutionis pastoralis de ecclesia in mundo huius temporis: Expensio modorum partis secundae* (Vatican City: Vatican Press, 1965), 37–38.
6. See, for example, Louis Janssens, "Artificial Insemination: Ethical Considerations," *Louvain Studies* 8 (1980): 3–29.
7. Franciscus Hürth, "La fécondition artificielle: Sa valeur morale et juridique," *Nouvelle revue théologique* 68 (1946): 413.
8. Franz Scholz, "Innere, aber nicht absolute Abwegigkeit," *Theologie der Gegenwart* 24 (1981): 170.
9. Brendan Soane, *Theological Studies* 43 (1982) 73, n. 13; Brendan Soane, *Clergy Review* 66 (1981): 265.
10. John H. Wright, "An End to the Birth Control Controversy?" *America* 144 (1981): 175–78.
11. ASRM Ethics Committee, *Ethical Considerations,* 15 and 25.
12. Joyce Poole, "Ethical Problems Arising from New Reproductive Techniques," in *Christian Ethics,* ed. Bernard Hoose (London: Wellington House, 1998), 301.
13. Congregation for the Doctrine of the Faith, *Respect for Human Life in its Origin,* 14.
14. *Catholic Standard,* 28 October 1982, 6.

15. ASRM Ethics Committee, *Ethical Considerations,* 335.
16. A good place to start a review of the debate is Lisa Sowle Cahill's report on the literature in "The Embryo and the Fetus: New Moral Contexts," *Theological Studies* 54 (1993): 124–42. After the appearance of Cahill's review article, Thomas R. Kopfensteiner published "The Role of the Sciences in Moral Reasoning," *Science et esprit* 50 (1998): 79–97. Following Klaus Demmer, Kopfensteiner believes the reluctance of theologians such as Thomas Shannon, Allan Wolter, John Mahoney, James Keenan, Lisa Cahill, Karl Rahner, and myself to attribute personhood to the preembryo is traceable to a prescientific notion of substance. Kopfensteiner argues that contemporary science emphasizes unified fields, not separated substances. Thus, substance must be understood in processual terms. "In this way, the personhood of the embryo is not linked to its individuality appearing at any one point . . . of its development" (Kopfensteiner, "The Role of the Sciences in Moral Reasoning, 95).

    Kopfensteiner's contention is built on several assumptions. First, it supposes that individuality (incommunicability) is a prescientific static feature of personhood. On the contrary, I would suggest that it derives from the common-sense conviction that two persons rubbing shoulders on an elevator will never become one person. Second, it assumes that the processual emphases of contemporary scientific theory have produced or can produce an adequate theory of personhood. Both assumptions are open to serious challenge.
17. Richard A. McCormick, "Who or What Is the Preembryo?" *Kennedy Institute of Ethics Journal* 1 (1991): 1–15.
18. Krauthammer, "The Ethics of Human Manufacture," 18.
19. Paul Lauritzen, "Pursuing Parenthood: Reflections on Donor Insemination," *Second Opinion* (July 1990): 57–75.
20. Lisa Sowle Cahill, "The Ethics of Surrogate Motherhood: Biology, Freedom and Moral Obligations," *Law, Medicine and Health Care* 16 (1988): 65–71.
21. Lauritzen, "Pursuing Parenthood," 64.
22. Ibid., 65.
23. Annette Baran and Rubin Pannor, *Lethal Secrets: The Shocking Consequences and Unresolved Problems of Artificial Insemination* (New York: Warner Books, 1989), 51.
24. Congregation for the Doctrine of the Faith, *Respect for Human Life in its Origin,* 24.
25. Ibid., 25.
26. Paul Ramsey, *Fabricated Man: The Ethics of Genetic Control* (New Haven, Conn.: Yale University Press, 1970), 39.
27. William J. Winslade and Judith Wilson Ross, *New York Times,* 21 February 1986, 27.
28. I have argued this way in registering my dissent against the use of third parties. See "Dissent on the use of third parties," in ASRM Ethics Committee, *Ethical Considerations,* Appendix A, 985.
29. Congregation for the Doctrine of the Faith, *Respect for Human Life in its Origin,* 26.
30. Ibid., 27.
31. *Donum Vitae* sees the "deprivation of proper perfection" in the separation of the unitive and procreative aspects of sexual expression. John Finnis regards as a foundational consideration in *Donum Vitae's* rejection of AIH the reduction of the child to the status of object. That may be Finnis's basic consideration, but I think it is secondary and supportive in the Congregation's text. See John Finnis, "The Consistent Ethic—A Philosophical Critique," in *Consistent Ethic of Life,* ed. Thomas G. Fuechtmann (Kansas City, Mo.: Sheed and Ward, 1988), 177, n. 44.

32. Congregation for the Doctrine of the Faith, *Respect for Human Life in its Origin,* 28.
33. Ibid.
34. Ibid., 32.
35. Ibid., 34.
36. Ibid., 35.
37. In this respect, see Leslie Griffin, "*Evangelium Vitae:* The Law on Abortion," in *Readings in Moral Theology No. 10: John Paul II and Moral Theology,* ed. Charles E. Curran and Richard A. McCormick (Mahwah, N.J.: Paulist Press, 1998), 92–108.
38. Krauthammer, "The Ethics of Human Manufacture," 21.

The Search for the Meaning of the Human Body

Judith Lee Kissell

HUMAN NONSUBJECT RESEARCH

Emerging biotechnology is producing a genre of cases that question, in an unprecedented way, the ethical meaning and significance of the human body in the practice of medicine. These cases span clinical practice and research, laboratory experimentation and public policy. Examples include the cultivation of human embryonic stem cells for various research purposes, including the generation of substitute body tissues and organs;[1] the selling of human tissue by not-for-profit research institutions to for-profit health product and pharmaceutical companies; the use of bone from a hip replacement for dental procedures; the accessing, for experimental purposes, of stored pathology specimens;[2] the patenting of genetic material;[3] and the transfer of human genes into sheep, cows, or pigs to produce human biological products.[4]

Genetic science and engineering, in particular, raise value questions that diverge in at least two important directions. On the one hand, these technologies have momentous significance for human subjects, an area that has long been the domain of ethical concern. On the other hand, the issues create a unique range of questions that are not quite about "human-subject research"—that is, they are not about *subjects*—but clearly engage the *human* with its concerns for respect and dignity. These cases constitute a type of scientific endeavor to which we might cogently attach the designation "human nonsubject research" (HNR).

Until now, however, ethicists have taken a scattershot approach toward these issues. Their analyses span some miscellany of questions linked by attempts to define the nature, and the moral status, of human body parts and materials. A glance at the literature reveals a chaotic groping about for the *real* nature of the human body and its components—as if this authentic meaning is out there waiting to be discovered, and we have only to locate it. One finds copious attempts to differentiate body tissues from body materials, body parts from body tissues, body products from body parts,[5] renewable materials from nonrenewable materials. Arguments abound about whether these parts, tissues, and materials should be considered the sacred vestiges of a person or as property—a sort of commodity or natural resource. If the body and its parts are property, does it belong to the individual, to the

177

society,[6] or to the person who *invests work* into it[7]—or is it merely abandoned refuse?[8] If it is property, can it be bought and sold? Is there a distinction between full ownership and some more limited meaning of property rights?[9] Might we not resolve the whole issue by a proper use of informed consent as justified by the notion of self-determination? Alternatively, in cases such as that of the sheep with human genes, ethicists ignore the issue altogether because no moral handle presents itself for an easy cognitive grip.

What we require is an adequate way to think about the problems that HNR poses, so I focus on the hermeneutic task of determining the meaning of the body rather than on a definition of the body itself. I seek to articulate an interpretive ethic that clarifies thinking about the different views on the body, about the relationship of the human to the material universe, and about the profound and literal meaning of *self-determination*. I criticize as insufficient thinking that would identify human body parts and materials merely as property and would resolve the issue merely as one of informed consent. Likewise, I dispute the adequacy of addressing the problem in essentialist terms about the *human*. The goals of an interpretive ethic are as remote from the moral calculus of rationalistic theory that determines whose interests and whose rights are to be protected as they are from an abstract metaphysics. Instead, interpretive ethics explores moral complexity—a task that can be accomplished only by bringing to bear on our experiences the full weight of the hermeneutic process: a bold, discerning, and imaginative confrontation with our history; our social, technological, and political culture; our language; and our convictions. The challenge for an interpretive ethic is to examine all of the deep implications of our relationship to the world.

I begin by exploring the drawbacks of the property and essentialist solutions to this problem. An adequate analysis requires the nuance and subtlety of an interpretive ethic, but even this hermeneutic approach does not suffice. Rather, we must confront the full meaning of humankind as self-determining creator of its own meaning, in light of the potential provided by ongoing advances in biotechnology.

THE CONCEPTUAL AND ETHICAL COGENCY OF THE PROJECT

To discover HNR's profound social, moral, and public policy implications, we require a scrutiny analogous to—but significantly different from—that with which we address human-subject research. We need conceptual clarity about the problem. We must re-examine whether concepts such as inviolability and respect for person—traditional guideposts in our concerns about human subjects—have a place in this new context. We begin by affixing the label HNR; this label enables us to develop a language and identify a framework for dialogue for reflecting on this issue as a first step toward its resolution. Doing so imparts a coherence to the inconsistency with which we currently view HNR's seemingly intransigent ethical problems.

HNR encompasses any experimentation or procedure that deals with human material that is separated from the donor's body—nucleic acid, genetic sequences, genes, cells, blood, organs, and so forth—and that does not, therefore, affect the personal-physiological functioning of its donor-source. The tissue, the stem cell, the cloned cell, the transferred human gene: These materials are human in origin, but they have only an ambiguous relationship to persons—that is, to subjects; thus, these materials fall within the category of the human but outside the aegis of human-subject research.

These cases are intriguing because they straddle traditional categories and produce ambivalence, confusion, and, indeed, a host of logical chimeras and conceptual hybrids. For instance, HNR includes research that may entail the proving of a hypothesis or the development of a nontraditional therapy, or something in between (as with genetic engineering). HNR cases involve organisms with which we have extensive familiarity, as well as some for which we lack categories. We know about human beings, cells, organs, and so forth, but what are we to make of tissue or organ banks: What are they, and what relationship or responsibility does the researcher or the clinician have to these tissues and organs and to the persons from whom they have been obtained? Can these materials—and should they—be treated as just another organic substance? How does tissue removed during circumcision differ from meat?[10] Moreover, HNR confounds a system of genus and species that has long constituted the basis of the Western world's biological science, as well as its value system. That system can now be altered by technological manipulation, causing us to wonder what identity to attribute to the human gene ensconced in the sheep.

The Short-Sightedness of the Property and Essentialist Solutions

Lawyers, scientists, health care professionals, and ethicists have addressed this complexity by regarding such research simply as an extension of human-subject experimentation and by continuing to observe human-subject protocols[11] in a kind of ultimate, but empirically grounded, dualism in which the subject determines what can be done with *its* body. Institutions—either out of conscientious concern or legal necessity—review such procedures through their institutional review boards and obtain informed consent from patients from whose tissue they might, for instance, develop profitable biological products.

HNR cases are exceptional because the personal risks or therapeutic options for the patient that have historically grounded our thinking about human-subjects is not an issue.[12] Tissue sold to the pharmaceutical company, for example, may "belong" (in a yet-to-be-determined way) to the donor, but its disposition presents no physical, health-related risk, nor any therapeutic choices, as we traditionally understand those concepts in medical treatment or clinical trials and about which the donors might make decisions. We must ponder why informed consent is relevant in the absence of risk and choice. Solicitation of consent suggests an awareness that continuity exists between personhood and human material, however obscure this connection. We must puzzle over how the scientist's treatment of tissue in a petri dish bears on the respect for autonomy, self-determination, and bodily integrity that the consent process suggests. We need to weigh how privacy, respect, and inviolability affect the disposition of human materials. We should mull over what "health care" could mean for the professional whose job requires him or her to tend stem cells being cultivated as future transplantation or research material.[13]

The safeguards and protocols peculiar to human subjects assume a certain legal/ethical paradigm. Yet that paradigm is not the one originally envisioned for human subjects. More important, the informed consent protocol effects a metamorphosis from the idea of risk and autonomous decision making on the part of the embodied person into the paradigm of body-as-property. The now-famous Moore case—in which a patient sued to defend his right to profit from his own body material—raises the issue of whether the patient's tissue should be considered his own property.[14] Although the courts ultimately rejected Moore's argument, the issue remains unfortunately central.

Even weightier ethical, epistemological, and scientific problems attend this new interpretation given to the body and its parts, however. As Henk ten Have and Jos Welie so astutely point out, the property paradigm may simply be a category mistake.[15] What could it possibly mean to alienate (in a legal definition) my tissue? Would the buyer then really *own* my stuff, and in what sense? How can my personal identifying factors—my DNA—become yours? If a patient makes an economic agreement to convey some of his tissue to another person,[16] in what way does the tissue belong to the purchaser and cease to belong to the seller? Is it even the patient's to convey? What of the fact that my genetic material also belongs to my family lineage?

Moreover, a single gene—though human and originating from a person—most often lacks individual-personal identity. Rather, most genes belong to the human race at large.[17] Furthermore, the ethical implications that attend the commercial alienation of tissue are many and various: Might the property paradigm create a rift between *gift* and *merchandise* having a detrimental effect on donation of tissue and organs,[18] thereby eroding human solidarity? Would selling the body (or its parts) be tantamount to treating it as a commodity, reminiscent of slavery?[19] Would allowing the sale of body parts exploit the poor, who might sell tissues and organs to sustain their lives?[20]

In his thought-provoking *Body Parts: Property Rights and the Ownership of Human Biological Materials,* E. Richard Gold cautions that the property model will be the default standard by which we regard and dispose of the body—but only if we fail to seize this problem and grapple with it.[21] Other options are not only available but desirable and necessary. To accept the definitional task as one of accepting or refuting the idea of body as property is already to have lost the battle.

Aside from these more practical concerns, the property paradigm stands in the way of more profound questions about the relationship of the human to the material world and about the meaning of *self-determination* that biotechnology provokes. The autonomy-driven property paradigm is rooted in a classical liberalism and contemporary clinical bioethics that insists on the individualistic designation of the good and the valuable that lacks any mutuality of responsibility and spirit of community. We use *self-determination* to mean that everyone can do what he or she wants with his or her body, including cloning it and selling it. Presumably, this meaning of the concept also includes designing the bodies of other persons—our offspring and the offspring of our offspring[22]—as in the realm of genetic engineering (particularly with regard to germ cells), simply because we want to, regardless of the effects on gender balance, or to increase the variety in the gene pool.

The trouble with classical liberalism and a bioethics fixated on autonomy, however, is that they do not go far enough. In a deeper sense, *self-determination* refers to the radical freedom[23] by which we create life plans, character, and moral destiny—not only as individuals but as a human race. For this sense of self-determination, the liberal model falls far short.

The seemingly obvious alternative to the property paradigm is to elucidate the meaning of *human* by locating some essentialist definition. We must, it seems, find a meaning of *human* itself that is distinct in important ways from *subject.* When are body parts, tissues, genetic material, or corpses, for instance, due respect because they are human? What do we mean in these cases by human? What do we mean by respect? Should we use body parts in this way at all? At the very least, threats to a person's privacy and rights may exist, and information garnered from the tissue might yet jeopardize the donor. An emphasis on the person and the personal seems necessary.

The hoped-for meaning is elusive, however. A search for *human* through the history of philosophy reveals a preoccupation (to this searcher's way of thinking) with *personhood*: with rationality, soul, reason, will, autonomy, sentience, communication, and interpersonal relating—in short, with *subjecthood*. Even attempts to overcome this dualism through discussions of embodiment confound us. The search for the meaning of the human, disengaged from the person and the subject, is indeed frustrating and seemingly unresolvable.

Besides, therapies and procedures that treat the body as a pharmaceutical ingredient can also facilitate skin grafts for burns or eliminate genetic diseases that, in principle, constitute the compassionate use of medicine. Although the gross materialism often present in the property arguments[24] are off-putting in the way they protect the medical-industrial complex, we cannot ignore the real medical benefits that these technologies provide. Neither the property paradigm nor the essentialist definition captures the whole picture.

THE SEARCH FOR MEANING

Until now, many ethicists have treated the problems of biotechnology and HNR as a quest for—or perhaps a rummaging through—definitions and conceptual systems to determine which frame of reference will win the battle over articulating this issue. Writers who reject the property paradigm turn to philosophical anthropology to explain the conditions under which persons have proprietorship over their bodies or to define the human, as opposed to the personal and subjective. Although a few thinkers acknowledge the multi-faceted notion of how our society views the body and the dangers of such a dualism,[25] this issue, for the most part, centers on the question of finding and then articulating the meaning of the human body.

The futility of this search is itself telling: Although the physically human has an inescapable, if nebulous, connectedness to the person, the nature of this connection continues to elude us. As long as *the human* and *the body* are regarded as concepts to be mastered and domesticated for our purposes, we are doomed to failure. If, on the one hand, we search for an instrumentalist ethic that calculates conflicting claims on body parts or a conceptual scheme that meets our social, cultural, economic, and entrepreneurial purposes, we misconstrue the task. If we seek ahistorical, essential meanings and ignore the therapeutic possibilities of the body opened up by biotechnology, we fall short. The search confounds us so long as we are blind to the dialogic nature of moral understanding about the body and the human. We require an interpretative and hermeneutic grasp of the problem that reveals the deeper meaning of human self-determination.

THE HERMENEUTIC TASK

Clearly the task of an interpretive ethic in regard to HNR must focus on the search for meaning itself rather than on a simplistic definition. The key to hermeneutics is the idea that meaning is dialogic. Meanings do not exist in the world to be discovered, nor are they merely conceptual schemes of knowers. Meanings include the several facets of the knower's world: the scientific, the political, the emotional, the cultural, the religious, the moral. Some of these facets relate to one's health condition, some to one's intellectual heritage, some to one's faith tradition, and so forth. The task of the interpretative ethic is consciously and deliberately to bring these meanings into dialogue.

Exploration of the problem of genetic engineering, for example, entails an objective knowledge of genetic science together with insight into the philosophy, and the ends, of medicine—that is, whether medicine's intrinsic purpose is healing, improving the gene pool, or some other goal. This exploration also encompasses our lived experiences—for instance, the experiences of physical limitation and illness brought about by the lottery of fate and the experience of attempting to surpass these constraints of the human condition through human ingenuity. Most important, it includes common beliefs and sayings—not of geneticists, physicians, and philosophers but of the person on the street—about the meaning and significance of bringing life into the world, belonging to a family, and being valued and accepted as the persons we are, as well as how this is to be done and whether a child should be the fruit of a loving relationship or the product of a technical process.

The problems of HNR and the issue of human body parts are similarly complex. They entail corresponding insight into the ends of medicine and scientific knowledge about the determination of individual characteristics through genetic manipulation, the possibility of reproducing a human being from a single cell through cloning, and the pharmaceutical uses of body materials. These problems also include our lived experiences—such as a patient's affliction with a disease that could be cured through genetic manipulation of human tissue or the reverence afforded to body remnants exemplified by Navy divers who, to provide closure for survivors, risk their lives to salvage the body parts of plane-crash victims from the ocean. Lived experiences include rituals of death and burial; efforts by the military to fingerprint its members genetically—at least in part because families need to know whether their loved ones have perished; the veneration afforded by many cultures to the placenta following a birth;[26] and the efforts of Native American tribes that strive to reclaim from museums the body parts of their ancestors.

Questions about the moral status of the human body involve knowledge of an economic culture that is motivated by profit-making and willing to convert almost anything into a commodity, as well as the knowledge that a slice of tissue could contain information rendering a person ineligible for employment or insurance. It includes a history of regarding as property human beings who cultivated our fields and raised our children—the repercussions of which haunt us still. It embraces the common beliefs and sayings of the person on the street about the meaning of being human, as exemplified by the symbolic importance of a loved one's lock of hair or the relic of a revered person: the arm bone of a saint or Kepler's finger, preserved in a church in Prague.

The interpretive process is a matter of discernment, a close relative of *phronesis*[27]—that "eye of the soul," as one translation of Aristotle calls it, that yields insight into the moral complexity of our lives. This vision eludes more rationalistic approaches, with their narrower meanings of autonomy and self-determination. Discernment is possible only because we are already rooted in a community and a tradition. We must nevertheless foster a more reflective appreciation of our community's beliefs and sayings. This process demands that we grasp the true meaning of freedom as part of human flourishing—or the good; it demands the richness of experience that comes with maturity. Finally, discernment is possible only if and when we possess the moral acumen that is the fruit of these other elements.[28]

Paul van Tongeren argues that ethics is—or should be—a hermeneutic of moral experience.[29] That is, ethics is a systematic and reflective appraisal of the moral events that constitute our lives as collective and individual agents, with a view to making us more sensitive and imaginative as conceivers of ideas and as decision makers. Furthermore, van Tongeren claims that "philosophical ethics . . . helps moral consciousness to attain clarity concerning itself."[30] The hermeneutic approach to ethics is more, however, than a process of retrieving and clarifying meanings previously created in and through experience. Ethical reflection is not simply an exercise in past-gazing or even of present-awareness. It also encompasses and projects meaning into the future. Just as the study of hermeneutics raises self-consciousness about our understanding of our *technocultural* evolution, we have become and must become more self-conscious and more proactive about our ethical assessment of our world. The hermeneutic task of determining the meaning of the body becomes a further stage of moral self-reflectiveness upon an already reflective capability for adaptation.

Adaptation and Technoculture

Interpretive ethics must take into account the literalness of *self-determination.* In its most profound sense, this concept refers to that future-oriented ability, and indeed *responsibility,* of human beings to define themselves, on a shared level, through technoculture. We have the capacity not only to secure a scientific and technical handle on our world but also to stand back, self-reflectively, from our knowledge. We are able to manipulate the world in adaptive ways:[31] We can and do create, modify, and orchestrate our existence. We are also able to assess, interpret, and evaluate our adaptations. Karl Rahner recognizes in biotechnology the human capacity for "categorial self- manipulation" that actually changes the direction of our biological evolution. Biotechnology has made us capable of producing radically new human things: Already we can develop body products such as insulin[32] and body parts, such as skin,[33] and we are, in principle, capable of producing human organs for transplant. We are closing in on the elimination of certain diseases and already have, in principle, the technology for cloning human beings. We are able to manipulate our very selves to radically affect our own nature so that we can actually redefine—redetermine—our human selves.[34]

Just as cultural adaptation is inherently bound up with technological change, so the genesis of values is an integral component of the evolution of technoculture. This evolution entails the creation of value-meaning as a constituent part of human self-reflectiveness and adaptation. That is, we not only have the capacity, we have an *essential* capacity, as part of our adaptive natures, for moral improvisation and acculturation:[35] We can—indeed, we *must*—attune our moral responses to our constantly new technoculture. For these reasons, the explanation of human body parts is much more than a matter of seeking out definitions. It is simultaneously and essentially, as hermeneutic task, the improvisation of value-meaning about being human in this current, if unfamiliar, world.

As part of discernment, rootedness in communities means recognition of this technoculture as adaptation. We are a technically optimistic society that believes the only problems not solved by science are those yet to be unraveled. To a remarkable extent, the advances of technology *are* our adaptation to the world; increasingly, this adaptation is biological and genetic. Philip Hefner, in his provocative and lucid *Being Human and Being Religious,* talks about adaptation as "surpassing":

> ... the experience of being human is the form of nature surpassing itself . . . a surpassing occurs: the radiation that accompanied the Big Bang became matter, stars, galaxies; in a primeval soup there emerged life. . . . If there is a process of surpassing or transcending, nature itself is the subject, as well as the object of that process.[36]

Hefner argues compellingly that healing, by its nature, has a symbolic and spiritual component. Healing points to our capacity to "surpass," and be redeemed from, the demons that beset us, and thus to come-to-grips-with. His insight into healing is key to our understanding of its importance in any society, and it is true for us. In our society, biotechnology is first of all a way of adapting to and of overcoming the obstacles presented by the world in order to survive. It is a part of technoculture.

Discernment, however, would have us distinguish between biotechnoculture as adaptation; healing in its spiritual and symbolic senses; and the lived experiences of disease, suffering, and hope for a cure. Adaptation and spiritual symbolism are critically important to reflection on our world, but their value lies in their universality and distance from our personal lives. Not only are genetic screening, contemporary reproductive techniques, and the pharmaceutical use of body materials expressions of adaptation and "surpassing"; they also aim at human flourishing. In the clinical—as opposed to the technological—setting, disease screening may constitute what a couple considers responsible parenting. They may ask themselves: Do we have a moral obligation to abstain from bringing into the world a child who would be exposed to great suffering? Would reluctance to have a seriously ill or disabled child make a statement about the worth, or relative lack of worth, of diseased or impaired persons? Does loving parenting mean the prevention of suffering by not having such a child, or attentive caretaking of him or her?

From the viewpoint of technoculture and adaptation, the production of insulin or the prediction of bipolar disorder presents one problem to the scientist (who views the body material as specimen), another to the entrepreneur (who sees it as property), and another to the ethicist (who aspires to determine its moral status). It presents yet a different problem to the patient and the physician—both of whom (though in different ways) confront a lifetime of suffering from diabetes or mental illness. Like the parents who must decide about bearing a child, the patient and his or her physician relate to these uses of human body parts as a lived experience. Human flourishing appears differently in the clinical setting, the home, and the patient's bedside than it does in the laboratory, the board room, or the ethicist's study.

Being rooted in community raises a particular set of issues for the Navy divers, the forensic scientist who identifies the body parts,[37] and the families of those killed in the plane crash who keep vigil. To them, the notion of body parts as property would be not only inappropriate and crass but abhorrent. Here technoculture in the form of diving and forensic expertise is part of the scenario. This expertise represents an authentic valuing of the body that is remote, however, from HNR. These practices also are manifestations of human flourishing in the way they honor the dead and benefit and console the living.

The Native American tribes who object to maintaining their ancestors' body parts in museums, the churches that keep Kepler's finger and other relics, the mother who keeps a lock of hair of all of her children in a scrapbook, and various burial rites testify to other ways of valuing the human body as vehicle of the person. This reverence for human fragments as representations of persons appear in various guises in diverse cultural settings, but the inherent link between body part and person is eminently real. That new technologies play a less important role in these instances merely testifies to the constancy and universality of our understanding of embodiment as a part of human be-ing throughout many cultures and many periods of time. Once again, these observances are ways of honoring the absent and the dead for the benefit of the present and the living.

A FINAL VIEW

As promised, I acknowledge that an interpretive probe into human nonsubject research yields neither meanings nor practical solutions. As an interpretive task, however, this exploration into the ethics of HNR—and of biotechnology in general—reveals the criticality of our radical human freedom. Human beings, with their technoculture, are part of a "surpassing" process that commences with the origins of nature itself. Because biotechnology has the capacity for "categorical self-manipulation," our "surpassing," adaptation, and self-determination require an entirely new level of self-consciousness and reflectiveness.

This radical human freedom, far from resembling the more limited classical liberal notion of autonomy and self-determination, is capable of doing far more than influencing, in a scientifically interesting way, the evolutionary course of the race. Because we are human, as Rahner reminds us,[38] we are at risk of making irretrievable biological and moral errors.[39] To view the body as commodity, to value it as property, to protect entrepreneurial endeavors at the expense of the beliefs and convictions of ordinary folk, to overlook how information contained in each piece of human flesh is a matter of personal integrity is to render sightless that "eye of the soul" of which Aristotle speaks and to walk at the edge of a moral cliff, courting what could be irreversible disaster. To serve individual preferences and economic interests while ignoring the outcome for the environment, the diversity of the gene pool, alteration of germ lines, or the balance of gender throughout the world could be to invite final tragedy for generations yet unborn. It need not be so, however. We must integrate our radical freedom and awesome technological capability with a correspondingly radical self-reflection and creation of value-meanings sustained by moral acumen.

The answer about which road we should take at this juncture—if there is an answer—is that value-meanings are created in dialogue. As bearers of discernment, as creators of meaning, and as determiners of our futures, we are not engaged in a simple win/lose situation: This discussion is not a contest in which either the body-person defenders or the body-property defenders are bound to win. We all stand to lose, or to flourish, together.

NOTES

1. John Gearhart, "Cell Biology: New Potential for Human Embryonic Stem Cells," *Science* 282, no. 5391 (November 6, 1998): 1061–62; James A. Thomson et al., "Embryonic Stem Cell Lines Derived from Human Blastocysts," *Science* 282, no. 5391 (November 6,

1998): 1145–47. See also A. Kimbrell, *The Human Body Shop: The Engineering and Marketing of Life* (San Francisco: HarperCollins, 1993).

2. Wayne W. Grody and Mark E. Sobel, eds., "Update on Informed Consent for Stored Tissue Research," *Diagnostic Molecular Pathology* 5 (1996): 79–80; J. Stephenson, "Pathologists Enter Debate on Consent for Genetic Research on Stored Tissue," *Journal of the American Medical Association* 275, no. 7 (1996): 503–04; E. W. Clayton et al., "Informed Consent for Genetic Research on Stored Tissue Samples," *Journal of the American Medical Association* 274, no. 22 (1995): 1786–92.

3. Mark J. Hanson, "Religious Voices in Biotechnology: The Case of Gene Patenting," *Hastings Center Report* (November-December 1997): 1–21; Baruch A. Brody, *Protecting Human Dignity and the Patenting of Human Genes* (New York: Oxford University Press, 1998).

4. Gina Kolata, "Lab Yields Lamb with Human Gene," *New York Times,* 25 July 1997, 1. Jos Welie raises the question about whether the insertion of the gene into an ape ovum, for instance, would be an instance of HNR (private correspondence).

5. Karen Wright, "Human in the Age of Mechanical Reproduction," *Discover,* May 1998, 75–81; Jos V. M. Welie and Henk A. M. J. ten Have, eds., *Ownership of the Human Body* (Hingham, Mass.: Kluwer Academic Press, 1998).

6. Anne Fagot-Largeault, "Ownership of the Human Body: Judicial and Legislative Responses in France," in *Ownership of the Human Body,* ed. Jos V. M. Welie and Henk A. M. J. ten Have, 115–42.

7. Margaret S. Swain and Randy W. Marusyk, "An Alternative to Property Rights in Human Tissue," *Hastings Center Report* (September/October 1990): 12–15.

8. *Nuffield Report* (London: Nuffield Council on Bioethics, 1995).

9. See, for instance, Diego Gracia, "Ownership of the Human Body: Some Historical Remarks," and Jos V. M. Welie and Henk A. M. J. ten Have, "Ownership of the Human Body: The Dutch Concept" (both in Welie and ten Have, *Ownership of the Human Body*).

10. Zbigniew Szarwarski, "Talking About Embryos," in *Conceiving the Embryo,* ed. D. Evans (Boston: Kluwer Law International, 1996).

11. Courtney S. Campbell, "Body, Self, and the Property Paradigm," *Hastings Center Report* 22 (September-October 1992): 34–42; Rhonda G. Hartman, "Beyond Moore: Issues of Law and Policy Impacting Human Cell and Genetic Research in the Age of Biotechnology," *Journal of Legal Medicine* (1993): 463–77.

12. In Tom L. Beauchamp and James F. Childress, *Principles of Biomedical Ethics,* 4th ed. (New York: Oxford University Press, 1994), for example, informed consent is based on risk and autonomous decision making. In *The Right to Die* (New York: Wiley, 1995), A. Meisel claims that the goals of informed consent are self-determination, patient autonomy, and the patient's therapeutic options.

13. Hanson, in "Religious Voices in Biotechnology," suggests that this tissue should be treated with respect, but the crux of the problem remains: What does respect mean here?

14. Sandra Blakeslee, "Patient Rights: Patient Sues for Title to Own Cells," *Nature* 311 (September 20, 1984): 198; Barbara J. Culliton, "Moore Cell Case Has Its First Court Hearing," *Science* 226 (November 16, 1984): 813–14.

15. Welie and ten Have, eds., *Ownership of the Human Body.*

16. According to Anthony M. Honoré, to *own* means the right to possess, to exclusively use, to manage, to enjoy income from, to gain capital from, to alienate, to consume, to waste or to destroy, to have immunity from expropriation from, power to bequeath and to prohibit harmful use of (Anthony M. Honoré, "Ownership," in *Oxford Essays in Jurisprudence,* ed. A. G. Guest [London: Oxford University Press, 1961].

17. Swain and Marusyk, "An Alternative to Property Rights in Human Tissue."
18. See Hartman, "Beyond Moore"; Patricia A. Marshall, David C. Thomasma, and A. S. Daar, "Marketing Human Organs," *Theoretical Medicine* 17, no. 1 (1996): 1–18.
19. Marshall, Thomasma, and Daar, "Marketing Human Organs."
20. Swain and Marusyk, "An Alternative to Property Rights in Human Tissue"; John Harris, *Wonderwoman and Superman: The Ethics of Human Biotechnology* (New York: Oxford University Press, 1992).
21. E. Richard Gold, *Body Parts: Property Rights and the Ownership of Human Biological Materials* (Washington, D.C.: Georgetown University Press, 1996).
22. Stephen G. Post, "Mark the Judeo-Christian Case Against Cloning," *America* 176, no. 21 (June 21, 1997): 19.
23. Karl Rahner, "Christian Coolheadedness in the Face of Man's Future," in *Theological Investigations,* vol. 9, trans. Graham Harrison (New York: Crossroads, 1972).
24. Hartman cites the Moore court's concern with the potentially devastating effects on economic incentives for scientific research (Hartman, "Beyond Moore," 475).
25. Lori Andrews and Dorothy Nelkin, "Whose Body Is It Anyway? Disputes Over Body Tissue in a Biotechnology Age," *The Lancet* (January 3, 1998): 53–56; Gold, *Body Parts.*
26. Victor Turner, *The Forest of Symbols* (Ithaca, N.Y.: Cornell University Press, 1967).
27. Aristotle, *Nicomachean Ethics,* rev. standard trans., ed. Jonathan Barnes (Princeton, N.J.: Princeton University Press, 1985), 1144a29.
28. Aristotle, *Nicomachean Ethics,* Book VI; Judith Lee Kissell, "Experience—the Key to Moral Judgment: A Comparative Study of Aristotle's *Phronesis* and Aquinas's Prudence" (unpublished manuscript).
29. Paul von Tongeren, "The Relation of Narrativity and Hermeneutics to an Adequate Practical Ethics," *Ethical Perspectives* 1, no. 2 (1994): 57–70.
30. von Tongeren, "The Relation of Narrativity and Hermeneutics to an Adequate Practical Ethics," 57.
31. Philip Hefner, *Being Human and Being Religious: GHI as Text for Theological Interpretation* (Berkeley, Calif.: Center for Theology and the Natural Sciences, 1993).
32. Such as human insulin and other enzymes.
33. D. Pascovitz, "Lab-produced Human Skin Just a Start, Researchers Say," *Omaha World Herald,* 11 December 1997.
34. Rahner, "Christian Coolheadedness in the Face of Man's Future."
35. Albert Jonsen, "The Ethicist as Improvisationist," in *Christian Ethics: Problems and Prospects,* ed. Lisa Sowle Cahill and James F. Childress (Cleveland: Pilgrim Press, 1996).
36. Hefner, *Being Human and Being Religious,* 9.
37. National Public Radio's *Morning Edition* interviewed a medical examiner who examined body parts rescued after a crash. The medical examiner related his difficulty in doing his job and how, because he lived alone, he valued the company of his dogs to escape the sadness and the pressure of his task. Without the dogs for companionship, he explained, he would not have been able to go on.
38. Rahner, "Christian Coolheadedness in the Face of Man's Future."
39. Ibid.

Healing the Dying: Spiritual Issues in the Care of the Dying Patient

Daniel P. Sulmasy, O.F.M.

In the final analysis, every dying person who retains the capacity to hear and to understand the call of death faces two important sets of questions: questions of *value* and questions of *meaning*. Whether the dying individual addresses or ignores these questions is totally up to the individual in his or her own freedom. The fact that some persons freely choose to ignore these questions does not vitiate their importance. Even if all persons freely chose to ignore these questions, they would remain important. Regardless of whether people confront these questions, they always present themselves as obvious questions for the dying person to address. Regardless of whether the dying person subscribes to some particular system of religious belief, these questions are aptly described as spiritual in character.

The first set of questions relates to value. At some level, the dying person must ask questions such as the following: Do I, as an embodied person, now dying, have any value here and now as *me* dying? Has my life, as I have lived it until now, had any value? Will there be anything of value about me that persists after I have died?

The second set of questions relates to meaning. At some level, the dying person must ask such questions as the following: Does my dying now, as an embodied person, have any meaning here and now? Has my life, as I have lived it until now, had any meaning? Has there been any meaning in what I have suffered? Will there be any meaning in my living and dying that perdures beyond the moment of my death?

In most contemporary discussions of caring for persons who are dying, these questions have been addressed obliquely, subsumed under a pair of words that have received far too little critical reflection. Questions of value have been subsumed under the word *dignity*; questions of meaning have been subsumed under the word *hope*. These words are invoked continually, as if everyone understood clearly what they mean. Yet the meanings of these words and the questions they evoke in discussions about the dying are rarely clear. These words have served, in some respects, as metaphorical rugs under which all the messy questions about meaning and value have been swept. One is left with the appearance of a technically correct, electronically controlled, antiseptically spiritual death: "At Acme HMO, we provide what consumers want: high quality, cost-effective care at the end of life, treating our patients with dignity and always reassuring them of hope." Very neat.

Even well-meaning persons concerned with improving the care of the dying have moved too quickly to package these concerns under very broad labels such as "spiritual suffering." Some have even dared to try to create quantitative scales to measure (and therefore to control) the spiritual experiences of dying persons. I wonder, however, whether this quantification is even possible. One can almost hear the echoes of questions raised long ago by the prophet Isaiah: "Who has held in a measure the dust of the earth, weighed the mountains in scales and the hills in a balance? Who has directed the spirit of the Lord, or has instructed him as his counselor? Whom did he consult to gain knowledge?" (Is. 40:12–14). Even the best health care professionals are sometimes far too uncomfortable with the idea of the unfathomable. Outcomes researchers concerned with care at the end of life try to reduce the spiritual to a check box. Even in the desire to serve the spiritual needs of dying patients, medicine is in danger of sterilizing the spirit right out of dying.

In criticizing some recent approaches to improving the spiritual care of the dying, I do not wish to imply that health care professionals cannot discuss these issues, grapple with them, and do a better job of facilitating the spiritual work of the dying. It seems obvious to sensitive persons who care for the dying that whenever dying goes awry (as it often does), it is frequently because the patient or the caregiver has paid insufficient attention to these questions of meaning and value. Health care professionals can and should do a better job. All I suggest is that empirical science will not give us the answers to these questions. Total Quality Management will not redress these deficiencies. The truly spiritual is frightfully unmanageable. Spiritual concerns are not resolved glibly by questionnaires. One cannot measure the unmeasurable.

Yet everyone has some intuitive sense of the nature of these spiritual questions, particularly as they relate to death. People fear that their own end might be undignified. They wonder if there is anything in which they will be able to hope when their own time comes. Too many health care professionals remain fearful, however, of discussing these issues in any depth with their colleagues—or with their patients.

DIGNITY

The phrase "death with dignity" has become a slogan for many people, but the real meaning of this phrase is anything but clear. Consider that the bill that legalized physician-assisted suicide in the state of Oregon was called the "Death with Dignity Act." Yet many people who opposed the legalization of assisted suicide in Oregon based their opposition on their belief that assisted suicide is always a violation of the dignity of the dying. Thus, parties to discussions about "death with dignity" mean different things by *dignity.* It therefore seems wise to get a bit clearer about what dignity means.[1]

One must begin by stating a principle: Moral words ought to be used consistently and coherently. This principle implies that whatever one says one means by *dignity* in discussions of death ought to be the same meaning one assigns to *dignity* in all spheres of human moral experience. This principle seems unassailably true and therefore provides a good place to start.

Dignity, at its root, means worth, stature, or value. Whatever has dignity has value. In the Middle Ages, when the idea of the "Great Chain of Being" dominated metaphysics, and cosmology, the situation was very simple. Everything had value, as created by God, and one's value was relative to one's place in the hierarchy of beings. Thus, plants had more dignity than rocks, animals had more dignity than plants, humans had more dignity than animals, priests had more dignity than lay people, bishops had more dignity than priests, popes had more dignity than bishops, angels had more dignity than popes, and God had more dignity than angels. People no longer think quite this way, however, about the universe or about human beings. In particular, the notion of human dignity has taken a much more egalitarian turn. Although most people would accept as true the notion that a human being has more value than an amoeba, few would accept the notion that a rich person has more dignity than a poor person does, or that a politician has more dignity than an unelected citizen does. Dignity seems to be something Western societies now attribute to all persons equally, regardless of their station in life.

The Civil Rights movement in this country made copious use of the word *dignity*. The point of these activists was elegantly simple, no matter how much it may have upset prevailing social assumptions. Their point was that all human beings have equal dignity. The color of a person's skin does not add to or decrease anyone's dignity.

The Rev. Martin Luther King, Jr., said that he learned this lesson from his grandmother.[2] She told him, "Martin, don't let anyone ever tell you that you're not a somebody." *Somebody-ness* captures the core of this notion of human dignity. Everybody is a *somebody*. Everyone has equal worth—at least in the eyes of the law, even if one does not believe in a God who views everyone equally.

DIGNITY AND DEATH

The relevance of this message to the care of the dying may seem obvious: Everyone ought to believe that the same is true of the dying—that the dying have no less dignity than the surviving. At least, one ought to believe this if one wishes to be consistent in one's use of moral terms. That is why it was important to begin this discussion by setting forth a principle of consistency.

Confusion seems to creep in, however, when people begin to talk about dignity in relation to death. This confusion can be explained if one takes note of a distinction between *attributed* dignity and *intrinsic* dignity.[3] The kind of dignity I have discussed is intrinsic dignity. People have this kind of dignity simply because they are members of the human family. This dignity is *intrinsic* to being human.

Intrinsic dignity may be contrasted with attributed dignity. Attributed dignity is the value or worth that one attributes to others or to oneself. Attributed dignity is based on one's power, prestige, function, productivity, of degree of control over one's situation. We attribute this sort of dignity to heads of state, for instance: We call them "dignitaries." This sort of dignity is situational: It depends on one's station in life. It differs from person to person, society to society. It changes over time. It can be completely subjective (i.e., how much dignity individuals are willing to attribute to themselves), or intersubjective (e.g., how much dignity a society is willing to attribute to its sanitation workers).

It is undeniably true that illness and death attack *attributed* dignity. Persons who are dying are robbed of their station in life. They become less productive or even unproductive. They lose control. They become dependent. They lose esteem in the eyes of others. Dying brings these changes upon them. The spiritual question about death and dignity, however, is whether such an assault is ultimately complete or whether there is, after all, such a thing as intrinsic human dignity that can be found even in death.

Donald Hall—husband of the late Jane Kenyon, a poet who recently died of leukemia—is himself a poet. Hall has written powerful poetry about his wife's death. His words capture the transcendent splendor of the mundane details of dying. The following is an excerpt from his poem "Last Days."[4]

> Incontinent three nights
> before she died, Jane needed lifting
>   onto the commode.
> He wiped her and helped her back into bed.
>   At five he fed the dog
> And returned to find her across the room,
>   Sitting in a straight chair.
> When she couldn't stand, how could she walk?
>   He feared she would fall
> And called for an ambulance to the hospital,
>   But when he told Jane,
> Her mouth twisted down and tears started.
>   "Do we have to?" He cancelled.
> Jane said, "Perkins, be with me when I die."

This poem is about dignity in death. It is about *intrinsic* human dignity persisting in the midst of assaults on attributed dignity. How is it that a human being seems to walk even if rendered physically incapable of standing? Regardless of whether it is literally true, it is always metaphorically true that the lame can walk in dignity.

Thus, this poem is a proclamation of the intrinsic sense of human dignity that is not lost when a person becomes powerless and dependent. It proclaims the dignity that is not lost as a person becomes disfigured. It proclaims the dignity that does not depend on how others view a person or even how individuals view themselves. It is about the dignity that all persons have—the dying no less than the surviving. This dignity is ineradicable. It does not admit of degrees. It does not depend on how productive one is. It does not depend on any function one might serve. It is the dignity all human beings have simply because they are human.

Nor can any individual decide what constitutes the intrinsic value of any human being, including the individual himself or herself. As Simone Weil somewhat shockingly observed, it is not what is most personal and unique about us that constitutes the basis of our dignity but what is most impersonal and common: "What is sacred in a human being is the impersonal in him."[5] What seems most trivially true about us—that we are all human beings—constitutes our dignity. This notion may come as a shock to Americans. Americans are so caught up in individualism and the language of rights that they may have trouble grasping that what is least individual in people constitutes the grounds for respecting individual freedom.

Human beings have respect for each other's rights because they all have dignity. The opposite is not true. People do not have dignity only to the extent that their rights are respected. When Martin Luther King, Jr., sat in an Alabama prison cell, his rights had been trampled. He had been robbed of his independence. Many people did not believe he had equal dignity. Yet despite what had happened to him and what others thought of him, his *intrinsic* dignity shone forth between the bars of his cell with all the brilliance of the sun.

SPIRITUALITY, DIGNITY, AND DEATH

Dying mounts an assault on human dignity. Ineluctably, dying raises questions about one's worth and value as one is dying; about the value of the life one has led up to the moment of death; and about whether anything that is of value perdures beyond the moment of one's death. The spiritual task of the dying is to reject, to discover, to recover, or to affirm their own grasp of their own intrinsic human dignity. As the grounds for *attributed* dignity fade (as they inevitably will for each of us), the question becomes: Is that all there is? Is there nothing more about me of value except how I feel, how I appear to others, how much I can do without anyone else's help, and how productive I can be? This questioning process may lead to further questions: If there is intrinsic value to my life, what is the source of that value? Can such a belief be validated? Does such value endure?

These questions are spiritual, regardless of whether they are raised in a religious context. One is free to choose not to grapple with these questions; nonetheless, they are the *obvious* questions. One can also choose to answer in the negative—to conclude that there is no intrinsic value to human life. To do so, however, one must be consistent in one's belief about the valuelessness of all human life. One should also bear in mind that such a response requires no less faith than belief in a divinity that creates, redeems, and sanctifies human life.

HOPE

The word *hope,* like the word *dignity,* has been haplessly muddled in discussions about dying. In fact, this muddled thinking has probably been true for centuries. The Hippocratic texts, for instance, talk of concealing information from patients so that they do not worsen on hearing bad news.[6] Writing in this tradition, Thomas Percival advised,

> A physician should not be forward to make gloomy prognostications. . . . For the physician should be the minister of hope and comfort to the sick; that by such cordials to the drooping spirit, he may smooth the bed of death, revive expiring life, and counteract the depressing influences of those maladies which rob the philosopher of fortitude, and the Christian of consolation.[7]

Clinicians often speak in such ways today. They whisper in dark corridors about "hopeless cases." Even with the best intentions, they write about the care of the "hopelessly ill."[8] Families sometimes hesitate to authorize discontinuation of treatment because it would signal that they had "given up hope."

Is anyone's dying necessarily truly hopeless? Do the dying have anything for which to hope? I think they do, and I urge health care professionals to choose their words with greater care and not glibly declare any patient hopeless.

What is hope, after all? Thomas Aquinas writes that hope is a specialized type of desire—a desire characterized by a special type of object. The object of hope must be clearly good, apparent in the future, difficult or arduous to attain, and yet regarded as possible to attain.[9]

A dying person might naturally *desire* not to die. Most of the people who survive them have this same natural desire. No one can really *hope* never to die, however; all persons are mortal. Because the object of such a desire is impossible, it would violate the fourth characteristic of a proper object of hope as set forth by Aquinas.

It might seem, then, that individuals who have exhausted all means of cure are properly said to be "hopeless." This assessment, however, would be true only if there were nothing more for a human being to desire than long life and the death of tumor cells, HIV virions, or tubercle bacilli. Most persons recognize, however, that human desire is far deeper. At the limit, a hope based on needles and pills dissolves into delusion. A proper object of hope must be attainable. Therefore, if one is dying, one's hopes must be deeper than death.

Death is the ultimate human limit. It cannot be avoided. It cannot be wished away. It cannot be prayed away. Christians believe that God the Father delivered this message to Jesus in the Garden of Gethsemane (Luke 22:42). This cup will not pass from any of us.

Ultimate hope, then, is not about a cure for cancer or AIDS. Although such goals are certainly good things to be wished for, they cannot be the source of ultimate hope. Ultimate hope is a transcendental virtue. Aquinas called it a "supernatural virtue." The object of ultimate hope must be located beyond the limits of finite, corporal, individual existence.

Meaning is such a transcendental object. The object of ultimate hope is a source of meaning, however this might be construed. For Christians, Muslims, and Jews, this transcendental object of desire is the one, holy, all-loving, and almighty God. For those of other faiths, or of no faith, this object of ultimate, genuine hope must be whatever source of meaning a person holds to be prior to or to transcend the limits of finite, corporal, individual existence.

To reject, discover, recover, or hold onto an ongoing source of transcendental meaning is one of the major spiritual tasks of the dying. The opposite of hope is despair, but *despair* is really just another name for meaninglessness. To suffer without any sense of meaning is abject hopelessness.

Jane Kenyon, whose husband wrote so movingly of the dignity of her dying, herself wrote a poem that speaks eloquently about the hope she found in her own dying. This poem is called "Let Evening Come."[10]

Let the light of late afternoon
shine through chinks in the barn, moving
up the bales as the sun moves down.

Let the cricket take up chafing
as a woman takes up her needles
and her yarn. Let evening come.

Let dew collect on the hoe abandoned
in long grass. Let the stars appear
and the moon disclose her silver horn.

Let the fox go back to its sandy den.
Let the wind die down. Let the shed
go black inside. Let evening come.

To the bottle in the ditch, to the scoop
in the oats, to air in the lung
let evening come.

Let it come, as it will, and don't
be afraid. God does not leave us
comfortless, so let evening come.

Hope for the dying lies beyond the limits of what is measurable in the space and time that they are allotted on this earth. Beyond the physical realities of suffering and death, either there is meaning or there is not. Evening will come. Each dying person must face the issue of whether there is any meaning beyond the horizon of human finitude.

SPIRITUALITY AND THE CARE OF THE DYING

Having discussed what I mean by questions of value (i.e., dignity) and questions of meaning (i.e., hope), I have an obligation to discuss what this analysis means for health care professionals who are caring for persons who are dying. The fundamental point is this: Health care professionals do not give their patients dignity or hope. This conclusion follows from the foregoing discussion. Dignity and hope are already present as givens in every situation of death. Value is already there, commanding respect. Meaning is already there, awaiting affirmation.

The task of the health care professional is to show respect and reverence for the dignity that all dying persons have simply because they are human, and to share their own hope that meaning transcends the dying process. They can do nothing more; they must do nothing less. Where possible, health care professionals can create an atmosphere that is conducive to the patient's own grasping of the dignity and hope that are already there to be grasped. Doctors, nurses, and their colleagues should be neither so naïve nor so arrogant as to think that dignity and hope are theirs to give. Health care professionals who think it is their responsibility to provide dignity and hope to patients will burn out. If they take upon themselves the tasks of offering dignity and hope, they are doomed to failure: Sisyphus *redux*.

Respecting the intrinsic dignity of dying patients does bring with it certain concrete moral responsibilities, however. Respect is dynamic, not static. The link between intrinsic and attributed dignity is forged in moral action. Respect for intrinsic human dignity demands action to build up, to the extent possible, the attributed dignity of human beings, provided this action does not undermine or contradict the intrinsic human dignity that is the ground of moral action. In other words, to respect someone's intrinsic human dignity demands that one show that respect in concrete ways. Respecting the intrinsic dignity of the dying requires that one assist them in their concrete needs. Respect for the dying is demonstrated by bathing them, feeding them, treating their pain, relieving their nausea, helping them to get out of bed. Respect for the dying is demonstrated by being with them and listening to them attentively, paying careful attention to what they can teach those who survive them.

More than this, however, respect for the dying requires attention to their spiritual struggles. Health care professionals can point out, by word and action, that dignity is already there to be grasped by the dying. People who are dying need to be reminded of their dignity at a time of fierce doubt. They need to understand that they are not grotesque, bothersome, or unvalued because they are unproductive or that they are unworthy of time, attention, and resources. Physicians, nurses, and others can help dying persons to grasp their own intrinsic dignity through concrete actions that thwart or mitigate the assault that the dying process mounts against their patients' attributed dignity.

Health care professionals also need to create an atmosphere in which persons who are dying can search for meaning. Doctors and nurses need to be open to discussions of spiritual issues and ready to refer to experts in pastoral care who, as part of the team, can assist patients in their struggles with these issues. Health care professionals can help the dying by pointing out, in words and in actions, that they themselves do not consider the state of the patient to be hopeless. Rather, doctors and nurses must somehow communicate to dying patients gratitude for the meaning and the hope that persons who are dying freely (and often unwittingly) give to those who care for them. Persons who are dying can teach nurses, physicians, and other health care professionals countless lessons about life and its meaning every day. Health care professionals have only to open their ears and their hearts.

In the end, then, hope has nothing whatsoever to do with prognosis. It has everything to do with the human spirit. Health care professionals can cultivate a spirit of genuine hope in their dying patients only if they themselves are in touch with their own spirits. Only in this way is it possible to heal the dying.

MORALITY, SPIRITUALITY, AND END-OF-LIFE CARE

As important as spiritual issues might be, one certainly ought never coerce a patient into addressing spiritual issues. Respect demands that patients be allowed the freedom to choose to ignore these issues—or even to answer the ultimate questions in the negative. Although this expression of respect is the right approach, it can be very painful to give someone the freedom to die believing that life has no intrinsic value and that the universe is absurd. This feeling is particularly difficult for people of faith. One can still believe in that dying patient's dignity and hold out hope for that person, however, even if they themselves do not. Believers must also remember that the freedom not to believe is exactly the freedom that God gives everyone. One should not usurp prerogatives that God has freely abdicated out of His love and respect for the persons He has created.

It is also important to recognize that there are "good" and "bad" deaths, just as there are good and bad persons. As Karl Rahner puts it, a person's "free, personal, self-affirmation and self-realization achieves in death an absolute determination."[11] Death is the punctuation mark on a person's life, as it were. A person may come to the moment of death full of bitterness, anger, fear, vanity, jealousy, greed, and pride. A life lived this way may lead to a death died that way.

Such patients can be very difficult to care for. Watching people die this way can be even more painful than watching patients die in pain. A person's physical pain ceases with death, but a person's free, personal self-affirmation and self-realization in death endure. This is what the dying finally say to those who remain behind. This is that into which they place themselves for all eternity. Yet simply because a person freely chooses to die in bitterness, anger, fear, vanity, jealousy, greed, and pride does not mean that this death is a good death. It is not good merely because it is freely chosen. Freedom is the context for morality, not the content of morality.[12]

On the other hand, watching patients die in dignity, hope, and love can be a remarkable event. Dying can clarify so much—stripping away all that is false and laying bare the pure figure of life's meaning. Caring for patients who die in this manner can be a profound experience and a rare privilege. That a person's self-affirmation and self-realization might irrevocably determine him or her in dignity, hope, and love says these things to those who remain behind.

Understanding that there are good deaths and bad deaths, one must also humbly recognize one's limitations in judging the souls of others. Persons who believe in a deity are better off leaving this judgment to God.

One should also be extremely careful not to manufacture an artificial "ideal" death and try to force patients to adopt some particular model of death or judge patients for not adopting it. Some dignified deaths are accompanied by wailing and tears; some are accompanied by stoic silence. Some hopeful deaths are founded on certain belief in the meaning given by traditional religious belief; some hopeful deaths are dogfights with doubt.

Finally, health care professionals who are concerned about the spiritual well-being of dying patients must not mistake personality or culture for spirituality. One can make judgments, but one ought not be judgmental.

The task of the health care professional includes attending to the spiritual needs of the dying patient. Death is the end of a long spiritual journey. Persons who are dying want company as they walk the way, and health care professionals can provide that accompaniment. Going the extra mile has its own rewards.

NOTES

1. Daniel P. Sulmasy, "Death and Human Dignity," *Linacre Quarterly* 61 (winter 1994): 27–36.
2. Garth Baker-Fletcher, *Somebodiness: Martin Luther King, Jr. and the Theory of Dignity* (Minneapolis, Minn.: Fortress Press, 1993).
3. Sulmasy, "Death and Human Dignity."
4. "Last Days," from *WITHOUT* by Donald Hall. Copyright 1998 by Donald Hall. Reprinted by permission of Houghton Mifflin Co. All rights reserved.
5. Simone Weil, "Human Personality," in *The Simone Weil Reader,* ed. G. A. Panichas (New York: David McKay, 1977), 313–39.

6. Hippocrates, "Decorum," XVI, in *Hippocrates*, vol. 2, trans. W. H. S. Jones (Cambridge: Harvard University Press, 1923), 296–99.

7. Thomas Percival, *Percival's Medical Ethics*, ed. C. D. Leake (Huntington, N.Y.: Robert E. Krieger, 1975), 91.

8. Timothy E. Quill, Christine K. Cassel, and Diane E. Meier, "The Care of the Hopelessly Ill: Proposed Clinical Criteria for Assisted Suicide," *New England Journal of Medicine* 327 (1992): 1830–34.

9. Thomas Aquinas, *Summa Theologiae* I-II, trans. J.P. Reid, vol. 21, Blackfriars ed. (New York: McGraw-Hill, 1963), q. 40, a.1.

10. "Let Evening Come," copyright 1996 by the Estate of Jane Kenyon. Reprinted from *Otherwise: New and Selected Poems* with the permission of Graywolf Press, Saint Paul, Minnesota.

11. Karl Rahner, *On the Theology of Death*, trans. C. H. Henkey (New York: Herder and Herder, 1961), 26.

12. Edmund D. Pellegrino and David C. Thomasma, *Helping and Healing: Religious Commitment in Health Care* (Washington, D.C.: Georgetown University Press, 1997), 77.

Prophet to the Profession: Healing and Physician-Assisted Suicide

Courtney S. Campbell

The ethos of medicine as a profession is under challenge and critique as never before. Under the influence of managed care and public policy regulations—and under the pressure of public image of medical professionals—physicians are asked and indeed demanded to deliver the highest quality medicine at the lowest possible cost to the greatest number of people. As patients increasingly become "customers" and "consumers," physicians find their roles undergoing a transformation to those of "retailers" and "providers" in the delivery of a market commodity—namely, health care. This context seems guaranteed to generate patient and political discontent with medicine as an ethical profession and make it especially difficult to maintain foundational images of the physician as friend and healer.

The fragmentation of the ethos of medicine is displayed no better, perhaps, than in societal and professional disputes over end-of-life choices—especially the ethical controversy of the decade: physician assistance in the suicide of a terminally ill patient. Advocates for terminally ill patients have asserted a moral "right" to the assistance of physicians in a patient's suicide (and thus a correlative duty of assistance by *some* physician); in some jurisdictions, such as the state of Oregon, this right has become legally recognized. The traditional goals of medicine have been disparaged as antiquated and irrelevant for this brave new world of professional practice in which deliberately hastening the patient's death is deemed permissible.[1]

In this morally confusing world that medicine has entered, few voices have been as clear and consistent on the goals and boundaries of medicine as that of Edmund Pellegrino. Pellegrino has articulated a vision of medicine's purposes and the lines medicine must affirm and maintain—lines it crosses only at the risk of compromising its integrity as an ethical profession. Pellegrino has offered an especially compelling case that medical professionals, in their care of the terminally ill, must not cross the line from "healer" to "killer," lest the constitutive values that identify a caregiver as "physician" be violated.

In this essay, I provide a brief overview of Pellegrino's discussion of the practice of assisted suicide and active euthanasia in medicine and then use this overview as a critical lens by which to interpret the fragmentation of medicine's ethical identity in the ongoing debate in Oregon to legalize the participation of physicians in a patient's suicide. In so doing, I seek to address questions central to Pellegrino's work, as well as the future of medicine in the twenty-first century: What becomes of the role(s) of physician in an ethical climate that is increasingly tolerant of patient (i.e., consumer) requests for hastened death? What implications are presented for the ethical integrity of medicine once the profession accepts physician assistance in patient suicide as one of several options it can provide to the terminally ill person? In this context, moreover, it is possible to argue that Pellegrino assumes a "prophetic" role for the medical profession, recalling the medical community to its foundational moral commitments.

"DOCTORS MUST NOT KILL"

In 1988, the *Journal of the American Medical Association (JAMA)* published a short, anonymous story titled "It's Over, Debbie" in one of its regular columns. The story related an episode in which a gynecology resident provided a lethal injection of morphine to an emaciated female patient who was suffering and dying from ovarian cancer.[2] The publication of the story provoked a firestorm of controversy within medicine, among bioethicists, and in the national media. Pellegrino joined three other distinguished physician-ethicists— Willard Gaylin, Leon Kass, and Mark Siegler—in a vigorous criticism of the resident's actions (as well as the editorial decision to publish the account).[3] Their commentary forcefully crystallized one position in what would turn out to be a diverse response by the medical (and bioethics) community to the story. Pellegrino and his colleagues maintained of "medical killing": "This issue touches medicine at its very moral center; if this moral center collapses, if physicians become killers or are even merely licensed to kill, the profession— and, therewith, each physician—will never again be worthy of trust and respect as healer and comforter and protector of life in all its frailty."[4] The seriousness of the issue was reiterated throughout the commentary: " . . . the deepest meaning of the medical vocation" had been violated by the resident in the "Debbie" story and by similar actions by other physicians throughout history; indeed, the authors claimed, "the very soul of medicine is on trial."[5]

The response by Pellegrino and his colleagues to the "Debbie" incident drew acclaim in part because of the distinctive way it framed the questions about the ethical integrity of medicine. The authors drew upon—and unified—utilitarian, deontological, and virtue-based concepts of ethics to mount a very compelling argument against this episode and future incidents of killing in the name of medicine. They invoked utilitarian themes to condemn such actions on the grounds that medicine will rend the fragile fabric of trust and respect upon which a healing relationship is based. The authors' appeals to medicine's "soul," "vocation," and "moral center" indicate that they believed the resident had violated values intrinsic to the identity of medicine as a *moral* practice. In addition, the influence of Pellegrino's philosophy of medicine is unmistakable in the commentary's observations about the character and integrity of the physician who participates in such actions: No longer a "healer" of disease-ridden patients or "protector" of vulnerable life, the image of the physician as killer is that of a "cold, . . . morally neutered technician."

To be sure, the commentary did not receive unanimous acclaim among the medical community or among bioethicists. The argument provided a moral touchstone, however, that subsequent discussions of the issue would have to address to be credible. The moral presumption, Pellegrino and his colleagues argued, lay not with patient autonomy but with a core vocational proscription against killing. If the medical community could not unite around *this* moral center, they seem to suggest, such a "community" ceases to exist; if medicine cannot affirm this principle as central to its vocation, its status as a moral practice and profession is irreparably diminished. The ethical integrity of medicine would be diluted to the point that its practitioners would be morally indistinguishable from plumbers, electricians, or computer repair persons—that is, the physician would be a technician who "fixes" an annoying problem but lacks an overarching sense of the human good that is to be served by his or her practice.

THE INTERNAL MORALITY OF
THE HEALING RELATIONSHIP

Pellegrino provided a fuller exposition for the purposes of medicine as an ethical vocation—and how that vocation is contradicted by physician assistance in suicide and participation in active euthanasia—at an international conference on medical ethics three years later. Even within that short time span, the medical and social context had evolved significantly from the "Debbie" controversy. Jack Kevorkian's assistance in the death of several terminally and chronically ill patients had raised nearly unanimous protestations, even among supporters of assisted suicide, but his actions had nonetheless riveted public attention on issues of technological prolongation of life, unbearable pain, and unnecessary suffering to which medicine seemed inadequately responsive. The public's receptivity to such an alternative was strikingly borne out by the best-selling book *Final Exit* by Hemlock Society founder Derek Humphrey.[6] Moreover, the conduct and advocacy of Dr. Timothy Quill offered the professional communities a public example of a conscientious and compassionate physician participating in the suicide of his patient.[7] The prospect of legalized "physician aid-in-dying"—a term that encompassed assisted suicide and lethal injections by physicians—had become a reality through a ballot initiative in Washington state, and proposed initiatives in California and Oregon sought to extend the trend.

In this changed context, Pellegrino's account of what he designated the "internal morality" of medicine provided a prophetic call to the medical community to reclaim its moral foundations and ethical integrity or risk ceasing to assume the responsibilities of medicine.[8] Pellegrino reiterated the claim in the *JAMA* commentary that the deliberate hastening of death by physicians through assisted suicide or active euthanasia (Pellegrino argues for the [im]moral equivalency of the practices) was not an issue toward which the medical profession could be morally indifferent; instead, it was a "defining" moral challenge about the meaning of being a physician. This is the case because of the nature of medicine and the goods internal to its practice that constitute its "internal morality."

For Pellegrino, medicine is fundamentally about "healing," which encompasses restoring the health of the patient, and seeking to make the patient "whole" as a person. In contrast to the common "fight or flight" response of medical professionals in the face of death—that is, to employ "aggressive measures" or "give up"—it is important for Pellegrino that the medical community recognize that healing can occur even in the dying process. As patients face the meaning of their morality and the significance of their life and achieve closure in their relationships, they can experience a wholeness and completeness to their life journey. This process is not solely the existential responsibility of the patient; Pellegrino argues that enabling a person to "die well"—free of pain, and in a manner consonant with the dignity of human beings—is an *obligation* of the physician. In this respect, there might be common ground between opponents and advocates of assisted suicide over the *ends* sought in care of the terminally ill, as suggested by Pellegrino's assertion that "a good death completes life with a finale befitting our true dignity as thinking, conscious, and social beings."[9] Thus, the dispute is largely over the *means* used to achieve these ends.

Pellegrino maintains that the achievement of healing, including a fitting and dignified end to a human life, presupposes a trusting relationship between physician and patient. This fiduciary relationship is fundamental to the meaning of the medical vocation, and Pellegrino is convinced that the relationship (and perhaps medicine as a profession) cannot survive accommodation of the practice of direct physician assistance or participation in a patient's death.[10] Although physicians must be more sensitive to the context and meaning of patient requests at the end of life—and less parsimonious in their use of medication to relieve pain—Pellegrino believes that the boundary between allowing patients to die from natural causes and causing the death of the patient through medical knowledge and expertise should not be crossed. Such actions, which are wrong in terms of general social morality and principles, also simply contradict the internal morality of medicine that defines it as a professional calling.

Pellegrino also questions assumptions held by advocates of assisted suicide and euthanasia regarding physician competence and character. Although physicians may be rightly criticized for doing too little in the face of intractable pain experienced by terminally ill persons, assistance in suicide or participation in active euthanasia asks too much of a human being committed to the vocation of healing. Such a possibility expands the enormous powers physicians already possess toward their patients, yet neglects the finitude and fallibility to which physicians are also subject. Indeed, Pellegrino notes, "the doctor is an ordinary human being called to perform extraordinary tasks."[11] Legalized power over life and death, coupled with the physician's ordinary limitations of finitude and fallibility, provide no confidence that such powers will not be abused.

As the debate over physician-assisted suicide has evolved over the past decade, Pellegrino's position has been a model of clarity, consistency, and integrity. Pellegrino has effectively articulated the central issues for the medical profession on the care and healing of terminally ill patients in the shifting economic and ethical contexts of the time. He has prophetically reminded his professional colleagues of their basic moral commitments, which seem incompatible with (popular) practices that bring the doctor to the threshold of death. I am inclined to agree with Pellegrino that assisted suicide and active euthanasia are defining issues for the internal ethos of the medical profession. In the remainder of this essay, I develop this claim further by looking at the way the debate within the medical community over legalized assisted suicide unfolded in one jurisdiction—the state of Oregon—in which the practice is lawful.

DEATH WITH DIGNITY AND DIMINISHED INTEGRITY

Citizen initiatives to legalize physician aid in dying were defeated in Washington state in 1991 and California in 1992, and proponents of legalization turned, for several reasons, to the initiative process in Oregon as a place to make both a last stand and a beach-head in their political effort.[12] A diverse group of advocacy groups united under the umbrella organization Oregon Right to Die drafted the Oregon Death with Dignity Act (DDA), with the intent to bring it before citizens of the state in the fall 1994 election.

The DDA contained some very significant changes from the failed predecessor initiatives. It did not use the expansive euphemism "physician aid-in-dying," instead opting for a legalistic description of acts that would be permitted under the law. The operative language of the DDA is that patients could make, and physicians could comply with, a "written request for medication for the purpose of ending [the patient's] life in a humane and dignified manner."[13] This language clearly limited the scope of the DDA to physician assistance in suicide and thereby rejected the attempt in the Washington and California initiatives to legalize active euthanasia.

The language of the DDA also made no reference to patient deaths carried out in accord with the statute as acts of *suicide*. Indeed, were the DDA to pass, "assistance in suicide" would continue to be prohibited based under existing Oregon statute. Thus, one euphemism—"prescribed medication to achieve a humane and dignified death"—replaced another ("physician aid-in-dying"). There was a simple political explanation for such language. Advocates of the DDA had discovered through preliminary polling data that when the language of *suicide* was used in interview questions, support for legalization proposals diminished by as much as 10 percent; this result tended to tip majority opinion against legalization.

In other words, the political strategy for making physician-assisted suicide publicly palatable was to describe it and define it so that it was conceptually, linguistically, and practically *continuous* with modes of caring for the terminally ill that were already accepted and embedded in medical practice. Thus, not only was there a deliberate effort to avoid bringing the DDA under the moral casuistry of *suicide*, the DDA was portrayed by its chief legal interpreter, Eli Stutsman, as an effort to "codify existing medical practice."[14] In short, the strategy of DDA proponents entailed denying that the DDA involved anything distinctive or novel for patients, physicians, or society. Consequentialist concerns about initiating slippery slopes could be rejected because medicine was portrayed as *already* engaged in practices similar to what the DDA proposed.

With the DDA initiative looming on the 1994 electoral horizon, the Oregon Medical Association (OMA) considered the DDA specifically, and physician-assisted suicide generally, in its annual delegates meeting in April 1994. This meeting proved indeed to be a defining moment for the OMA—although not in a way Pellegrino would welcome. The debate was initiated by a proposal from physicians opposed to the DDA that the OMA reaffirm its opposition to physician-assisted suicide and specifically declare opposition. A variety of perspectives on medical assistance in suicide ensued among the delegates; after several hours, it became clear that no resolution was possible. Finally, the participants agreed to a motion indicating that the OMA would "neither oppose nor endorse physician-assisted suicide." This result enhanced the prospects of passage for the DDA.

The debate process, despite its acrimony and polemics, indeed supported Pellegrino's contention that assisted suicide and active euthanasia concern the very core of the moral meaning of medicine. A debate of such intensity does not occur over peripheral issues or minutiae. Nonetheless, the outcome of the debate—the passage of the "neither . . . nor" motion—has all the hallmarks of what gives compromise a bad name: It was politically expedient, noncommittal, and evasive, and it lacked integrity. It reflected an avoidance or even abandonment of the moral conscience of medicine.[15] One need not agree with Pellegrino's position on killing in the name of medicine to claim that organized medicine has the resources in its ethical traditions to generate *some* kind of substantive and constructive position on the question. These substantive commitments and resources were compartmentalized, however, for the sake of procedural consensus. Yet—and here Pellegrino's earlier critique seems prophetic and prescient—if the substantive values that have guided medicine historically are relegated to the periphery, it becomes important to examine what constitutes and binds together physicians in a "community" or professional association.

For the OMA, the principle of autonomy replaced the historical ethical traditions of medicine. As the association's president said after the debate, Oregon physicians "need to hear from our patients on this. We need to hear from the people of Oregon what to do."[16] The principle of autonomy and self-determination is certainly a legitimate ethical concern, and it has often served as a moral corrective to the paternalistic pretensions of physicians. It is not a sufficient ethical condition for moral action, however. Moreover, in these particular circumstances, the OMA was not appealing to autonomy as a corrective for a paternalistic ethic but invoked it as a substitute in the absence of *any* ethic. Indeed, I know of no other realm of medicine in which physicians have been so willing to cede their power and professional authority to public preferences. This attitude makes the public the authority for determining the standards of good medical practice.

Pellegrino is harshly critical of what he calls "plebiscite ethics"—that is, of deciding weighty moral matters through the ballot box. After citing several examples of immoral laws and popular approval of violations of basic human rights, he argues, "Something more philosophically cogent than public opinion, national sentiment, or law is needed to make a cogent case for the moral acceptability of euthanasia."[17] Yet the professional organization responsible for developing and implementing practices of good medicine in Oregon seemed quite willing to let a fundamental matter of medical ethics be resolved by the *vox populi*. In this respect, the appeal to patient and citizen autonomy appears to be nothing more than moral evasion.

Although the "neither . . . nor" motion effectively kept the OMA on the sidelines during the political campaign to pass the DDA, its effects were neither politically nor morally innocuous. Offering a (noncommittal) resolution to the public is one thing; public *interpretation* of the resolution is another matter, especially if the statement expresses moral ambivalence or implies moral and professional indifference. As the campaign entered the weeks immediately preceding the public vote, the OMA's reticence about opposing physician assistance in suicide clearly was viewed as tacit and indirect acceptance of the practice as a possible option within medicine. Indeed, given the public status and stature of organized medicine in society, such an interpretation is readily understandable. That is, public discourse implied that if the organization authorized by society to determine standards of good and appropriate medical practice could not come to a conclusion about the professional status of something as significant professionally as participation in suicide, it would seem that professional assistance and/or cooperation with the practice could not violate any intrinsic value or internal morality of medicine.

This kind of public interpretation, and the practical evolution of its implications, is why Pellegrino and others are quite right to emphasize the value of trust in the healing relationship. To be sure, Pellegrino is most concerned to emphasize the necessity of trust within individual healing relationships, which cumulatively generates trust in the profession as a collective body. My point is that precisely because medicine as a profession is regarded as a social institution worthy of public trust, its pronouncements and actions are not only influential for practitioners but also carry some authority with the public and with patients. Thus, when the medical profession opts out of a public controversy, it gives the impression that it can live (and die) with whatever resolution the nonmedical sectors of society decide on. I believe that that is a mistaken conclusion to draw in the case of physician assistance in suicide, but it was nonetheless frequently drawn in public discourse and electoral rhetoric.

The DDA passed in November 1994, making Oregon the first jurisdiction in the world in which physicians could legally assist in the suicide of their patients—albeit by prescribing medication to bring about a humane and dignified death. The stance of the OMA in this circumstance must be assessed as a moral and professional failure, and Pellegrino's interpretation of what is at stake for medicine in the assisted suicide issue helps explain why such an assessment is warranted. First, the OMA discounted the ethical traditions of medicine. Physicians may not agree about whether these traditions proscribe physician participation in suicide in the way that Pellegrino claims, but discarding the traditions in favor of majority rule is simply mistaken. Instructively, in the waning weeks of the campaign for passage of the DDA the OMA president publicly broke with the stance of the American Medical Association and rejected its condemnation of the DDA on the grounds that "since [the DDA] is an Oregon issue, it would have been appropriate for [the AMA] to stay out of it."[18]

Somehow, the accidents of geography and membership in a political society took precedence over fidelity to the ethical traditions of the profession; the organization's pledge to affirm these traditions at a national level was now disparaged by the term "outsider." Ironically, whereas Pellegrino and others have vigorously argued for a morality that is *internal* to medicine, these traditions were deemed external or outside the professional parameters of the OMA. The implication of this position is that medicine is bereft of any ethical content; it reflects precisely the stance of the "morally neutered technician" about which Gaylin, Kass, Pellegrino, and Siegler had issued their warning. The professional can no longer claim the title of *healer;* instead, the physician is simply a *technician* who carries out the requests of the patient, whatever they may consist in, and oversees their implementation.

A corollary of the "neither . . . nor" motion regarding assisted suicide is a lack of concern about the goals and purposes of medicine as a profession and the goods internal to its practice. Pellegrino has offered one interpretation of these goals that focuses on promoting health and healing; certainly, other interpretations are possible—some of which may not be as incompatible with physician assistance in suicide as Pellegrino's. The OMA approach, however, implies that there is no internal morality to the medical profession; such morality as the OMA can claim is entirely extrinsic, defined by patients and citizens. The moral status of the profession has been surrendered to the claims of self-determination. Such an account cannot provide any ethical integrity for medicine; it leaves medicine at the whim of arbitrary social customs that fluctuate and change over time.

Finally, the OMA statement overlooks the centrality of trust in the physician-patient relationship. The culmination of this neglect was a significant misinterpretation in public discourse of what the OMA actually intended by the "neither . . . nor" motion. It is ironic that the OMA opted for professional silence and indicated the need to listen to the preferences of voters to get its professional cues. Patients and their families had long presented complaints about the inadequacy of care for the terminally ill. In particular, organized medicine was popularly perceived as failing to be responsive to continued objections to technological over-treatment and palliative under-treatment. Thus, the professional silence of the OMA followed a longstanding professional deafness as well. Such an approach does little to cultivate trust in the profession or in individual practitioners. It violates the fiduciary relationship that, for Pellegrino, is at the moral core of medicine.

PROFESSIONAL FRAGMENTATION

As a result of legal challenges, the DDA was enjoined from taking effect for nearly three years, until October 1997. This delay offered medical professionals an opportunity for considered reflection on some common goals of medicine and principles of ethics. The outcome of this deliberation, however, was fragmentation of the profession—as Pellegrino had anticipated several years previously.

During this three-year period, the OMA's "neither . . . nor" position made it the only medical association in the United States on record as not opposed to physician-assisted suicide. As the litigation dragged out, however, and a re-vote of the DDA was contemplated, a coalition of OMA physicians formed a new group, Physicians for Compassionate Care. This new group persuaded the delegates to the April 1997 OMA meeting to adopt (by a 121–1 vote) a resolution that described the DDA as "seriously flawed"—though it stopped short of condemning physician-assisted suicide in all circumstances,

What led to this change? The coalition of physicians that developed and successfully passed the 1997 resolution cited a controversial study from the Netherlands on lingering deaths from oral administration of barbiturates.[19] This evidence was coupled with arguments that assisted suicide would inevitably lead to euthanasia by lethal injection, perhaps as a recourse for patients in drug-induced comas. Although American physicians in general seem to favor the concept of assisted suicide for terminal patients—and a majority appear willing to participate in prescribing the needed medication—physicians clearly are less comfortable personally and professionally with administering lethal injection. Thus, the 1997 resolution seemed designed to undermine support for the DDA by raising the more fearsome specter of regularized lethal injection.

One consequence of the 1997 resolution was the beginning of professional fragmentation. The passage of the resolution was the catalyst for the formation of a second group, Physicians for Death with Dignity, who claimed (with some justification) that a vote of 122 persons should in no way be taken as the conclusive last word for a professional body with more than 5,700 members. It soon became clear—through exchanges in newspaper editorials, for example—that the membership of the OMA was not at all united behind the new resolution expressing condemnation of the DDA; indeed, it is not evident that the resolution represented a majority position within the OMA.[20] These patterns of internal dissent and professional fragmentation characterized this second round of medical debate over assisted suicide.

Paradoxically, whereas the "neither . . . nor" motion had effectively relegated the OMA to the political sidelines during the 1994 vote on the DDA, now two groups claiming to represent the ethical perspectives of medicine on assisted suicide presented themselves in public discourse as legislative support for a re-vote began to galvanize. Needless to say, their competing views only sowed confusion about whether medical professionals as an organized constituency had anything constructive to contribute to the public discussion. No one could claim that the profession was constituted by an "internal morality." Moreover, the unified front that Pellegrino and his colleagues had urged the profession to adopt in the wake of the "Debbie" case had been clearly and irreparably breached. The defining issue had turned out to be a divisive issue.

A brief consideration of the kinds of arguments presented by physicians opposed to the DDA in the second vote over the legalization of assisted suicide is important. A coordinator and spokesperson for the Compassionate Care physicians dismissed ethical arguments on the issue as "tangled territory" that could not be resolved or would be preempted by appeals to autonomy.[21] Instead, the group made its case for opposition on the basis that the DDA contained "fatal flaws" for medical practice, including:

- the failure of prescribed medication to hasten a peaceful death in many cases (a claim based almost entirely on anecdotal information);
- the immunity of physicians from liability in such cases, which was viewed as lowering the required standard of medical care or expressing abandonment of patients;
- the risks of error in physician diagnoses of terminal illness, raising the prospect of premature and unnecessary deaths (a study of more than 2,700 Oregon physicians indicated that 50 percent could not confidently predict that a terminally ill person would die within six months);[22]
- the risks that physicians would not diagnose depression accurately (28 percent of the physicians could not reliably diagnose depression)[23]—thus depriving some patients of counseling and raising questions about involuntary or possibly incompetent requests for medication.

Most of these "flaws" are procedural rather than substantive. These flaws could have been remedied by legislative action; indeed, most were discussed in the course of legislative debates. They are also largely speculative, matters of possibility rather than probability or actuality, inasmuch as they focus on what *might* happen should the law be implemented. The accuracy of these risk assessments could be evaluated only by permitting the practice to occur, perhaps under some "controlled" experimental conditions.

The "flaws" also speak to the fallibility of the physician—a point that Pellegrino has emphasized. This is a supporting reason for Pellegrino, however, not a decisive one. For him, the decisive reasons turn on ethical principles and the internal ethics of medicine. By contrast, the strategy adopted by the Compassionate Care physicians implicitly conceded the medical legitimacy of assisted suicide in many cases. Having opted for moral disarmament by dismissing substantive ethical arguments as "tangled territory," the group could argue that in individual *acts* of assisted suicide, things could go badly for the patient from a medical standpoint. It presented very little in the way of a compelling case, however, about a *practice* of assisted suicide.

The effort to repeal the DDA was decisively defeated by a vote of 60 percent to 40 percent in November 1997. This result left the OMA struggling to articulate practice guidelines for its members within the new medical world of legally sanctioned assisted suicide. Despite the OMA's "public" support of repeal and the internal dissent and fragmentation that the April resolution had prompted, the OMA was obliged to formulate some common ground for its fractious membership. To this end, the OMA issued a "statement of philosophy" and a "compliance checklist" following the vote. The philosophy embodied in these documents reiterated the association's support for comprehensive, palliative care at the end of life; the OMA also indicated, however, that it would provide physicians with resources to practice medicine—including the provision of assisted suicide in accordance with the law. The OMA pledged to undertake to protect the "sanctity of the doctor-patient relationship," particularly from regulatory intrusions.[24]

Although the OMA advanced the "statement of philosophy" rather late in the day, it at least finally tried to situate professional perspectives and roles in physician-assisted suicide within a concept of the object of medical practice. It is impossible, however, for a professional association to affirm positions of "neither . . . nor" (1994 to spring 1997), then "opposition" (spring to fall 1997), and then "compliance" (November 1997 onward) on something as critical to professional identity as assistance in suicide and still retain its ethical integrity and credibility. The change of position implies a malleable medical ethic, rather than a firm moral center, in the manner that Pellegrino and his colleagues sought to defend.

Moreover, it is difficult to know what to make of the "sanctified" status of the medical relationship. Although Pellegrino and others have affirmed the vital nature of the physician-patient relationship for medicine, they have used the language of *healing* rather than *sanctity* to describe the relationship and to prescribe moral norms internal to the relationship. A sanctified relationship, by contrast, refers to a relationship that is set apart, sealed off and inviolable from external intrusion. It is not evident, however, what internal moral norms should guide a medical relationship so demarcated—other than that of patient autonomy in the context of requests for assisted suicide.

As distinct from its confusing meaning, the *function* of the appeal to sanctity has become clearer as the DDA has been incorporated into medical practice over the past year. Such a relationship is intended to be a shield from public scrutiny for physician and patient alike. It carves out a relational sphere within which the relationship is deemed autonomous and asserts a claim of nonintervention. It is, in short, a version of an appeal to guarantees of privacy and medical confidentiality. Why, though, is that common language not used, instead of *sanctity?* Such language inevitably invokes an aura of religious meaning around the relationship—indeed, as though the intent is to prescribe a model of priest-penitent. Such a model again highlights the stringency of confidentiality in the relationship; given the practical actions to which the language grants moral and public dispensation, however, it seems especially inappropriate: a rhetorical appeal without substance.

CONCLUSION: RECLAIMING MEDICINE'S INTEGRITY

Pellegrino has maintained that the end-of-life controversies that currently embroil the medical profession place the soul of medicine on trial. At least in the case of Oregon— the only jurisdiction where physician assistance in suicide is legally sanctioned—a fair verdict would find the soul of medicine lacking in integrity, highly skilled at technical specialization but empty of ethical substance. The medical profession has ceded its leadership position in the care of terminally ill patients to task forces and regulatory subcommittees because it is a fragmented community, riven with internal dissent. By denying that there is any morality intrinsic to the practice of medicine, the profession has experienced a substantial diminishment of its credibility and has opted for an ethic of procedure defined by the political process.

The understanding of the physician as healer, even in the midst of the dying process, seems completely overlooked in the context of medical assistance in suicide. Although it is not accurate to see the role of participating physicians transformed to that of killer—because in this setting, the patient ultimately decides whether to use the lethal medication and thus bring about death—it is appropriate to refer to the physician as a technician who facilitates the autonomous choices of the patient. To paraphrase Max Weber: Specialists without spirit, technicians without conviction, the medical profession in Oregon believes it has blazed a groundbreaking path in the care of terminally ill patients.[25] Yet, as Pellegrino reminds us, medicine has traversed this trail of tears before, with horrific professional and social consequences.

I have described Pellegrino as a prophetic voice to the medical profession, seeking to call the community back to the fundamental moral commitments of the vocation of healer. Yet prophets do not only critique; they also propose alternatives that should be pursued. It is important to recognize that Pellegrino does not deny that there are understandable grounds for patient requests to have their death hastened. The remedy, however, does not lie in a resort to assisted suicide or active euthanasia. The moral recourse instead is in an unequivocal affirmation of the physician's obligations to "practice competent analgesia, to understand why the patient requests death, and to deal with and remove those reasons in a program of palliative care."[26] Insofar as physicians are reticent about using methods of pain control, reluctant about engaging the patient and his or her family in substantive discussions about the meaning of their requests to die, or unwilling to refer patients to hospice lest that be interpreted as surrender to the enemy of death, there is substantial space for physicians to build on and improve their current modes of caring for the dying. These new modes of caregiving could enable the profession to preserve its ethical integrity and warrant the term *healer* for the physician.

NOTES

1. P. Singer, *Rethinking Life and Death: The Collapse of Our Traditional Ethics* (New York: Oxford University Press, 1995).
2. "It's Over, Debbie," *Journal of the American Medical Association* 259 (1988): 272.
3. W. Gaylin, L. R. Kass, E. D. Pellegrino, and M. Seigler, "Doctors Must Not Kill," *Journal of the American Medical Association* 259 (1988): 2139–40.
4. Ibid., 2140.
5. Ibid., 2139.
6. D. Humphrey, *Final Exit: The Practicalities of Self-Deliverance and Assisted Suicide for the Dying* (Eugene, Ore.: Hemlock Society, 1991).
7. T. Quill, "Death and Dignity: A Case of Individualized Decision Making," *New England Journal of Medicine* 323 (1991): 691–94; T. Quill, *Death and Dignity: Making Choices and Taking Charge* (New York: W. W. Norton and Company, 1994).

8. E. D. Pellegrino, "Doctors Must Not Kill," in *Euthanasia: The Good of the Patient, The Good of Society,* ed. R. I. Misbin (Frederick, Md.: University Publishing Group, 1992): 27–41.

9. Ibid., 31.

10. Ibid., 34.

11. Ibid.

12. C. Campbell, "The Oregon Trail to Death," *Commonweal* 12 (1994): 9–11.

13. Oregon Revised Statutes, *The Oregon Death with Dignity Act,* ORS 127.800–ORS 127.995 (Salem: Oregon State Legislature).

14. C. Campbell, "The Oregon Trail to Death," 9.

15. C. Campbell, "When Medicine Lost Its Moral Conscience: Oregon Measure 16," in *Arguing Euthanasia: The Controversy Over Mercy Killing, Assisted Suicide, and the "Right to Die,* ed. J. Moreno (New York: Simon & Schuster, 1995): 140–67.

16. Ibid., 146.

17. Pellegrino, "Doctors Must Not Kill," 33.

18. C. Campbell, "When Medicine Lost Its Moral Conscience," 148.

19. Royal Dutch Society for the Advancement of Pharmacology, *The Administration of and Preparation for Euthanasia* (The Hague: Royal Dutch Society for the Advancement of Pharmacology, 1994).

20. C. Gordon and R. Loomis, "Doctors Protest OMA Not the Majority View," *The Oregonian* (Portland, Ore.), 15 October 1997, B9.

21. G. K. Hill, "Californian Will Lead Suicide Repeal Law Fight," *The Oregonian* (Portland, Ore.), 15 September 1997, A1.

22. Melinda A. Lee, Heidi D. Nelson, Virginia P. Tilden, Linda Ganzini, Terri A. Schmidt, and Susanne Tolle, "Legalizing Assisted Suicide—Views of Physicians in Oregon," *New England Journal of Medicine* 334 (1996): 310–15.

23. Ibid.

24. Oregon Revised Statues, *Oregon Death with Dignity Act.*

25. M. Weber, *The Protestant Ethic and the Spirit of Capitalism* (New York: Charles Scribner's Sons, 1958).

26. Pellegrino, "Doctors Must Not Kill," 32.

The Role of Reason, Emotion, and Aesthetics in Making Ethical Judgments

Erich H. Loewy

Medicine must wear a human face and make human judgments. Indeed, the question of how judgments are made is tacitly present throughout any work on philosophy of medicine in clinical medical education or, more recently, bioethics. To be a sentient being is to make judgments; to be a physician or medical educator is to make judgments that may critically affect many others. In this essay, I examine the role of various components of judging and the process by which judgments are made.

INTRODUCTION

What is the role of emotion in making ethical judgments? Should we, as Kantians would suggest, make such judgments on purely rational grounds, setting aside and ignoring our emotions, or should we—as care ethicists have proposed—make such judgments through personal involvement and caring? Many writers in the field of ethics have thought the latter approach to be unavoidable—although in the instance of care ethics, it seems anti-intellectual. Philosophers from Hutchison and Hume to Ayer have felt emotion to be central to the moral life.

In this essay, I argue that the division between emotion and reason in our thought processes—including the formation of ethical judgments—is an artificial dichotomy. Furthermore, I claim that aesthetics invariably will play some part in the final judgment. This is evident in medical practice. In medical practice, judgments are affected not only by the emotions a particular situation or patient engenders. Judgments, if they are to be useful, must not only be the product of careful thought and thorough analysis. Judgments invariably are—and perhaps ought to be—affected by the aesthetics of the situation.

I not only emphasize the combined roles of reason, emotion, and aesthetics but show the central role that curiosity and imagination play in the process of making judgments. By "making a judgment," I mean judgments that we make (consciously or unconsciously) and that we may never express, as well as judgments that we consciously or unconsciously make and express. Such judgments are expressed in evaluative terms of "good" or "bad," "ugly" or "beautiful," "interesting" or "boring," "valuable" or "worthless." These dichotomies could be called *evaluative areas*. A given judgment may partake of many of these "subjudgments" and be informed by several of these evaluative areas. Thus, we may say that X is a good thing (or a good person) but that X is ugly or boring, and that, all things considered, X has some particular as well as some general value. Note that the first set of terms tends to reflect an ethical judgment, the second an aesthetic judgment, the third an affective judgment, and the last a more global or overall judgment. Strict separation of these concepts or evaluative areas is not really possible. A global judgment is a composite expression of these other judgments or evaluative areas.[1]

EVALUATIVE INTERACTION

Making a judgment about anything (especially about anything of importance) entails a host of subjudgments. Each of these steps addresses one of the evaluative expressions or evaluative areas already mentioned. Such evaluative areas cannot be entirely separated from one another. The object, event, person, or proposition as well as the past, present, or contemplated course of action being judged are multifaceted. Each is judged evaluatively not only as good or bad but also as ugly or beautiful, interesting or boring, valuable or worthless (or as something lying between these evaluative poles).

Furthermore, these evaluative terms tend not only to overlap but to affect each other. What is considered to be ethically good or bad does not occur in pure culture; its being judged as ugly or beautiful, interesting or boring (and more) enter into the global judgment of its ultimate value or into the ultimate overall or global judgment made about it. Moreover, although we judge a situation, object, person, or proposition or past, present, or contemplated courses of action as good or bad, we are not uninfluenced by their being ugly or beautiful, interesting or boring—or, for that matter, appealing or not appealing to us. These judgments interpenetrate. Much as we try to prevent their affecting one another, they will inevitably—to a variable extent—intrude and intermingle with one another.

We do not make judgments one at a time. Even if we attempt to keep evaluative areas of judging separate, they inevitably affect one another. When we judge a person and say that person is good or bad ("blameworthy" or "praiseworthy," to use another set of evaluative terms), we are trying to strip away the aesthetic and affective terms as well as attempting to discount the overall usefulness in making these judgments. In an analytic sense, stripping away all but one evaluative area has great value (if it could ever be done). Although focusing on a given evaluative area and attempting to exclude others has great value as part of the overall process of judging, it is not entirely possible—nor does it constitute making a global judgment about the problem at hand. The result of such an analysis (necessarily stripped, as much as possible, of context or personal meaning) is only partial; without further work, it cannot lead us to making a judgment—either an abstract judgment or a judgment as to whether we will or will not act.

NARROWING EVALUATION

The process of stripping away all but one evaluative area can be exemplified by judgments made in a medical context. When physicians diagnose or decide on a course of treatment, they generally claim that they have done so purely on the "facts" known to them—both the facts of the patient and the facts as currently available in the pertinent medical literature. Even here, however, emotion and aesthetics are not entirely excluded. Physicians cannot escape past judgments and their consequences, and they cannot totally evade an emotional or aesthetic commitment of a particular diagnosis or course of treatment. Nor can they entirely exclude the initial appeal of a particular case or the context in which it presented itself. Physicians will—as best they can—try to put aside the very evident fact that the patient is an attractive and well-spoken woman or, on the other hand, a disheveled and foul-mouthed man. This is not entirely possible to do, and because judgments about a given case ultimately must address all of the features of a case and the context in which it presents itself, doing so is not entirely desirable.

In the real world of judging, the attempt to focus on only one evaluation area and exclude others is neither entirely possible nor entirely desirable. Hard as we may try not to be affected by beauty or ugliness at the same time we are determining whether a given object, event, person, or proposition or a past, present, or contemplated course of action is ethically laudable or blamable, we will not entirely succeed. Even if it were possible to make a judgment purely within one particular evaluative area, the result would be disconnected not only from the world in which we must live and to which the ethical question of how we ought to act must ultimately address itself but also from the essential features of the problem itself.

As such, basing a judgment on one evaluative area alone, without consideration of the other evaluative areas, cannot guide us in our everyday lives. Each subjudgment is necessarily affected by judgments within other areas. Psychopaths may have the capacity to separate areas by virtue of being blind to ethical judgments.[2] During the Italian invasion of Abyssinia, Ciano spoke about the aesthetic pleasure of gunning down helpless natives from his airplane; he may truly have seen only aesthetic beauty in his actions—though I doubt it—or he may have made a judgment about the weight each of these areas should carry in this instance and come to the conclusion that the suffering he inflicted was of little account. Such a judgment would be the one worth examining and eventually condemning.

The notion that our judgment will be entirely unswayed by the affective elements of our likes and dislikes is not only unlikely but perhaps even distinctly wrong. These components of judging, much as we try—and, indeed, ought to try—to separate them, will affect each other. The best we can do is to be aware of, examine, put into context, and deal justly with the effect they have on us and, therefore, on our ultimate judgments. When we need to make judgments, our personal likes and dislikes will inevitably intrude. Many times such "prejudices" can be harmful—especially when we deny them or fail to sufficiently examine and evaluate them; at other times, after thorough examination we may conclude that, in a given situation and context, the prejudice is quite appropriate and proper. Obligations are determined at least in part by prior relationships: The concept of *friend, spouse, teacher, doctor, trustee,* or *enemy* is defined in part by the obligations these relationships entail. Many of our relationships are not merely rooted in contract (as some fiduciary relationships may be) but more often are based on deep feelings one for another. To discount such relationships when making a judgment is not only impossible in fact, I would argue, but is likewise even undesirable in theory. Inevitably, the relationship itself is one of the pertinent considerations.

Instead of pretending that we are immune to all but rational and logical decision making, we must become aware of how different evaluative areas and relationships inevitably affect, fit into, and mix with one another. By being honest with ourselves, we can more clearly judge effectively, fairly, and (ultimately) well. In part this intermingling and interpenetration of various evaluative areas explains how a scene that we recognize as evil (such as mowing down natives) can appeal to someone because of its beauty. It may be the case that when we become aware of this discordance, we find the evil particularly repellent and the beautiful, perhaps, especially appealing.

JUDGMENT AND ACTION

When a judgment can be acted upon, a decision to act or not to act must be made. Our decision not to act in a set of circumstances in which we might do so is a form of acting, in an important moral sense—that is, given the option, we have no choice but to choose action or nonaction (usually a moral equivalent). If acting is possible, making a judgment will involve us in some course of action.

Before we act or fail to act, we must decide on the merits of the contemplated action. Similarly, we often judge past courses of action separately from the judgment that informed the question of "ought I" or "ought I not" act. We may agree with our friend Joe that Myrtle's hat was ghastly but disagree with his speaking to her about it; or we may agree that our friend Jim behaved like a boor but disagree with Henry when he strikes Jim. Many Germans in Nazi Germany were appalled at the anti-Semitic program of the Nazi state—and we can agree with their judgment. Yet many of the same people who found the program unacceptable nevertheless tacitly accepted it and did not act on their judgment. Depending on the particulars, we may agree or disagree with their failure to act on their convictions.

Consider an example. When a physician must decide to treat a critically ill patient or let her die, this judgment is not made by "reason" alone. Obviously there are some empirical "facts" that must inform the decision. Such facts, however, also come within the embrace of values: When the physician decides that there is virtually no chance of returning the patient to acceptable function, the physician not only makes a value judgment about what is and what is not "acceptable" (and, we hope, makes such a judgment on the patient's terms); because one can never have absolute certainty, the physician must decide about what counts as "virtually no chance." Such a value judgment is not made only in terms of "good" or "bad." The fact that the judgment involves a lovely and appealing lady rather than a chronically inebriated derelict will play a role, regardless of whether it should.

Another example involves physician-assisted suicide or active voluntary euthanasia. A physician may search his or her soul and conclude that it would be kindest to help a patient to end his or her life. Factors that enter into such a judgment are not simply those that can be expressed in terms of "good" or "bad"—though that is how physicians usually express these judgments. Decisions of "ugly" or "beautiful" will, perforce, have some effect; the fact that the patient's room has an offensive and ineradicable stench or that the patient is a particularly pretty young girl cannot help but enter into the equation. Having made such a judgment, the physician must then make an entirely separate judgment: to act or not to act. If a physician fears that to act might entail criminal liability, his or her decision will be affected by far more than the good/bad or ugly/beautiful judgment. Evaluative terms that deal with self-interest and utility will inevitably enter the judgment. Furthermore, even if the physician judges that helping patients to die is morally offensive, extreme pity for a particular patient may motivate a quite different decision with regard to acting.

These examples are not intended to provide a particular answer. I offer them to illustrate the complexity of such a situation and to show the virtual impossibility—as well as the moral problem—of separating such evaluative areas. Again, the way we ultimately act clearly is informed by a complex range of decisions that are not made out of context but are necessarily intimately entwined with one another.

AFFECTIVE ELEMENTS

Emotions (the "passions," as Aristotle and Hume would have it) have been defined as the affective part of consciousness. Because *affective* is defined as what appeals to our emotions, the definition is circular. In neurological terms, the limbic system is what deals with our emotions—but that description merely serves to localize physically that which we have failed to define. For the purpose of this discussion, I use the term *emotion* as something that relates to states of feeling. Reason, on the other hand, deals with the faculty that some have termed the "faculty of the mind." *Mind* or *thought* inescapably has "brain" or "central nervous system" as the necessary condition of its existence. It relies on the same general (albeit not specific) substrate as emotion. I use the term *reason* to denote the capacity of comprehending, sorting out, and differentiating. This term includes the capacity to remember (memory) and to integrate that which has been sorted out and differentiated into that memory. Last, but not least, the term *reason* includes the capacity to use logical processes to arrive at tentative conclusions.

Saying that reason and emotion have the central nervous system as the necessary condition for their existence does not reduce either reason or emotion to biology or anatomy. I am merely making the claim (supported by innumerable observations and experiments) that having emotions or reasoning requires the presence of certain parts of the central nervous system. Dividing emotion and reason from one another is a useful heuristic device. Dividing them into entirely watertight compartments creates a dualism that does not stand up to systematic inquiry. I argue that emotion and reason are resident in the same general substrate (reason in the neo-cortex, emotion in the limbic system); that they consequently must be—and in fact are—interconnected and mutually interactive; and that, in fact, in everyday existence they can effectively complement each other as we deal with our scientific as well as our moral problems.

By *aesthetic,* I mean a judgment made that something is beautiful or ugly—in other words, a judgment depending on taste. An aesthetic experience is a consequence of an explicit, internalized, or tacit judgment. Such a judgment and such an experience depend on emotion *as well as* reason.

When we contemplate any action, "What ought I do?" is the central question. This question is as important for an action dealing with a technical question ("What ought I do when I want to change this tire?") as it is for a moral question ("What ought I do when I must decide whether to tell the truth or to lie?"). Finding a proper answer to any of these questions implies far more than merely a rational exercise: It requires *judgment.*

This situation obtains with regard to questions of ethics, technical questions, or—as is most frequently the case—questions that have technical as well as moral aspects. Judgment (also called "discernment") is the capacity to make choices and differentiate between different courses of action, options, offerings, or relationships; it is a complex act that is not reducible to any one of its components. Making a good judgment means making a judgment that has picked from among an array of different factors the action that, all things considered, is the most appropriate for the particular context within which the choice is made. This process obviously is a complex task; it depends on experience with similar cases in the past. Furthermore, discerning what is most appropriate requires experience and a definition of appropriateness—a separate judgment that likewise has a variety of components.

In seeking to answer questions and make judgments about ways of acting that we recognize as being in the "moral" realm, different thinkers have appealed to different components of this composite. Some, such as Hume, have sought to find answers in our emotions—not necessarily because they felt that following our emotions was "right" but because following our emotions was all that we were capable of doing. Indeed Hume goes so far as to claim that not only is following our emotions what we do when we confront such problems but that it is what we by rights *ought* to do. Hume's assertion that "Reason is and by rights ought to be the slave of the passions," modified somewhat in his later writings, exemplifies that position.

> Nothing can oppose or retard the impulse of passion, but a contrary impulse; and if this contrary impulse ever arises from reason, that latter faculty must have an original influence on the will, and must be able to cause, as well as hinder any act of volition. But if reason has no original influence, 'tis impossible it can withstand any principle, which has such an efficacy, or ever keep the mind in suspense a moment. Thus, it appears that the principle which opposes our passion, cannot be the same with reason, and is only called so in an improper sense. We speak not strictly and philosophically when we talk of the combat of passion and of reason. Reason is, and ought only to be the slave of the passions, and can never pretend to any other office but to serve and obey them.[3]

In this view, reason is employed as a tool of the passions: The passions give us the goal; reason, at best, can give us only the means.

At the other extreme are thinkers such as Kant who look at emotions (the passions) with fear or with hostile skepticism: Although emotions and the inclinations to which they lead are not necessarily evil, they are quite apt to corrupt judgment and ought not be allowed to enter into moral decisions. Our task is not only to bridle but indeed to suppress our passions entirely and to let reason control them completely. Reason and reason alone should set the goal. Reason also should choose the means; the passions are likely to mislead us.

Such thinkers feel that, at best, our inclinations may coincide with what reason tells us—the more so when reason has carefully schooled the passions. Yet just as often our inclinations will lead us down the wrong path. It follows that persons who resist their inclinations to follow the voice of reason are acting meritoriously or in a praiseworthy manner. For Kant, following one's inclination when duty and inclination coincide is neither blameworthy nor praiseworthy.[4] Suppressing our inclinations to adhere to a duty prescribed for us by reason *is* acting in a praiseworthy manner.

Hume does not claim that the passions are superior to reason in making judgments—merely that in the way we are built, the primacy of the passions is inevitable. Kant, on the other hand, does not deny the importance the passions can have in influencing our judgments but claims that if we are to act prudentially or ethically reason not only can but must have the final upper hand. Under this view, the more our judgments are the product of reason and the more we discount our emotions, the more our judgments will be truly ethically appropriate.

It would be wrong to claim that Kant failed to find some place for emotion in the making of ethical judgments. Kant is right when he claims that one cannot have an obligation to feel an emotion. Having or not having an emotion or an inclination is beyond our immediate control: Emotions just are. As skeptical as Kant was of the role of compassion (*Mitleid*) and as much as he denied a central role to it, he nevertheless acknowledged the importance of compassion. Indeed, he went so far as to claim that although we do not have a perfect duty to cultivate the feeling of compassion, we do have an imperfect duty to do so:

> Even though it is not in itself a duty to experience "*Mitleid*" (suffering because of the suffering of another) and so also "*Mitfreude*" (joy because of the joy of another), it is a duty to participate actively in the fate of another. Hence we have an imperfect duty to cultivate the sympathetic natural (aesthetic) feeling in us. . . .[5]

AESTHETICS AND MORAL JUDGMENT

Another factor to which I have already alluded is often overlooked and can play a significant role in motivating our judgments and consequent actions: aesthetics—an appreciation of the beautiful (or a realization of the ugly) rather than an appreciation of the "true" (or "false") or the "good" (or "evil"). Aesthetic appreciation partakes of both reason and emotion. It may, at times, be regarded as mediating between these two.

As Dewey already remarked and as all will readily recognize, we frequently use aesthetic language when describing moral actions.[6] On the other hand, we may use terms usually used in moral evaluation to describe aesthetic experience. We describe the raiding of the ghetto in *Schindler's List* or attacks on minorities on our streets as ugly; we describe the saving of a child or the lives of persons who have devoted themselves to the service of others as beautiful. We instinctively use aesthetic language to describe ethical judgments. Likewise, we use the terms *good* and *bad* (and the various terms in between) to describe a performance of Beethoven's *Eroica*. We unhesitatingly use aesthetic language to describe ethical judgments. We likewise—albeit less clearly and less commonly—describe aesthetic experience in language usually used for moral evaluation. Whether one concludes that these were originally the terms of aesthetic evaluation that have become used in the moral sphere or terms initially used in moral evaluation that have been transposed to the moral sphere—or whether one concludes that these are terms initially used in moral evaluation that have been transposed to the aesthetic realm or whether one concludes that these are terms that denote any kind of approbation or disapprobation of anything—the conclusion remains unchanged: Intuitively, we accept these as fitting terms in both spheres. Thus, there is at least one common thread—that of approbation or disapprobation of whatever we are evaluating.

In this regard, if someone remarks on the aesthetic beauty of watching a fire devastate a village of thatched huts, we feel a strong and troubling dissonance between what is aesthetically appreciated and could well be counted—absent the context in which it occurs—as beautiful in terms of color or power and what is, in fact, happening in moral terms. We are appalled when a soldier finds the sight of an exploding tank "beautiful" for the very reason that what is aesthetically beautiful must be evaluated within its own context and not bereft of its own context. Dewey is quite clear about the connection between the moral good and the aesthetically beautiful:

> One of the earliest discoveries of morals was the similarity of judgment of good and bad conduct with the recognition of beauty and ugliness in conduct. Feelings of the repulsiveness of vice and the attractiveness of virtuous acts root in aesthetic sentiment. . . . The sense of justice, moreover, has a strong ally in the sense of symmetry and proportion. The double meaning of the word "fair" is no accident. . . . The modern mind has been much less sensitive to aesthetic values in general and to those values in conduct in particular. Much has been lost in direct responsiveness to right. The bleakness and harshness often associated with morals is a sign of this loss.[7]

Like all other capacities that are components of consciousness, aesthetic feelings—defined as the appreciation of the beautiful or ugly—are resident in the central nervous system. More than other components of consciousness, however, aesthetic feelings are prone to social and experiential conditioning. When we perceive a given object, person, or event in the present or in the past, as well as when we evaluate a particular course of action, we inevitably and inescapably use reason and emotion, as well as, in some way, our aesthetic sense. These components of judgment are inseparable. When we make judgments, they inevitably affect each other.

Aesthetic appreciation appears to have evolved quite late. Although there is ample evidence that animals endowed with fairly well-developed central nervous systems can "reason," feel pain, and have emotions, there is little evidence that animals have aesthetic appreciation (except, perhaps, for a rudimentary form of aesthetic appreciation in primates). Nor, except for primates, is there any evidence that animals have a sense of wonderment. They appear to use "reason" to solve practical problems, but they are unlikely to wonder about the nature of the problem they are solving: They seek to determine where a light is coming from but do not appear to wonder about the nature of the light itself.

REASON, EMOTIONS, AESTHETICS

In this section, I attempt to demonstrate that the process of making moral judgments entails interactions among at least these three components and that experience helps us to find a balance among them. I claim that the relationship among reason, emotion, and aesthetics is not a relationship in which one can properly be allowed to dominate the others. I suggest instead that such a complex relationship is best envisioned as a homeostatic balance. In a practical sense, this balance is mediated through our experience, which occurs within a community of others.[8] I argue that the balance is socially mediated: In part, at least, our social nexus determines how much weight we give to one or the other.

Making judgments—whether these judgments are about ethics or about other matters—is, above all, a learning experience: Our experience grows as our discernment becomes more refined, and our judgments, which are never absolutely good, become better. Such learning takes place in the embrace of community. Although such judgments are not determined by our community, at the very least they are modulated by the community and by our understanding of our relationship with it and with all others within it.

Our understanding of ethics, like our understanding of anything else, can never be complete. We hope to do less badly tomorrow what we did not do well today or do better tomorrow what we did reasonably well today. As our understanding of ethical judgments evolves, moreover, so does our understanding of what we mean by "reasonably well."

To understand how reason, emotions, and aesthetics operate, I also turn my attention to two other capacities that all sentient beings share: curiosity and imagination. I claim that these two capacities are necessarily prior to our reasoning, feeling emotion, or having an aesthetic experience.

Curiosity and Imagination

I define *curiosity* as an urge to investigate and to know. These two urges are not the same. If investigation is to lead to at least tentative "knowing," it must be connected by a series of steps. The first step is to engage the imagination. Imagination offers hypotheses that reason subsequently tests. Each step along the way is stimulated by curiosity, much as enzymes or catalysts facilitate or speed up reactions. Although neither curiosity nor imagination can be defined as entirely emotional or as reason, they are ultimately connected to and serve to interconnect both. In a sense, curiosity is affective: That is, it is a feeling leading to action.

Curiosity is an inborn trait of all higher beings that obviously is essential for and precedes meaningful cognition. Curiosity causes us to investigate our sense impressions; it leads us to seek out their essence and look for their meaning. Curiosity is present in all higher species and is evident almost from birth. Infants examine their toes, puppies examine the edge of their bedding, and birds flap their wings and peek outside the confines of their nest. All wonder about what something is before they start to explore and conjecture. Curiosity leads to wonderment, and wonderment ultimately connects curiosity to imagination. Moreover, curiosity has distinct survival value: If human and higher nonhuman animals failed to investigate their sense expressions, random appearance or movement would fail to be translated into appropriate action.

Imagination refers to the ability or faculty of forming mental images. Common to reason and imagination is the capacity to see analogies. Imagination engages feelings if only because it is energized by the affective part of curiosity. Imagination, however, has more of a rational component of comprehending, sorting out, and suggesting. It presents reason with a number of possible hypotheses that reason then tests. Reason linked to, stimulated by, and challenged by curiosity and imagination is not entirely separable from emotion.

I do not argue that reason, emotion, aesthetic experience, curiosity, and imagination are arrayed in a linear arrangement; I claim that they are interactive, that they are mutually fortifying and corrective, and that the relationship can be conceptualized as homeostatic. These components of judging are not in conflict with one another but in balance, and they are mutually corrective in pursuit of the common goal of a proper and equitable judgment. The metaphor of the compost heap springs to mind. Stuart Hampshire has pointed out that our life experiences are not an aggregate—like a heap of stones that remain separate as one is piled on another—but organic, like the components of a compost heap: They do not stand alone but mingle, interpenetrate, and interreact with one another until a new whole is produced. Although that new whole consists of its components and these components are the necessary condition of a particular compost heap, they are no longer readily recognizable.[9] When I claim that reason, emotion, aesthetics, curiosity, and imagination interact when we make judgments, I am not merely making an observation. I not only claim that this is the case but indeed make the more radical claim that moral judgments not only are but ought to be affected by all of these components.

Essentially—especially in health care ethics—we make two types of judgments. One deals with "identified" (known) lives and the other with "unidentified" (statistical) lives. Physicians and other health care professionals customarily make the former judgment at the bedside; a judgment about terminating life support serves as an example. Judgments about unidentified or statistical lives are made remotely. They are made in boardrooms or other settings in which decisions about groups of people must be made. An example might be hospital policy regarding "do not resuscitate" policy or, on a communal level, decisions about rationing of scarce resources.

Such a differentiation between judgments about identified and unidentified lives is not peculiar to ethics: When physicians choose a given treatment for a given patient, they are dealing with identified lives; when they write books or articles and make recommendations for the treatment of a particular condition, they are making recommendations for unidentified lives. Nor is this differentiation peculiar to health care: When judges judge defendants, they deal with identified persons; when legislators make laws, they deal with unidentified lives. If such judgments are to be well made, both reason and emotion must play a part in them.

When we deal with identified lives (persons we know or about whom we know), our emotions are aroused first. The emotion is likely to be compassion (the capacity to feel "with" someone his or her joys or woes) but may, if the person is an enemy, be the converse. Here reason must interpose between our emotion and our action. Acting on emotion alone can cause us to do destructive things: A physician who feels uncontrolled compassion for a patient in pain may fail to do an essential but very painful task. Acting from uncontrolled emotion may lead persons to do unjust things to their enemies. I call this tempering of compassion by reason "rational compassion."

On the other hand, when we deal with statistical or unidentified lives (persons we do not know or of whom we have no personal knowledge or future persons), we tend to address their problems with reason alone. When that happens, we may make inhumane decisions: Welfare recipients may suddenly be cut off from benefits and their children made hungry; aliens may be deprived of certain benefits and, therefore, thrown into abject poverty in their old age; brutal rationing decisions that negatively affect many persons who lack recourse may be made. Here reason must be modified by compassion. I call this process "compassionate rationality."

In both cases, curiosity and imagination connect reason and imagination. Imagination offers us several hypotheses about what is the case, as well as about contemplated courses of action, that reason then tests. Thus, a physician may decide to inflict pain on a patient to save his or her life; on the other hand, one may decide not to harm an enemy one hates and whom our emotions would impel us to harm. With regard to compassionate rationality (or, if you will, emotion directed by reason), curiosity and compassion mediate. When we make judgments about unidentified lives, curiosity and imagination work together—curiosity to ask the question, "What would it be like to be in the shoes of that person?" and imagination to go at least part of the way toward finding an answer. Curiosity and imagination allow us to realize that unidentified lives are not merely statistical but very real (past, present, or future) lives that we simply have not identified.

Aesthetics

If we were to make judgments about identified or unidentified lives guided purely by reason or emotion alone, unfortunate results would occur. Where does aesthetic feeling fit in? Aesthetics obviously does play a role in our everyday decision making. When we are confronted with concrete problems in health care ethics, the fact that one course of action is ethically repellent whereas another is not inevitably enters into our judgment. Such a state of affairs, however, describes but does not morally justify such a situation. Whereas I have claimed that emotion and reason not only do but ought to interact in making sound ethical judgments, the role of aesthetics in such judgments is far more tenuous.

The problem of the role of aesthetics in ethical judgments can be called the *Schindler's List* problem. In one scene, while the ghetto is devastated and its inhabitants savaged, the camera flashes to an SS officer sitting at an old piano playing Bach—and doing so beautifully. We know that Eichmann relaxed from his labors by playing Mozart sonatas with a friend. What role, if any, does aesthetics play in our moral life? What role did it play in theirs?

Beauty for Kant, as Dewey put it, is "remote from all desire, action, and stir of emotion."[10] Therefore, the question of what the SS man heard and the question of the influence of aesthetics on ethical judgments is moot: Ethical judgments are (or at any rate ought to be) free of empirical or emotional influence.

My argument is not only that aesthetics invariably play a role in individual as well as general judgments, not only that the function of aesthetics must be as conscious as possible, but also—far more radically—that aesthetics is part of the moral life and that without it, the moral life would be severely impoverished.[11] That argument, however, does not answer our *Schindler's List* problem: It fails to explain how monsters such as Eichmann or the SS officer in *Schindler's List* could appear to appreciate Bach or Mozart and still commit atrocities or cause them to be committed. Following Dewey, I claim that the cultural and personal context in which an aesthetic experience takes place conditions not only the way the experience is perceived and the way it is understood but, most importantly, the way it is interpreted and utilized. Human beings endowed with normal senses will undoubtedly hear the notes, sequence, and rhythm of what the SS man plays in the same way. A person coming from a similar cultural context as the SS man (a central European context, in that case) is likely to perceive the experience of Bach similarly: Such a person would not only hear the same notes, sequence, and rhythm but would find them pleasing, if not beautiful. Persons within that same context, because of personal differences in their own history, may associate different things with this same piece of music: They may be put into a mood similar to that when they first heard it with their grandparents or experience a mild return of grief if their past experience exposed them to this particular piece at a sad time of their lives. The SS man and Albert Schweitzer might or might not react in similar ways.

For some persons, an aesthetic experience (say, a Mozart symphony) is only a way of whiling away their time—a form of amusement that does something for them but not to them. For others, an aesthetic experience enables a state of transcendence in which we are taken "out of ourselves" and our everyday mundane concerns. Such an experience does not occur to the same person in the same way every time he or she experiences a given work of art; much depends on the setting and context. When it occurs, however, it takes such a person beyond his or her immediate concerns.

It is quite possible that the SS man gained more from playing Bach than a finger exercise or an amusement. Terrible as that is to realize, he seems to have experienced a form of transcendence not altogether different from what Schweitzer may have experienced playing the same piece. They diverge in the ultimate state to which they are brought by that music. They may both experience transcendence, both be brought out of themselves; the difference, one suspects, may lie in what they are brought to—in what they *do* as a result of this state. The precise difference may lie here, and that difference is intimately connected with the specific cultural, historical, and personal context of each person. The SS man came out of a society that had become distorted, a society in which what was formerly considered right had abruptly been labeled wrong, and what was formerly considered good had become bad. In such a truly diseased society, persons not endowed with a strong inner core of uprightness were easily perverted. For persons who shared in the disease of their culture, everything else they did, thought, or were brought to was affected.

Persons who are "brought out of themselves" cannot be entirely brought out of their cultural context. In a sense, we are brought out to something similar from whence we came: That is, our vision of what is greater than we, what we strive for, and what we emulate depends in large measure on the very culture, context, and personal experience from which we started. Persons taken beyond themselves in a Nazi culture were apt to be taken to the place from whence they came—a place in which the parochial vision of particularism, of blood, soil, and race, prevailed. The universal vision for which Schweitzer strove and was considered admirable in his particular day and culture was now despicable. In both cases (the SS officer's, as well as Schweitzer's), transcendence supported their prior commitment.

When all is said and done, aesthetics may play a role in the moral life by taking persons "out of themselves" and giving their thoughts, feelings, and passions free reign. In so doing, art and aesthetic experience may create a free space for persons affected by it that allows them the sort of reflection that is difficult to carry on while they are in immediate contact with the more mundane world. Furthermore, aesthetic experience may act as a catalyst to strengthen sensitivity and connect us to our fellow beings. What we do with this space is very much a product of our deepest self and of its prior conditioning. Ultimately, our aesthetic experience may say more about us as human beings than it does about the particular experience itself.

MAKING JUDGMENTS

The initial sorting out of a judgment tends to take place on an abstract level. The process of translating or not translating a judgment into action takes place at a more concrete level. All things being equal, the more abstract a judgment, the more it will be influenced by reason; the more concrete (and the more personal) a judgment, the more emotion and aesthetics may enter in. Abstract judgments may be about statistical or unidentified lives or, on a lower level of abstraction, about a particular situation or a particular action in an abstract situation. Judgments about acting or refraining from acting in concrete situations are very much about identified lives—the life of the actor as well as that of the person or situation acted on. Even abstract judgment is not bereft of some emotional and some aesthetic components. Persons have certain feelings about certain subjects—even about abstract judgments. When scientists work in the laboratory, they often relate feelings that are very much aesthetic feelings. The evaluative terms they use underline such a statement: Scientists often speak of "a beautiful solution" to a scientific problem or "a lovely theory"—and with good reason.

Making a judgment does not necessarily denote concrete action or even the possibility of concrete action. When we judge a historical event or person we often cannot act, except to praise or condemn the event or person publicly. When we judge a work of art before us, the only action we might take is one of overt expression. When the possibility of concrete action exists, however, a judgment to act or to refrain from acting must connect the initial judgment with the ultimate action or nonaction.

When we must make a judgment about a situation, object, event, person, or proposition or the ethical status of a past, present, or contemplated course of action (even whether it can be considered to have been wise), we necessarily invoke an admixture of various evaluative areas. When we judge a concrete situation, the types and strength of the particulars that compose such a situation will determine the preponderance of one evaluative area within the composite: The more personally involved we feel, the more emotive and aesthetic elements play a role; the farther the situation is from us, the less the force of emotion or aesthetics will be. Past courses of action, likewise, are easier to judge if they are remote; not only are we likely to feel less emotion about them, we also are apt to succeed in getting and accepting more diverse information. Present or contemplated courses of action are nearer to us and therefore are more likely to have greater emotive and aesthetic evaluative areas mixed with the rational.

This analysis explains why historical writing needs what we have come to call "proper perspective"—a perspective that is sufficiently distant from the event and in which the writer is not personally involved. On the other hand, such an approach also has problems: The very act of having oneself been involved allows one to see in a way in which the so-called dispassionate (or, at least, more dispassionate) observer cannot. Both approaches have advantages and disadvantages; both are needed for a real appreciation of a historical event. The value of oral history lies exactly in the intimate contact of the person speaking with the event he or she describes. Alternatively, relative lack of emotion, remoteness and distance, is as valuable to the inquiry as the presence of emotion is when a person who was involved is relating the story.

In general, when we make judgments about predetermined goals we make more concrete judgments than when we make judgments about the goals themselves. For example, we can think more easily, more clearly, and more "rationally" (by which we generally mean "unemotionally") about our medical goals than we can think about the means we might need to employ to gain these goals. Often—but not invariably—choosing means (ventilators, surgery, chemotherapy) involves more emotion than does choosing goals.

The fact that emotion often plays a greater role when we choose means than it does when we choose goals is evident when patients are asked to formulate "advance directives"—to make determinations in the fullness of their decision-making capacity about options for a time when such decisional capacity might be lost. In general, patients will quite readily describe what kind of quality of life or lifestyle they might consider acceptable and which they might consider to be a "fate worse than death itself." They may tell you that nursing home existence would be quite acceptable, provided the nursing home was decent, or they might decide the contrary. Such judgments, of course, are not made entirely by reason alone; after all, much depends on how they "feel" about the options, how much the aesthetic qualities of such an existence enter into the judgment, and so forth. Such decisions, however, are apt to be less emotional than are decisions about the use of some means, especially a means held to be particularly unpleasant or aesthetically particularly repellent—for example, the use of a mutilative surgical procedure or a ventilator, resuscitation, or chemotherapy. Some analysts will argue that such a judgment is not about an ethical problem; others will find it rich in ethical content. Assuredly, it is a value judgment in which a variety of evaluative areas have to interact and find their proper balance.

ETHICAL JUDGMENT

Consider what most persons would consider a strictly ethical judgment: the generic judgment about whether to continue life support when consciousness is permanently gone. Such a generic judgment will be informed by far less emotion than will any judgment involving discontinuing a ventilator or discontinuing a feeding tube in a particular patient at a particular time and place. Part of the reason may be that a judgment made about goals seems more remote than a judgment made about the means to be used to attain those goals, but that explanation can be only part of the reason.

In a sense, judging an abstract situation means concretizing it—that is, through the power of our imagination we render it "visible" to our inspection. Before we can do that, curiosity must have prompted our examination. Even when we deal with mathematics—perhaps the most abstract human activity—this "making things visible" takes place. To say that two and two are four or that a given proposition in calculus is such and such requires one to apprehend these propositions in terms we can visualize and therefore understand. To say to someone that he or she should "envision" something is to invite that person to do just that. When composers work on a score and can "hear" it as they work, they are rendering the abstraction of the notes concrete—in this case, audible. They do this through their imagination, disciplined and fortified by memory. Composers such as Beethoven, who became deaf as an adult but composed great works of music, are engaged in this activity whenever they compose, perform, or conduct. Had Beethoven been born deaf, his imagination alone would hardly have sufficed: Imagining sounds when one is entirely deaf, or light or color when one is entirely blind, is possible only by an act of recall—an amalgam of imagination dipping into the source of memory. By dipping into the storehouse of memory, such persons can imagine the abstract notes cast against the background of sounds remembered.

When ethicists ponder the various courses of action in a given problematic situation, they make that situation "visible" in much the same way. Imagination allows them to concretize the situation by dipping into a storehouse of memory and imagining the particular cast against the background of the abstract. Curiosity prompts them to do so.

Different persons dipping into different experiences concretize things in different ways. When they come together in dialogue to share this experience and to converse and communicate, a new, shared, experience emerges. This shared experience helps us formulate communal judgments. Such shared experiences and interchanges cannot be reduced to their individual parts. What emerges cannot be reduced to the summing of individual opinions, viewpoints, or judgments. Although this conversation inevitably is a social activity, it need not be verbal. It happens when we "really" read, when we write meaningful letters to one another, or when we exchange various forms of artistic expression. Intellectual life is not possible without this dialogue. Without this dialogue it would never even start, except as a very primitive shadow of itself, and without its nourishment it would be impoverished and ultimately would wither and die. Such dialogue is what teaching and learning—as well as reading and writing—are all about.

CONCLUSION

Making ethical judgments is complex. Like all other judgments, ethical judgments are informed by a variety of factors. I have argued that these factors (reason, emotion, aesthetics, curiosity, and imagination) not only do but ought to act and be allowed to act together if a judgment that we and those affected by it can live with is to be made. Yet even if we grant that our judgments are and even, perhaps, ought to be informed by such factors, questions remain: Which of these components, and under what circumstances, should take the lead role? How can these components of judgment fit together?

I have argued that the various components of our judgments (reason, emotion, aesthetics, curiosity, and imagination) act together and form a compost heap. The "evaluative areas," even though they may initially be conceived as separate entities, likewise intermingle and form such a mélange. The question of what role each of these components and judgment areas should play remains. The answer to this question obviously will differ depending on the nature of the judgment to be made; perhaps at least as important, the answer to the question depends on the community in which it is made. As individual judges, we are socialized and conditioned to judge in certain ways. Our past experiences (which we must rely on to balance the various components and evaluative area of judgment) are conditioned and, in a sense, translated to us by and through the community of which we are an integral part.

I do not claim that as decision makers we are prisoners of society or automatons programmed to judge in certain ways. I do claim that the role of socialization is significant and must not be overlooked. If we wish to encourage good judgments (judgments that all individuals within a community can live with, as well as judgments that the community can live with), we need to pay more attention to the structure of the community and the education such a community affords to its members. Judgments made on a personal level and for known lives (those, for example, made by physicians at the bedside) are directed by and made within the context of judgments that have been made for unknown lives: The known lives that physicians deal with today are the unknown lives that they dealt with yesterday.

Furthermore, and most important, both of these types of judgments are made within the embrace of a particular society and conditioned by the values and attitudes of that society. This society ultimately is a mix of all of its members—a compost heap. The particular attitudes and viewpoints of those community members intermingle. From that mix emerges something akin to what Rousseau referred to as the *volonté générale*—a general will that, of necessity, sees its own will only in the embrace of the community of willers.[12] The process of making such judgments, of allowing this important interplay, and of learning from it not only underwrites the judgment itself but tells a great deal about us as human beings and about our society.

When a society functions in a truly democratic fashion (when, in other words, not only a political but a real democracy that is underpinned by personal, economic, and educational democracy exists) such a mix, changing and evolving over time, will occur.[13] Therefore, our task is not only to learn to be good judges but likewise—and perhaps more important—to help create a society in which equitable processes underwrite the judgments we make. In this way, moral judgment in medicine can advance.

NOTES

1. Two works of mine are basic to this essay. One is a book I am currently writing that deals with the problem of emotion, reason, and aesthetics in making ethical judgments. The other is Erich H. Loewy, "Curiosity, Imagination, Compassion, Science and Ethics: Do Curiosity and Imagination Serve a Control Function?" *Health Care Analysis* 6 (1998): 286–94.
2. This capacity to separate evaluative areas from one another is similar to what Lifton calls doubling: "the division of self into two functioning wholes." Lifton claims that this phenomenon allowed many Nazi doctors to go about their tasks without being troubled. This behavior was largely a Faustian bargain. Much doubt has been cast about the ability of "normal" humans to really carry this off. R. J. Lifton, *The Nazi Doctors: Medical Killing and the Psychology of Genocide* (New York: Basic Books, 1986).
3. David Hume, *A Treatise of Human Nature,* ed. L. A. Selby-Bigge (Oxford: Clarendon Press, 1968), 415.
4. Immanuel Kant, "Grundlegung zur Metaphysik der Sitten," in *Immanuel Kant: Werkausgabe Band VIII,* ed. W. Weischedel (Frankfurt am Main, Germany: Suhrkamp Taschenbuch, 1968).
5. Immanuel Kant, *The Doctrine of Virtues,* trans. Mary J. Gregor (Philadelphia: University of Pennsylvania Press, 1964), 126. This quotation is from section 35 of this work in its original German ("Tugendlehre") and in the translation. I have taken the liberty of making a few slight changes in the translation. The concepts of *Mitleid* and *Mitfreude* are difficult to translate; roughly speaking, they refer to the sorrow or joy we feel in contemplating the joy or sorrow of another.

6. John Dewey, *Ethics, John Dewey: The Later Works,* vol. 7, ed. J. A. Boydston (Carbondale: Southern Illinois University Press, 1989), 221.

7. Ibid.

8. The way I use the concept of homeostasis in this work can be further understood by reference to Erich H. Loewy, *Freedom and Community: The Ethics of Interdependence,* (Albany: State University of New York Press, 1995); Erich H. Loewy, *Moral Strangers, Moral Acquaintance and Moral Friends: Connectedness and Its Conditions* (Albany: State University of New York Press, 1997).

9. The metaphor of the compost heap was first used by Stuart Hampshire in another context. I have found it to be a most useful metaphor with many applications. See Stuart Hampshire, *Innocence and Experience* (Cambridge, Mass.: Harvard University Press, 1989).

10. John Dewey, "Art As Experience," in *John Dewey: The Later Works,* vol. 10, ed. J. A. Boydston (Carbondale: Southern Illinois University Press, 1989), 257.

11. Dewey, *John Dewey: The Later Works,* vol. 7, 221.

12. The concept of the general will as Rousseau uses it entails that each member of a well-functioning community is willing not so much to subjugate as to envision his or her own interests in the context of the interest of a flourishing community. This concept entails the realization that our individuality outside a community that supports it is empty and that a community without vigorous individuals is not viable. For an excellent discussion of this concept, see: G. D. Cole, "Preface," in *J.J. Rousseau: the Social Contract and the Discourses* (New York: Everyman's Library, 1993).

13. John Dewey, "Creative Democracy: The Task Before Us," in *John Dewey: The Later Works, 1939–1941,* ed. J. A. Boydston and A. Sharp (Carbondale: Southern Illinois University Press, 1991), 224–30; John Dewey, "The Public and Its Problems," in *John Dewey: The Later Works, 1925–1953,* ed. J. A. Boydston and B. A. Walsh (Carbondale: Southern Illinois University Press, 1991).

The Contribution of Philosophical Hermeneutics to Clinical Ethics

Lazare Benaroyo

In this essay, I explore the significance of philosophical hermeneutics for medical ethics. I claim that hermeneutics is the philosophical framework within which the ethical core of the healing act comes into being.

My assumption is that healing is oriented toward restoring or improving the patient's good. On this view, medical morality is grounded in the patient's desire to be delivered from the burden of suffering. According to Pellegrino and Thomasma,[1] the ethical core of this encounter is an alliance, a caring pact, based on mutual trust. Physician and patient are united to fight against disease and to relieve suffering: "Healing is a mutual act that aims to repair the defects created by the experience of illness," writes Pellegrino.[2]

To realize the *telos* of medicine, the physician's clinical judgment is based on *phronesis*—the capacity, in a given set of circumstances, to discern what course of action is most conductive to the good of the patient.[3] *Phronesis* is oriented toward understanding the extent to which the patient's own experience of illness is lived as an assault on his or her sense of self-worth—in other words, the extent to which illness is the source of the patient's wounded humanity. In this respect, Pellegrino states, "Illness is the perception of the change in existential states that forms its central experience. It is an altered state of existence arising out of an ontological assault on the humanity of the person who is ill."[4] Understanding the nature of this ontological assault is the essential feature of the moral authenticity of the healing act: "The promise implicit in the act of profession, the promise of the healer, and the expectation the patient derives from that promise can be aligned properly if the assault of illness on the person of the patient is fully comprehended and ameliorated."[5]

Drawing on this assumption, I explore how understanding the patient's experience of illness proceeds. Building mainly on Hans-Georg Gadamer's philosophical and hermeneutical reflection, I investigate how philosophical hermeneutics opens the horizon of this understanding and how this hermeneutical approach helps to ameliorate the patient's state of wounded humanity.[6]

PHILOSOPHICAL HERMENEUTICS

A brief description of hermeneutics will clarify my analysis. Very broadly, hermeneutics is defined as the practice or study of interpretation. The term was first employed within a seventeenth-century theological context. Theologians sought rules and principles for interpreting sacred scripture, giving rise to a biblical hermeneutics. In the nineteenth century and at the turn of the twentieth century, Friedrich Schleiermacher and Wilhelm Dilthey pointed out that hermeneutics has a wider import than its classical definition as an art of interpretation: It was a theory of human understanding. On this basis, Martin Heidegger developed an influential conception of this concept; as Richard Bernstein puts it, in Heidegger's view, "Hermeneutics is no longer conceived of as a sub-discipline of humanistic studies . . . but rather as pertaining to questions concerning what human beings are. We are 'thrown' into the world as beings who understand and interpret—so if we are to understand what it is to be human beings, we must seek to understand understanding itself, in its rich, full, and complex dimensions."[7]

Hermeneutics, then, is the necessary condition of our knowledge of other human beings. The two major versions of twentieth-century contemporary hermeneutics—Gadamer's and Paul Ricoeur's versions—are strongly influenced by Heidegger's conception. Both of these authors have sought to complete Heidegger's conception by examining the moral dimension of the hermeneutic process: They point out that hermeneutics is a practical knowledge based on moral values such as attention, solidarity, and responsibility. According to Gadamer and Ricoeur, this moral framework especially shapes one's understanding of other human beings, as well as the constitution of the self.

Gadamer's contribution is interesting for our questioning because it helps elucidate the link binding hermeneutics and understanding. For Gadamer, understanding is not merely a concern of scientific rationality but part of a total experience of the world. This analysis draws on Gadamer's view that rationality cannot free itself from its historical context and horizons: Reason is itself historical or situated, and it always gains its distinctive power within a living tradition. In Gadamer's eyes, this situation is not a limitation or deficiency of reason but its essence, rooted in human finitude—an essence that is cosubstantive with the historicity of all understanding. In this respect, every act of understanding involves interpretation, a hermeneutical experience. Philosophical hermeneutics is the type of judgment or reasoning involved in all understanding. Like Gadamer, Charles Taylor defends the idea of an unavoidably hermeneutical component of the sciences of mankind.[8]

A basic theme of Gadamer's philosophical hermeneutics is the constitutive role of prejudices and prejudgments in understanding: In all understanding, fore-having, foresight, and fore-conception play a positive role in shaping the meaning of what the interpreter seeks to understand. Prejudices and prejudgments have a threefold temporal character: They are handed down to us through tradition; they are constitutive of what we are now (and what we are in the process of becoming); and they are anticipatory—always open to future testing and transformation.

Gadamer's thesis is that prejudices and prejudgments belong to the very possibility of understanding (and hence that the Enlightenment project of objective knowledge is an illusion). He develops this thesis in relation to Heidegger's notion of the hermeneutic circle. The hermeneutic circle describes a process that is basic to all understanding: the to-and-fro movement between part and whole. We attempt to comprehend the whole on the basis of what we already understand. For Heidegger, this circle refers to a mode of being in the world that precedes any methodological distinction between subject and object. Gadamer retains this insight, conveying it through his notion of "effective-historical consciousness" (*wirkungsgeschichtliche Bewusstsein*). As Gadamer sees it, we belong to a tradition before the tradition belongs to us: What we are, regardless of whether we are explicitly aware of it, is always being influenced by tradition and culture, leaving traces and sedimentations. The task of effective historical consciousness is to bring to awareness this historical affinity that influences what we consider worthy of investigation, how we go about investigating, and how we achieve an interplay with "others."

Heidegger and Gadamer's hermeneutic circle clarifies the relationship between the interpreter and what he or she seeks to understand, thus providing the interpreter with an alternative to objectivism and relativism. Gadamer suggests that both positions misconstrue the common hermeneutic experience; he argues that from a phenomenological viewpoint, the event of understanding is more appropriately described as a dialogue between interpreter and what the interpreter seeks to understand. A dialogue always presupposes that no matter how foreign the other's world view, there always exists some shared history or common basis—or, at least, that a common basis can be created—that can provide a point of departure for further understanding. On this view, hermeneutics is a form of reasoning that is appropriate to praxis; it deals with what is variable, it always involves a mediation between the universal and the particular, and it requires deliberation and choice. For Gadamer, the type of judgment and reasoning exhibited in hermeneutical understanding is a form of *phronesis*. In this sense, he contends that hermeneutics is a practical philosophy.[9]

IMPLICATIONS FOR CLINICAL ETHICS

I turn now to the significance of philosophical hermeneutics for medical ethics. Building on Gadamer's conception of hermeneutics, I suggest that in the medical setting, *phronesis* is a form of hermeneutical experience. In this experience, understanding is not detached from the healer but becomes constitutive of the healer's praxis. Thus, a first task of *phronesis* is to find resources in the healer's language and experience of the world that enable the healer to find—or create—a common belongingness (*Zugehörigkeit*), a fusion of horizon, that unites the healer and the patient. This task sets the healer's task for effective-historical consciousness to bring to explicit awareness the historical affinity or belongingness with the patient. Once this common belongingness is located or created, the ground is set for a communicative, trustful environment in which the patient's personal values and meanings may come to light.

This trustful environment may potentially open the horizon of a second task of *phronesis*—namely, to restore the patient's sense of self-worth. Two sets of factors that deal with the structure and the function of narrative participate in implementing this task.

According to Howard Brody, the setting of a common communicative, trustful environment structurally elicits a positive change along three perspectives. First, in this environment, the sufferer perceives that he or she "is surrounded by, and may rely upon, a group of caring individuals." Second, in this environment, suffering may be given "an explanation of the sort that will be viewed as acceptable, given the patient's existing belief system and worldview." Third, in this context, the sufferer may achieve "a sense of mastery or control over the suffering experience, either by feeling personally powerful enough to affect the course of events for the better or by feeling that his [or her individual] powerlessness can be compensated for by the power of some member or members of the caring group."[10]

According to Larry and Sandra Churchill's work on the function of narrative, storytelling has the power of refiguring the world of suffering in a threefold way. First,

> Narration is the forward movement of description of actions and events which makes possible the backward action of self-understanding. . . . When stories are told about ourselves, about our lives, narration becomes a way of taking up again our own past and also pondering, ordering, or interpreting the meaning of what may come.[11]

Second, distance and intimacy characterize storytelling. To tell our own story is to recount events and actions from a reflective posture, as an observer looking in from the outside. The temporal gap between one's actions and the telling allows the narrator to assume a distance about his or her actions as narrated in the story that creates a space for recognizing actions as good or bad, better or worse. This space provides the reflective ground for change. Third, "The dialectic of distance and intimacy is what makes storytelling distinctive as a mode of self-knowledge" in the realm of clinical dialogue. "Storytelling is one way persons cross the threshold from individual interpretation of the actions and events of their lives to make contact with a larger range of trustful common experience." In this respect, telling stories "manifests trust in the possibility of making connections" with a world made up of shared values where the self may be recognized as a person.[12] This refiguring function of narrative has been described in depth by Ricoeur in his theory of threefold mimetic activity at work in the narrative.[13]

In the wake of this ethical analysis, Warren T. Reich has studied the dialectical process of suffering and compassion.[14] Reich shows how compassion—which requires sharing in the suffering of another person—entails, in a hermeneutic perspective, entering into a dynamic process with the sufferer, who searches for meaning and is capable of undergoing a transition from meaninglessness to meaning, from pain to satisfaction. Reich describes three phases of the experience of suffering that are morally linked to three phases of compassion. Phase 1, mute suffering, is the experience of being speechless in the face of one's own suffering, which Reich links to silent empathy, silent compassion. In Phase 2, expressive suffering, the sufferer seeks a language to express his or her suffering—which is linked to expressive compassion, a way of helping find a voice for the voiceless. Phase 3 is the new identity in suffering: having a voice of one's own, which is linked to having a compassionate voice of one's own. In this phase, the healer experiences a constructive silence and a reverberative empathy, thus speaking the compassionate word that brings meaning to another's suffering. Reich's analysis ultimately shows that the positive interaction of compassionate solidarity with the patient's experience of suffering can produce a profound change in the sufferer. He writes that at the end of this dynamic process,

> the sufferer can find and accept a voice of his or her own, the new voice of the suffering self. . . . Solidarity with compassionate others enables the sufferer to "inter-

cept and work on" his or her suffering within the framework of narrative. When that suffering is accepted by another with caring compassion, the suffering can be radically transformed.[15]

CONCLUSION

Building on these ethical resources, I suggest that philosophical hermeneutics is an essential part of the groundwork on which the healing act lies. Its contribution to medical ethics is threefold: First, understanding the meaning of the patient's suffering requires effort and care, imagination and perceptiveness—which are directed to the healer's pathos of opening himself or herself to what he or she seeks to understand. Second, and correlatively to caring, understanding the meaning of the patient's suffering is an interpretive process that takes place in a dialogue. The phronetic resolution of the tension between strangeness and familiarity, which entails finding or creating a common belongingness between the healer and the patient, elicits understanding. To this end, understanding calls on the healer's effective-historical consciousness to allow the patient's suffering to speak to the healer. Third, building on these premises, the hermeneutical process may potentially remediate—on the ground of a trustful communicative environment—the afflicted state that illness represents.

On this view, *phronesis*—as a form of hermeneutic experience—is a practical-moral knowledge that is constitutive of caring in the dual sense of care-as-anxiety and care-as-solicitude; this dual sense calls on the metaphor of the "wounded healer." I therefore contend that hermeneutic experience is the way along which the ethical core of the healing act comes into being.

NOTES

1. Edmund D. Pellegrino and David Thomasma, *A Philosophical Basis of Medical Practice* (New York: Oxford University Press, 1981).
2. Edmund D. Pellegrino, "Being Ill and Being Healed: Some Reflections on the Grounding of Medical Morality," in *The Humanity of the Ill,* ed. V. Kestenbaum (Knoxville: University of Tennessee Press, 1982), 157.
3. Edmund D. Pellegrino and David C. Thomasma, *The Virtues in Medical Practice* (New York: Oxford University Press, 1993), 84.
4. Pellegrino, "Being Ill and Being Healed," 157–58.
5. Ibid., 161.
6. Hans-Georg Gadamer, *Truth and Method,* trans. and ed. G. Barden and J. Cumming (New York: Seabury Press, 1975).
7. Richard J. Bernstein, *Beyond Objectivism and Relativism: Science, Hermeneutics and Praxis* (Philadelphia: University of Pennsylvania Press, 1983), 113.
8. Charles Taylor, "Interpretation and the Sciences of Man," in *Philosophy and the Human Sciences, Philosophical Papers 2* (New York: Cambridge University Press, 1995), 15–57.
9. Hans-Georg Gadamer, "Hermeneutics as Practical Philosophy," in *Reason in the Age of Science* (Cambridge: MIT Press, 1990), 88–112.
10. Howard Brody, *Stories of Sickness* (New Haven, Conn./London: Yale University Press, 1987), 6.

11. Larry R. Churchill and Sandra W. Churchill, "Storytelling in Medical Arenas: The Art of Self-Determination," *Literature and Medicine* 1 (1982): 73.
12. Churchill and Churchill, "Storytelling in Medical Arenas," 74.
13. Paul Ricoeur, "Mimesis and Representation," in *A Ricoeur's Reader: Reflection and Imagination,* ed. M. J. Valdés (Toronto and Buffalo: University of Toronto Press, 1991), 137–55; Paul Ricoeur, "The Narrative Function," in *Hermeneutics and the Human Sciences,* ed. J. B. Thompson (New York: Cambridge University Press, 1981), 274–96.
14. Warren T. Reich, "Speaking of Suffering: A Moral Account of Compassion," *Soundings* 72 (1989): 83–108.
15. Ibid., 93.

Money, Medicine, and Morals

William S. Andereck

One problem that individuals venturing into the health care debate encounter is the multiplicity and complexity of special interests, each representing something different and contradictory to the whole. To seek order in this chaos, it is easier to start from the perspective of the big picture—global budgets, competitive health care purchasing groups, refocusing physicians on primary rather than specialty care—rather than address personal stories and needs.

My perspective on health care delivery was forged in the trenches; I have seen the advent and proliferation of the preferred provider organization (PPO) phenomena, lived with Medicare, and for nine years managed a small physician-held corporation that I helped form. One of my early interests in the nature of physician reimbursement involved the concept of "fee-splitting." In the early 1980s, as a young member of the San Francisco Medical Society's Professional Relations and Ethics committee, I frequently heard my older colleagues refer to the term "fee-splitting" as a standard of unethical behavior. Yet its definition was never clearly stated. It became apparent that there were as many meanings of the term as there were discussants.

My own inquiry into the origins of the concept began with the early nineteenth century work of Percival, *Medical Ethics*, in which he wrote about fees from apothecaries:

> Two practices prevail . . . which ought to be discouraged. One consists in suffering prescriptions to be sent to the druggist for the sake of a small savings in expense. The other in receiving an annual stipend, usually degrading in its amount, and in the services it imposes for being consulted. . . .[1]

The proscription against fee-splitting first appeared in the American Medical Association's (AMA) Code of Ethics in 1903:

> It is derogatory to professional character for physicians to pay or offer to pay commissions to any person whatsoever who may recommend to them patients requiring general or special treatment or surgical operations. It is equally derogatory to professional character for physicians to solicit or to receive such commissions.[2]

The drive to abolish this practice was led by the American College of Surgeons throughout the 1920s. Internists and general practitioners—who were the recipients of referral fees from specialists—opposed abolition, of course. In *Medicine, Money, and Morals,* Mark Rodwin suggests that the practice of fee-splitting was not eradicated until the Internal Revenue Service declared that the referral fee was no longer a deductible business expense.[3]

Always resourceful, however, practitioners of medicine and surgery collaborated to develop the concept of a second assistant who separately billed a percentage of the surgical fee. Instead of giving the referring physician a direct payment for sending a surgical case, the surgeon would now invite the general practitioner to participate in the operation. Often this second "assistant" would simply hold retractors or help close the wound. Although such assistance could often be provided by a less-trained individual, the general practitioner's attendance would allow him or her to bill a separate fee, which was set at 20 percent of the primary surgeon's fee. Although this fee was not "money for nothing"—as the original practice of fee-splitting was—the arrangement generally provided reimbursement beyond the effort expended or expertise required. Second assistant fees were often a substantial part of a general practitioner's income until managed care stepped in and abolished the practice (except in cases in which the services of two skilled surgeons were clearly indicated based on the complexity of the specific procedure).

In this regard, references to fee-splitting last appeared in the AMA's Principles of Medical Ethics in 1971.

> Section 6: A physician should not dispose of his services under terms or conditions which tend to interfere with or impair the free and complete exercise of his medical judgment. . . .

> Section 7: In the practice of medicine the physician should limit the source of his professional income to medical services actually rendered by him, or under his direct supervision, to his patients. His fee should be commensurate with the service rendered and the patient's ability to pay. He should neither pay nor receive a commission for referral of patients. Drugs, remedies or appliances may be dispensed or supplied by the physician provided it is in the best interests of the patient.[4]

The 1980 version of the AMA's Principles of Medical Ethics was condensed from ten to seven sections. The two foregoing sections were among the deleted sections.

Failure to include the idea of referral fees in current codes of ethics does not mean that the AMA has ignored the issue, however—nor have insurance companies and government. Recent developments in ownership and contractual relationships with payors have so changed our thinking on these matters that, perhaps, no coherent statement concise enough to be considered a principle can be produced.

One of the reasons things are so murky is that we continue to try to resolve the tension between allowing doctors to engage in activities that can have significant potential for conflict of interest and promoting an honor system to ensure that patient welfare will always come first. Experience suggests that this tension will not always be resolved in the patient's favor.

The relationship between financial incentives and patient care is too important to be ignored, however. The ways in which physicians have handled these incentives have played a major role in determining their overall prestige in society. The challenge is to recognize the financial incentives in medical practice and develop them in a manner consistent with the rich tradition that has evolved over 2,500 years. Financial incentives such as fee-splitting have been present in medical practice for years. Controls such as judgments about ethics are the way the profession has acted to restrain or control the practice.

THE MEDICAL VALUE SYSTEM

Medicine does not exist in a vacuum. The larger society has undergone tremendous upheavals in social thought. Likewise, the values that physicians recognize as the fundamental principles of their profession are not static. Failure to understand that value systems, like everything else, change leads to the intellectual sin of dogmatism.

Certainly a doctor's main responsibility has always been to the patient, but our attitudes toward that responsibility have undergone an evolution that we may not fully appreciate. The ethical basis of medical practice has been described as entailing four principles: nonmaleficence, beneficence, autonomy, and justice.[5]

In this section, I step back to put the idea of financial incentives in perspective. I claim that sensitivity to justice issues in medicine is very new in comparison to duties of nonmaleficence and beneficence. Readers of this volume will be well aware of the "Georgetown mantra" of bioethical principles. Thus, they will not need more exposition on the nature of the four principles.

Historically, the first principle or value of medicine was nonmaleficence. The Greek physicians of Kos were inspired by Hippocrates (460–380 B.C.), who taught a system of observation for the purpose of diagnosis and prognosis. Therapeutic treatments were less emphasized, and the general sentiment of the Greek age was consistent with the adage, "Above all, do no harm."

The principle of beneficence was incorporated into the medical ethic sometime later. During the Middle Ages, Arabic translations of Greek medical writings began to filter into Europe through Cordoba, Spain. The works of Averroes, Avicenna, and other Muslim scholars greatly influenced the intellectual development of western Europe by introducing it to Aristotelian philosophy and ethics, tempered with their own commentary and cultural obligations to benefit others.

Autonomy is a relatively new value in medical consciousness. Although the Supreme Court in 1914 recognized an individual's right to determine what happens to his or her own body,[6] autonomy was not accepted into everyday medical practice until the last quarter of the twentieth century.[7]

Even more recently, physicians have been asked to include justice in their decision making. By applying this principle, we are being asked for the first time to contrast benefits in much larger terms than the effect on our own patient.

Rising health care costs during the past 15 years have focused our society's attention on how fairly and wisely we are distributing the world's health care resources. Justice issues—particularly distributive justice issues—have been thrown in the face of the medical establishment. Government and the private sectors are turning to us in frustration to say,

"You can't control costs—and if you don't do it, we will." This threat, as well as a genuine effort to eliminate waste and inefficiency, has generated a shift on the part of physicians to incorporate justice when we think about how to care for our patients. By subjecting patient care to standards of economic justice, we introduce a principle that defines responsibilities for the physician that are not determined solely by the patient's interests. We need to consider carefully the very real conflict in a physician's responsibility to a patient-centered ethic and competing responsibilities to preserve society's resources. We are talking about the doctor's job description: what the patient can expect from the person in a white coat.

I concur with the proposition that a physician has a responsibility to justice, particularly at the level of the "statistical individual." In the rush to embrace duties to contain costs, however, physicians seem increasingly willing to be more open about their thinking on justice when they are deciding whether a patient will get a magnetic resonance imaging (MRI) scan or some other "big-ticket" procedure. Recently, a resident said to me, "We've spent $100,000 on this patient; isn't it time to quit?" The reality was that we probably had spent $100,000 on the patient, and it was indeed time to quit. What disturbed me, however, was that the resident thought the two things were directly related—that the patient had used up her "allotment" of health care resources.

Physicians should not be expected to accept justice as a valid concern when they make decisions about individual patients, as opposed to dealing with justice at a policy level or "statistically." Practicing distributive justice at the bedside without any clear societal consensus or bioethical standards beyond "this just isn't worth it" can become a very arbitrary process that depends largely on the value system of the person assigning worth. Even if physicians were to accept the responsibilities of resource distribution in a fair and just manner, what principle would determine distribution? The possibility that individual physicians will regard themselves as "lone rangers of distributive justice" introduces the potential for an arbitrary financial decision-making process by physicians that will place the public health in even greater danger than what we have now.

The process of involving doctors in decisions of justice shifts their allegiance ever so slightly. Duties to justice may conflict with a physician's duty to seek an individual patient's best interest. Most patients who are able to make a truly informed choice would opt for a doctor who is 100 percent on their side.

APPROPRIATELY DEALING WITH JUSTICE ISSUES

We may clarify our understanding of the physician's role in matters of distributive justice by considering two separate types of application. One application is the "statistical individual": Norman Normal, the 70 kg man with a blood pressure of 120/80, pulse rate of 72, and temperature of 37°C—the patient none of us has ever actually met. The other application is the "identifiable individual," the patient at the bedside: Mrs. Judy Ross, the woman in room 438 with ovarian carcinoma. Physicians' duties in considering justice are quite distinct depending on whether they are working in the realm of the statistical patient or the identifiable patient.

Helping to establish guidelines for utilization review or serving on a hospital capital budget committee are examples of statistical applications or distributive justice. Although these decisions eventually will affect real people, it is safer for physicians to consider and evaluate rationing decisions prospectively and across-the-board than to try to sort things out at each individual's bedside.

The alternative approach—considering the financial ramifications of medical treatment on the basis of the particular resources of each identifiable individual—exemplifies the hodgepodge system that is rapidly falling apart all around us. Medical treatment decisions at the level of the identifiable individual have many unique characteristics that are heavily influenced by the personal values of the decision maker—whether that is the doctor or the patient. If physicians are truly willing to move beyond the patient-centered ethic and introduce responsibilities to others into their medical decision making, they should be very careful about applying these duties arbitrarily at each bedside. This consideration is especially important as financial incentives are introduced and fostered.

One thing that separated priests from physicians in antiquity was that the physicians developed a socially acceptable way to charge a fee for the "magic" provided, whereas the priests did not. Since that time, doctors have been allowed to earn a livelihood in the practice of medicine. Therefore, financial incentives have always been present in medicine. How doctors are paid significantly determines the care they render to specific patients. Thus, involving physicians financially in the process of their decision making automatically brings rationing to the bedside.

Understanding how medicine got into the financial mess it is in is not too difficult. The fee-for-service system of reimbursement for medical services played a large role. Patients, physicians, and hospitals reaped the consequences of an unrestricted system of reimbursement with no controls on costs and, in particular, insufficient personal responsibility to face the price tag by either the patient or the doctor. As the patient increasingly was removed from the financial consequences of treatment, there often was no discussion of costs at the microeconomic level of the doctor-patient encounter. In short, positive financial incentives drove the provision of medical care. This "blank check" approach to financing ran costs through the roof.

Initial efforts to stem costs did not start with financial incentives; they took the stick approach: utilization review (UR). The record of success demonstrated by most of these efforts has been just shy of dismal. Tragically and ironically, one of the fastest-growing segments of health care expenditures is administrative costs for insurers to process paperwork and otherwise try to "manage" the system. Many initial efforts toward UR tended to foster an adversarial relationship between doctors and reviewers that encouraged doctors to "stand up" for their patients—especially if there was no untoward financial effect on the physician.

The history of all these "stick" approaches to cost containment has been one of guerilla warfare. For every better cost-containment mousetrap, doctors have devised ways to "beat the system" and frustrate legitimate goals. The flaw inherent in many of these efforts may be that they try to exert a direct effect on an identifiable individual. Exhortations to reduce costs out of duty have not been efficacious, and trying to drive doctors with a stick only compounds their resistance.

A business school analysis recognizes that doctors generate the expenditures not just in their own charges but in the tests, consultations, and treatments they prescribe. Less than 0.5 percent of our society controls more than 12 percent of our gross national product (GNP). Changes in the behavior of a relatively small number of individuals can have tremendous economic consequences. The marketplace offers financial incentives for physician cooperation; the catch-phrase here is "sharing the risk." Transferring financial risk to the provider, as insurance carriers began to do in many creative ways, creates a disincentive to provide care if that care could ultimately cost the physician. If the financial disincentives are large enough, there may no longer be a need for a utilization review committee. Capitation is a good example of one such creative idea: Choosing not to provide care directly increases a doctor's earnings.

Thus, financial incentives have been reintroduced to medicine, but with a twist. Instead of rewarding a physician for performing a service, the system could be construed as treating the service as a penalty for letting the patient get sick in the first place. What was a positive incentive has become a negative one.

Clinicians confront a smorgasbord of insurance programs daily. A brief overview of the financial incentives being introduced illustrates the scope and significance of reimbursement formulas in routine clinical decisions.

The traditional model of fee-for-service exemplifies the positive financial incentive. Each patient seen generates a payment that is determined roughly by the time spent and the procedures performed. Until recently, these costs were unchallenged. Increasingly, however, even fee-for-service patients are not required to pay full charges. The development of PPO contracts maintains the positive incentive of fee-for-service, at a discounted fee.

After a short while, the doctor figures out that he or she is making only about 60 percent of the usual charges per patient seen. The solution often is that the doctor spends only 60 percent as much time with each patient. I once asked an insurance executive how the physicians in our hospital community were expected to deal with deep discounts in office visit reimbursement. Her reply was firm and clear: "We have all the lives, doctor. After you sign our contract, you can make it up in volume."

Some PPO contracts are beginning to blend fee-for-service incentives with less direct incentives that still have significant financial impact. One example is the concept of "subspecialty pools." Primary care doctors, as well as specialists, are paid on a discounted fee-for-service basis. To augment their reduced fee-for-service income, primary care doctors are offered subspecialty pools. In this type of program, an insurer sets aside a predetermined pool of money that is intended to pay for all of the referral specialists required by the members of the plan. All specialists are paid from the pool, and the primary care physicians—affectionately known as "gatekeepers"—are clearly informed that any monies left in the specialty pool at the end of the year will be offered to them as a bonus for cutting referrals. Such incentives are intended to prevent unnecessary referrals. *Unnecessary* is a slippery word, however—especially when all referrals have the same financial disincentive regardless of whether they are "necessary" or "unnecessary." The participation of a primary care physician in an arrangement such as this can be considered a modern form of fee-splitting.

Not surprisingly, individual physicians attempting to deal with large "take it or leave it" payors are usually overwhelmed. Independent practice associations (IPAs) have been a natural and necessary outgrowth that enable physicians to contract in concert with one another and face giant corporations. Contracting together also allows physicians to share risk together.

In the early IPAs in San Francisco, 15–20 percent of a practitioner's income was not paid immediately but held "at risk" to cover the expenses of the IPA. Individual physicians are now forming groups in which all, or at least a majority, of the reimbursement is at risk of loss from poor financial performance by the group. The direct fiscal effect of poor economic performance can be targeted to one's group or physician category. It can even be based on individual performance. Physicians who perform poorly in this economic sense are identified and targeted and can be dropped by the others for inappropriate financial performance.

For example, I was one of the original founders (and eventually president) of a nine-doctor IPA during the 1980s. Each doctor also had an independent private practice. For this venture, we were brought together by the hospital administration specifically to provide physician services for one of their capitated contracts. Ninety percent of the income for our IPA was received as a capitation payment of about $109,000 on the first business day of each month. With that money, my eight colleagues and I were expected to provide or subcontract the medical care for approximately 3,000 people. Our capitation check covered all outpatient visits (except for a $4 copayment), all outpatient diagnostic tests, and all specialist fees. We paid administrative and malpractice costs for the IPA, staff salaries and benefits, and all other facility costs. The monthly payment did not include responsibility for hospital charges or drugs. Emergency room charges also were not paid out of our capitation. (This aspect of the arrangement explains why we never seriously considered a Saturday or evening clinic that would have been developed at our own expense.) At the end of each quarter, after all the bills had been paid, we divided the remainder of the money as our salary for the previous quarter's work. Some paychecks were better than others. The pressure on each of us to cut costs was enormous.

The resulting conflict between patient care and income is illustrated by the case of a tall, thin, thirty-seven-year-old man who saw me for a routine physical. He had no complaints. Yet routine auscultation of the heart revealed a grade I diastolic murmur. My first thought was, "Oh no, this is going to cost $10,000." My next thought was, "That's more than $1,000 apiece!" Soon, I found myself thinking, "Maybe I don't hear anything." Only then did I catch myself and order the echocardiogram, which demonstrated significant aortic insufficiency. The ensuing surgery cost our group more than $10,000 in specialist fees and prehospitalization work-up. Our paychecks were affected, and I was teased good-naturedly about my hearing.

Thus, physicians are becoming involved in health care plans, programs, and payment schemes that have the potential to compromise their historical fiduciary role for the patient. Some physicians are becoming uncomfortable and have refused to comply. Others say they can still practice in an honorable way. When people become involved in systems that tend to influence allocation of care, however—especially where dollars are involved—compromise can seem quite attractive. Making a few "adjustments" becomes easy.

To return to my example: While I was working part-time in this capitated IPA, I began to realize that my decision making was being clouded by an environment in which financial and medical decisions were too close for comfort. I began to appreciate the idea of "level of application" of financial incentives. A system might work well if the consequences of one person's actions are spread over a large number of individuals, but moving this model into a smaller practice such as our nine-member IPA was fraught with danger.

Direct negative incentives can make the doctor-patient relationship adversarial instead of a relationship based on common trust. The patient may want procedures or tests that we do not want to provide, and we may resent them. Seldom are these situations so clear-cut, however. For instance, we may have chronic headache patients or patients who have nonspecific abdominal pain—"worried well people." The physician may decide that these patients have nothing "wrong" with them and are wasting the physician's time and money. The resentment could build up gradually over a period of clinical care.

Measures that cause an individual physician to look beyond the needs of an individual patient and deny those needs, particularly for financial gain, will destroy the trust inherent in the relationship. When the doctor-patient relationship turns into an adversarial situation, the physician's ability to comfort and heal will be severely diminished. In these situations, the "adversary" is no longer the utilization reviewer but the patient.

Should physicians resist this model and remain helpless in stemming the costs of medical care? No, but they should be cautioned against balancing the budget at the bedside. Replacing positive financial incentives with negative ones may have an immediate attraction for payors who are merely interested in reducing costs. The ethics and principles that govern the insurance industry are the ethics of the marketplace. The fiduciary responsibilities inherent in the patient-centered ethic of medicine are not as stringent in the business ethics mode. Therefore, we should carefully explore the specific impact of this motivational change for physicians and patients before we commit the majority of our medical delivery system to it.

HEALTH CARE STRATEGIES

Because positive and negative incentives have potential for abuse, physicians should develop health care strategies that neutralize the more intrusive financial incentives; they also should recognize and disclose the ones that remain. Managed care strategies have been portrayed as good for patients in that they prevent unnecessary procedures. Disclosure of the financial disincentives that may influence a physician's judgment about what is "necessary" is more difficult to find in the marketing literature.

A negative incentive such as capitation works effectively if the financial risks of decision making are distributed among a large enough number of doctors. Physicians in large health maintenance organizations (HMOs) may not worry as much about costs when they order MRI or computed tomography (CT) scans for their patients. Individual patient decisions are unlikely to directly affect the decision maker's income.

Changing the "level of application" to one person caring for the entire plan, however, can make that incentive overwhelming. There may be certain incentives that should not be offered because the conflict of interest inherent in the smaller practice is too great— not that there are good or bad physicians. Physicians should clearly define some of the practices that may influence us to act in ways of which we might be ashamed. Likewise, in the fee-for-service system the positive incentive to overutilize services is strong for a physician who owns his or her own CT or MRI scanner, x-ray machine, physical therapy department, or laboratory. Numerous studies confirm that ownership of a facility is associated with increased referral patterns to that facility.[8]

One payment mechanism that removes most financial incentives from individual patient care is the salary model. Some degree of financial incentive can be beneficial to the practice and to patients. Despite concern about inappropriate financial incentives, I appreciate the value of these incentives if they are aligned in concert with appropriate goals. Removing all financial incentives for performance might produce physicians who do no more than their share. Most of us recognize a need to reward work well done in a field that is difficult to quantify. The current trend, however, is to regard physicians as interchangeable parts, each providing a service of equal value. Such a perspective fails to recognize the unique skills of individual practitioners.

OBSERVATIONS AND SUGGESTIONS

Some physicians are perceived as promoting change in medical practice, others as resisting it. The complexity of competing needs and abilities is staggering. Everyone is trying to guess what will develop. Like most physicians, I am not interested in reversing things; that is how we arrived at this perilous state. I also am not looking forward to the continued transformation of medicine that seems inevitable. Solutions eventually develop out of social crisis, although living through the remodeling required will be difficult. Through this haze, I offer a few observations:

First, we have a social obligation to provide at least some basic level of health care to all people. This obligation does not extend to providing everyone with a "Cadillac" plan, however; we could afford that only at the expense of all other social services. We need to define a basic health care system, one I might call the "Yugo plan"—a plan that is open to everyone and should be very large to fairly distribute the risks of illness in the community. At this very basic level, I would add a national system—a safety-net level with wide distribution of negative incentives that are not applied directly at the level of the individual decision maker. This system might provide physicians with a workable setting for continued dedication to beneficence in the context of justice.

For some percentage of society, alternative health care should be available; patients could purchase this health care out-of-pocket or share in the cost through tax credits, deductions, rebates, or even vouchers. This arrangement makes more sense than giving the government our money and having it returned to us in the form of a health care program. There is no better way to increase individual responsibility for sound decision making than by requiring patients to contribute some of the physician reimbursement. Such options will create a two-tiered system, but it would be more honest to admit that we have a multi-tiered system of health care than to deny that it exists.

This second tier of medicine might more closely resemble a fee-for-service system; it would promote a form of "free market" physician economy. Physicians would be competing on the basis of their skills, as well as how a patient feels when he or she leaves the office. We need to understand that we are motivated by financial incentives, and we need to create a system that takes the financial incentives of society, physicians, and patients into account.

Physicians also need to be honest with their patients. Physicians should explain the health care system to patients in a way that promotes high-quality medical care. Patients need to understand what kind of health insurance they or their employers are selecting. Insurance companies have done a wonderful job of marketing these new forms of managed care while disguising the restrictions to access. Often, the physician is placed n the role of the "bad guy" when treatment authorization is required.

In exchange for the removal of the hassle-factor of government and insurance company oversight and interference, physicians should give something up in exchange: the selling or receiving of profit on anything except their own personal diagnostic and therapeutic skills. Doctors would eliminate some of their alternate income streams—such as laboratories, the sale of durable medical goods, or in-office x-rays—except where patient convenience is a real issue.

Finally, physicians have to engage the public in a dialogue about the distribution of health care resources. This process has already occurred in Oregon and many other states and communities. Dealing with health care financing by simply assigning it a percentage of the GNP—and then expecting the participants to fight it out—is not only cruel but unsound. Where would we be now if we had focused on the percentage of the GNP going to the computer industry in the 1960s or the auto industry in the 1920s?

CONCLUSION

Rationing happens. It may be impersonal and cold. It may be chaotic. It can be aimed at individuals or groups. It can be subtle or oppressive. It might also be fair and just. We should push for the latter model. One way we can do so is to recognize the financial incentive structure that is built into medical practice and work to develop a distribution system that neutralizes inappropriate inducements. Limitations to access to medical care should be based on publicly recognized parameters that are developed at the level of the statistical individual. These parameters should emphasize not only a reduction of waste but solid research into the indications and effectiveness of all medical interventions.

A distinguished professor of bioethics once disagreed with my contention that health care economics is a valid topic for ethical analysis. Ethics, according to this gentleman, more appropriately addresses topics such as brain death, withdrawal of life support, or informed consent. I believe that ethics is really about values: what our values are, and how we act on those values. One of our values concerns financial arrangements. The way we practice medicine based on financial incentives has as much to do with ethics as how we practice medicine based on our respect for life. Events have vindicated this view. We need to do much more.

NOTES

1. C. Leake, *Percival's Medical Ethics* (Huntington, N.Y.: Krieger, 1985), 117.
2. Ibid., 255.
3. Mark Rodwin, *Medicine, Money, and Morals* (New York: Oxford University Press, 1993), 32.
4. American Medical Association Judicial Council, *Opinions and Report* (Chicago: American Medical Association, 1971).
5. Thomas Beauchamp and James Childress, *Principles of Biomedical Ethics,* 2nd ed. (New York: Oxford University Press, 1983).
6. *Schloendorff v Society of New York Hospitals,* 211 NY 125, 127, 129; 105 N.E. 92, 93 (1914).

7. David Novak, R. Plumer, and R. Smith, "Changes in Physician's Attitudes Toward Telling the Cancer Patient," *Journal of the American Medical Association* 241 (1979): 897–900.

8. J. Mitchell and J. Sunshine, "Consequences of Physician Ownership of Health Care Facilities—Joint Ventures in Radiation Therapy," *New England Journal of Medicine* 327 (1992): 1479–1501; A. Swendlow et al., "Increased Costs and Rates of Use in the California Worker's Compensation System as a Result of Self Referral by Physicians," *New England Journal of Medicine* 327 (1992): 1502–06; H. Luft, "Economic Incentives and Clinical Decisions," in *The New Health Care for Profit: Doctors and Hospitals in a Competitive Environment,* ed. B. Gray (Washington, D.C.: National Academy Press, 1983).

Theology and Bioethics[1]

Richard A. McCormick, S.J.

As we enter neighborhood homes, many of us have been quickened with the peculiar hospitality of a sign that reads: "Beware of Dog." Many people undoubtedly believe that an analogous hospitable sign is in place when a theologian is present with people who gather to discuss the ethical dimensions of biomedicine. Theologians just may bite. Perhaps worse, they may not. At worst, they are regarded as extremely dangerous; at best, they are harmless— that is, useless. For these reasons, they should be out of sight, or at least on a short leash. Alisdair MacIntyre may have had something like this in mind when he concluded one of his essays on medical ethics as follows: "Theologians still owe it to the rest of us to explain why we should not treat their discipline as we do astrology or phrenology. The distinctiveness and importance of what they have to say, if it is true, make this an urgent responsibility."[2]

I confess to being terrorized when my task is described as an "urgent responsibility," and my terror is not diminished when I read what I have done. MacIntyre's ultimatum clearly implies the conviction that theologians have not successfully articulated the "distinctiveness and importance of what they have to say." Unless I misread him, MacIntyre faintly implies that theologians really cannot articulate their importance because they do not have much to say. An urgent task is thus transformed into an impossible one—and under threat of relabeling as *disciplina astroligica*. I like neither the odds nor the possible outcome. To avoid the latter, however, I must risk the former.

To avoid unthreatening generalizations and verbal incontinence, I must explicate and narrow both terms in the title of this essay. I begin with theology.

Theology starts when faith begins to reflect on itself. This definition pirates that of Anselm of Canterbury: *fides quaerens intellectum* (faith seeking understanding). Two points should be noted at the outset. First, there are many different faiths (Catholicism, Judaism, Islam, and so forth). Second, the communities in which these faiths originate exist in history; therefore, they must continually reappropriate their inheritance in changing times and diverse circumstances—and often with different purposes in view. Moreover, with regard to the first point, an individual faith community clearly can comprise radically different theologies—a fact reflected in the varying theologies of the New Testament authors. Thus, how theologies can relate to bioethics can differ in a variety of ways from community to community, as well as within the same community at varying times.

To narrow the proportions of my "urgent responsibility" (impossible task), I note that I write as an adherent of the Catholic faith (the only one I know from experience) and therefore understand theology as reflection on that faith only; furthermore, I make no claims that my reflections are *the* theology or the *only* theology of that faith. Such claims are blasphemous in their pretensions that God can be adequately caught (really strait-jacketed) in human concepts. My reflections should be regarded as one possible way of approaching the subject. Clearly, this narrowing is not meant to detract from the validity or beauty of any other faith or theology.

Such narrowing is not enough, however. I also must make explicit the implications of the statement that theology is reflection on *faith*. The danger in our time is that the term "faith" will be collapsed into bloodless, intellectualized acceptance of creedal statements. When "I believe" is sterilized into mere affirmation of propositions, faith has lost its heart and soul. In this sense Johannes Metz states, "Christ must always be thought of in such a way that he is never merely thought of."[3] Merely to "think of" Christ is to trivialize Him, to reduce Him to one more observable historical event (among many)—an example of humane benevolence. For a person of Christian faith, Jesus Christ is God's immanent presence, His love in the flesh.

I borrow from the late Joseph Sittler at this point. Sittler has noted that the theme of the biblical narratives is God's "going out from Himself in creative and redemptive action toward men." He refers to "God's relentless gift of God," "God's undeviating will to restoration," the "history-involved assault of God upon man's sin," "the gracious assault of his deed in Christ."[4] Jesus Christ is no less than God's self-giving deed.

The response of the believer to this person-revelation is the total commitment of the person—which is known as faith. Thus, Sittler writes,

> It is not possible to state too strongly that the life of the believer is for Paul the actual invasion of the total personality by the Christ-life. So pervasive and revolutionary is the displacement and bestowal that terms like influence, example, command, value are utterly incapable of even suggesting its power and its vitally recreating force.[5]

The believer's response to this specific, momentous, and supreme event of God's love is total and radical commitment. For the believer, Jesus Christ—the concrete enfleshment of God's love—becomes the meaning and *telos* of the world and of the self. God's self-disclosure in Jesus is the self-disclosure of ourselves and our world. "All things are made through him, and without him was not anything made that was made."[6] The believer's response to this personal, divine outpouring is not a dead "amen" by an outside observer; it is a faith-response that is empowered by the very God who did the redemptive and restorative deed in Jesus Christ. This faith-response is utterly and totally transforming—so much so that St. Paul must craft a new metaphor to articulate it. We are "new creatures," plain and simple. Faith is the empowered reception of God's stunning and aggressive love in Jesus.

Theologian Walter Kasper summarizes this description of faith as follows:

> Faith is not simply an intellectual act or an act of the will. It includes the whole man [*sic*] and every aspect of the human reality. . . . It embraces the whole of Christian

existence, including hope and love, which can be seen as two ways in which faith is realized.[7]

Faith, then, is the proper term "to point to the total commitment of the whole person which is required by the character of the revelation."[8] I use the term *theology* (as it relates to bioethics) as a reflection on that sense of faith. I emphasize this usage because many influences tempt us to treat theology primarily as a reflection on creedal statements hammered out as communicative and protective vehicles of a more profound and original happening (God's self-communication and our response to it). It is much easier to deal with creedal statements because faith itself, as a response to God, exceeds the reach of human language. Moreover, the historical religious communities that provide the context of the faith-response have myths and symbols that differentiate them, which raises the temptation to confuse these symbols with faith itself. Finally, the temptation becomes almost irresistible when these myths and symbols lead to distinct ethical codes.

My second introductory qualifier concerns the term *bioethics*. Bioethics is a subspecies of ethics. There has been a tendency to equate ethics with "quandary ethics."[9] Symbols of this view abound. We are fascinated and fixed by the tangled casuistry of plug-pulling, palliation decisions, proxy determinations. Such newsworthy, eye-catching cases are amenable to legal resolution. Thus, courses in bioethics are loaded with names and issues such as Quinlan, Jobes, Fox, Storar, Chad Green, Conroy, Baby M, Jehovah's Witnesses, pregnancy reduction, testing for seropositivity, triage decisions, dilemmas about confidentiality. (Readers can test this assessment by picking up an issue of *The Hastings Center Report*.) We do not diminish casuistry by noting that such cases do not constitute the entirety of ethics —especially an ethics that calls itself Christian and most especially an ethics that claims to be *theological*.

An ethics that claims to be theological will root itself in God—that is, in God's actions and purposes. Its primary referents will be God's relation to us and ours to God. This relationship will be the prime analogate (to use scholastic language) of the term "morality." The most basic—though not the only—language of theological ethics builds on the notions of *goodness* and *badness* rather than the rightness and wrongness of actions because the goodness-badness scale is basically vertical and has its aortal lifeline to the God-relationship.

In slightly different words, a Christian theological ethics is founded on the fact that something has been done to and for us—and that something is Jesus. This prior action of God is revelatory and response-engendering. This prior action of God is reflected in the Pauline "therefore," which states the entire grounding and meaning of the Christian ethic.

In and through Jesus, we know what that God-relationship is: total self-gift. That is what God is, and we are created in His image. If we miss this point, we leave the realm of Christian ethics.

Another aspect of the notion of "ethics" (and therefore bioethics) requires mention here. There are four levels at which *ethics* can be understood with regard to the rightness or wrongness of conduct.[10] These distinctions are not made often, but they are essential if we are to gain precision in analyzing the relationship of theology to bioethics.

First is what we might call an *essential* ethic. This term designates norms that are regarded as applicable to all persons, whereby one's behavior is but an instance of a general, essential moral norm. Examples of this essential ethic relate to the rightness or wrongness of killing actions, contracts, or promises, as well as actions whose demands are rooted in the dignity of persons.

Second is an *existential* ethic. This term refers to the choice of a good that the individual should realize *as individual:* the experience of an absolute ethical demand addressed to the individual. For instance, an individual might conclude that his or her own moral-spiritual life cannot grow and thrive in the health care environment and therefore that he or she ought to abandon this work. Alternatively, because of background, inclination, or talent, an individual might choose to concentrate time and energy on a particular aspect of health care.

Third is *essential Christian* ethics. This term refers to ethical decisions that a Christian must make precisely because he or she belongs to a community to which the non-Christian does not belong. These choices are moral demands made on the Christian *as a Christian*—for instance, regarding fellow workers as brothers and sisters in Christ (not just as autonomous, to-be-respected persons), providing a Christian education for one's children, belonging to a particular worshiping community. These important ethical decisions emerge only within the context of a Christian community's understanding of itself in relation to other people.

Fourth is *existential Christian* ethics. This term relates to ethical decisions that Christians must make *as individuals* (e.g., to undertake the ministry of the priesthood).

I introduce these distinctions because the relation of theology to bioethics is only an instance of a larger theological discussion that has been occurring for years: the dispute about whether Christian ethics is a *Glaubensethik*—or, to use shorthand, functions autonomously.[11] The discussion has been lively, even heated at times, especially in Germany. Although the discussants appear to disagree, in fact they often are not discussing the same question: They are often talking past each other.

The four distinctions noted above would prevent much of this confusion. More concretely, we should readily grant that revelation and our personal faith do influence ethical decisions at the latter three levels (existential, essential Christian, existential Christian). An individual's choice of issues, as well as the dispositions and motivations he or she brings to these issues, can be profoundly affected by his or her personal appropriation of revealed truth (*faith*, in the sense explained), by his or her prayer life, and by the community in which these aspects develop. Proponents of an autonomous ethic do not discuss these levels, however. Instead, they emphasize the level of essential ethics only—a point that is fudged unless the distinctions noted above are kept in mind.

With these introductory notes on faith and ethics as background, I now turn to theology and bioethics.

I begin by citing James Gustafson:

> For theological ethics . . . the first task in order of importance is to establish convictions about God and God's relations to the world. To make a case for how some things really and ultimately are is the first task of theological ethics.[12]

I agree with Gustafson's description of the first task of theological ethics, though clearly we would disagree significantly about "how some things really and ultimately are." How, then, are they, "really and ultimately"? In its *Declaration on Euthanasia,* the Congregation for the Doctrine of the Faith made reference to "Christ, who through his life, death and resurrection, has given a *new meaning to existence.*"[13] If that formulation is true (and Christians believe it is), to neglect that meaning is to neglect the most important thing about ourselves, to cut ourselves off from the fullness of our own reality.

"A new meaning to existence": Those words are powerful. If Christ has given "a new meaning to existence," presumably that new meaning will have some relevance for key notions and decisions in the field of bioethics. At this point it is fair to ask: What is this new meaning?

Theological work in the past decade or so has rejected the notion that sources of faith are a thesaurus of answers. Instead, they should be regarded above all as narratives, as a story. From a story come perspectives, themes, and insights—not always or chiefly direct action guides. The story is the source from which the Christian construes the world theologically. In other words, it is the vehicle for discovering and communicating this new meaning.

At this point, we must attempt to disengage some key elements of the Christian story, and from a Catholic reading and living of it. One might not be too far off with the following summary:

- God is the author and preserver of life. We are "made in His image."
- Thus life is a gift, a trust. It has great worth because of the value He is placing in it.
- God places great value in it because besides being author He is also the end, the purpose of life.
- We are on a pilgrimage, having here no lasting home.
- God has dealt with us in many ways. His supreme epiphany of Himself (and our potential selves), however, is His Son, Jesus Christ.
- In Jesus' life, death, and resurrection we have been totally transformed into "new creatures," a community of the transformed. Sin and death have met their victor.
- The ultimate significance of our lives consists in developing this new life.
- The Spirit is given to us to guide and inspire us on this journey.
- The ultimate destiny of our combined journeys is the "coming of the Kingdom"—the return of the glorified Christ to claim the redeemed world.
- Thus, we are offered eternal life in and through Jesus Christ. Just as Jesus has overcome death (and now lives), so will we who cling to Him, place our faith and hope in Him, and take Him as our law and model.
- This good news—this covenant with us—has been entrusted to a people, a people to be nourished and instructed by shepherds.
- This people should continuously remember and thereby make present Christ in His death and resurrection at the Eucharistic meal.
- The chief and central manifestation of this new life in Christ is love for each other. This love is not a flaccid "niceness" but a love that shapes itself in the concrete forms of justice, gratitude, forbearance, chastity, and so forth—especially for poor, marginal, sinners; these sinners were Jesus' constant companions.

For the Catholic Christian, this summary describes "how some things really and ultimately are." In Jesus we have been totally transformed. This new life or empowerment is a hidden but nonetheless real dimension of our persons—indeed the most profoundly real thing about us.[14] The biblical materials present the history of the world in terms of creation, fall, redemption. As Thomas Clarke has noted, this triad also describes our personal history and is mirrored in Johannine and Pauline imagery: light-blindness-enlightenment; freedom-bondage-liberation; integrity-brokenness-reintegration; health-sickness-healing; peace-estrangement-reconciliation.

From the perspective of faith, we are in the process of being redeemed, and that process takes the form of enlightenment, liberation, reintegration, healing, reconciliation.[15] I have suggested that the integrating shape of our lives from this faith perspective is the self-gift of *agape*. We must be progressively healed, enlightened, liberated, reconciled, and reintegrated into the fullness of this original empowerment. In the concise words of St. Thomas, charity is the form of the virtues. Our lives are the struggles of pilgrims to render this central vitality ever more dominant, facile, and spontaneous. As exegete L. Cerfaux puts it, "Charity is the normal occupation of the Christian."[16]

What does this discussion have to do with bioethics? I reject two possible extremes from the outset. The first extreme is that faith gives us concrete answers to the problems of *essential* ethics. Josef Fuchs is surely correct:

> Medical ethics is theological, and hence Catholic-theological, ethics if it proceeds from faith, i.e., from the Catholic faith. This faith is ultimately not the assertion of the truth of certain faith propositions, but an act, in the depth of the person, of giving and entrusting oneself to the God who reveals and imparts himself to us. Naturally, no concrete ethics— and therefore no medical ethics—can be developed out of faith understood in this way.[17]

By "concrete ethics" I understand Fuchs to be referring to what I have called essential ethics.

The second extreme is that faith has no influence whatsoever on bioethics. It would seem passing strange indeed if what Sittler calls "the invasion of the total personality by the Christ-life" had no repercussions on one's dispositions, imagination, and values.

How, then, does faith exercise its influence? I take my lead from the Second Vatican council. In an interesting sentence, *The Constitution on the Church in the Modern World* states, "Faith throws a new light on everything, manifests God's design for man's total vocation, and thus directs the mind to solutions which are fully human."[18]

Here we have reference to a "new light." The nature of this "new light" is that it reveals human existence in the fullest and most profound dimensions ("God's design for man's total vocation"). The effect of this new light is to "direct the mind." To what? "Solutions which are fully human." The usage "fully human" I take to mean a rejection of any understanding of "a new meaning to existence" that sees existence as foreign to the human and radically discontinuous with it.

The Catholic tradition has encapsulated the way faith "directs the mind to solutions" in the phrase "reason informed by faith." Reason informed by faith is neither reason *replaced* by faith nor reason *without* faith. It is reason shaped by faith. Vincent MacNamara renders this concept as follows: "Faith and reason compenetrate one another and form a unity of consciousness which affects the whole of the Christian's thought and action."[19] What is the effect of such a Christian consciousness? MacNamara uses several phrases: "people who see things in a particular way, because they are particular sorts of people";[20] "it [faith] determines, to some extent, one's meanings, what one sees in the world, what are the facts of life, and what among them are the most prominent and relevant facts."[21] MacNamara also refers to the "total background out of which judgments and choices are made"[22] and a Christian's "interpretative self-awareness."[23]

In summary, the phrase "reason informed by faith" is shorthand for saying that the reasoner (the human person) has been transformed and that this transformation will have a cognitive dimension through its invasion of consciousness. The more profound the faith, the greater and more explicit will be the Christian consciousness—which is a way of saying that the way faith (and theology) affects ethics can be seen best of all in the saints. Even we non-saints ought to be able to give an intelligible account of theology's influence, however. Yet that account is destined to be incomplete, to some extent, because the transformation worked by faith is at a very profound level that is not totally recoverable in formulating consciousness.

With that analysis in mind, I suggest that theology can relate to bioethics in three distinct but overlapping ways: *protective, dispositive,* and *directive.*

PROTECTIVE

Moral philosophers, following St. Thomas, have identified basic inclinations toward goods that define our well-being or flourishing. Although these inclinations can be identified as prior to acculturation, they are culturally conditioned. We tend toward values as perceived. The culture in which we live shades our perceptions of values—a point made by Philip Rieff in *The Triumph of the Therapeutic* when he referred to "reasons that have sunk so deeply into the self that they are implicitly understood."[24] Rieff argues that decisions are made and policies set not chiefly by articulated norms, codes, regulations, and philosophies but by these "reasons" that lie below the surface. Our way of perceiving basic human values and relating to them is shaped by our whole way of looking at the world.

An example from bioethics will help here. In relating to basic human values, Daniel Callahan has pointed out that several images of human beings are possible.[25] In the power-plasticity model, nature is alien, independent of humans, possessing no inherent value. It is capable of being used, shaped, and dominated by humans. We see ourselves as possessing an unrestricted right to manipulate nature in the service of our goals. Death is something to be overcome or outwitted. In the sacro-symbiotic model (in its religious forms), nature is regarded as God's creation, to be respected and heeded. Nature is a trust; we are not masters but stewards. In secular forms, humans are regarded as a part of nature. Nature is a teacher, and we must live in harmony and balance with it. Death is but a rhythm of nature, to be gracefully accepted.

The power-plasticity model seems to have sunk deep and shaped our moral imaginations and feelings—as well as our perception of basic values. We are corporately *homo technologicus.* The best solution to the dilemmas created by technology is more technology. We tend to eliminate the maladapted condition (people who are defective, retarded, etc.) rather than adjust the environment to it. This is our cultural bias.

We can argue persuasively that the peculiar temptation of a technologically advanced culture such as ours is to view and treat persons functionally. All too often, our treatment of the aged is a sorry symptom of this tendency. Elderly people may be the most alienated members of our society. More and more of them spend their declining years in homes for senior citizens, in chronic hospitals, in nursing homes. We have shunted them aside. Their protest against a basically functional assessment of their persons is eloquent because it is helplessly muted and silent. We use the term "maladapted" to describe *them* rather than the environment. This behavior represents a terribly distorted judgment of the human person.

Faith can be protective against such a collapse. It should and, I believe, does sensitize us to the meaning of persons—to their inherent dignity, regardless of functionability. In this sense, faith aids us in staying human by underlining the truly human against cultural pressures to distort it. We might say that by steadying our gaze on the basic human values that are the parents of more concrete norms and rules, faith can exercise this protective function.

I have noted that the single, dominating, all-pervasive vitality in Jesus was the God-relationship. The human goods that define our flourishing (life and health, mating and raising children, knowledge, friendship, enjoyment of the arts), though desirable and attractive in themselves, are *subordinate* to this structural God-relationship.[26] Yet it is characteristic of the redeemed but still messy human condition to make idols—to pursue these basic goods *as ends in themselves*. This is the radical theological meaning of secularization: the loss of the context that relativizes and subordinates these basic goods and prevents us from divinizing them. The goods are so attractive that our constant temptation (our continuing enslavement, our bondage to the world, our constant need for liberation) is to center our being on them as ultimate ends, to cling to them with our whole being.

Jesus' love for us, of course, is primarily empowerment. In its purity and righteousness, however, this love also is the standard against the collapse known as idolatry. Whatever he willed for us and did for us, he did within the primacy and ultimacy of the God-relationship. Because this relationship is our very being and destiny, his love took the form of a constant reminder of this momentous dignity to people hell-bent on their idolatries.

Jesus' love, as standard, suggests the shape of our Christian love for each other. It is conduct that reminds others of their true dignity, reminds them of their being and destiny, and therefore pursues, supports, and protects the basic human goods *as subordinate*. Perhaps Barth had something like this idea in mind when he stated that the first service of others is witness—because the most urgent need of others is God himself.[27]

Vincent MacNamara has summarized what I have called the protective function of faith:

> It seems to me that the fact that union with God is the most important component of welfare or happiness will affect choice both for oneself and for one's service of others. One's own flourishing will mean preserving that relationship above all: this will relativize some goods that a non-believer might regard as important and highlight some which he would regard as unimportant. It will mean that choices which will lead to a weakening of one's sense of the relationship or which will endanger it will be regarded as morally undesirable.[28]

DISPOSITIVE

The Christian of profound faith will reflect in his or her dispositions the very shape of that faith. That shape, as I have noted, is the self-gift we call charity, love of God in others, charitable action. In an illuminating study, Edmund Pellegrino shows how the central dynamism of charity can shape moral choice within medicine. Pellegrino argues that charity will influence the way the three dominant principles of medical ethics (beneficence, autonomy, and justice) are interpreted, the way the physician-patient relationship is construed, and the way certain concrete choices are made.[29] Where beneficence is concerned, for instance, Pellegrino argues that some form of benevolent self-effacement (arguable on mere philosophical grounds) is a *minimum* obligation in an agapeistic ethic. The Christian physician sees himself or herself as called to perfection, to imitate Jesus' healing. In this perspective, appeals to exigency, fiscal survival, self-protection, and the canons of a competitive environment are morally feeble, even totally unacceptable.

Similarly, where justice is concerned, faith-full Christians will go beyond the strict calculus of duties and claims and exercise a "preferential option" for the very persons whose moral claims on society are difficult to establish: the poor, the outcast, the sociopath, the alcoholic, the non-compliant in the care of their own health.

Turning to the physician-patient relationship, Pellegrino argues that a charity-based ethic would reject notions of health care as a commodity transaction and the physician as a businessperson. Likewise, this ethic would reject the notion that the physician-patient relationship is a contract for services or is primarily for profit. The covenantal model is most consistent with the perspectives and dispositions generated by charity. Pellegrino does not argue for a fanatical devotion to medicine that would exclude other obligations to family, self, society, or country. Instead, charity disposes us to place these facets of medical practice in a morally defensible order.

Consider another aspect of an ethic rooted in Christian faith that also may be considered dispositive: the paschal mystery, the death-resurrection of Christ. Christians are accustomed to viewing aging, suffering, and dying within these perspectives.

Consider aging as an example. The most prominent quality of the lives of the elderly may be dependence. As Theodore Minnema points out, however, we are notoriously resistant to the idea of dependence.[30] Our national consciousness is shaped by the Declaration of Independence, and similar perspectives frame our individual attitudes. Dependence is vulnerability. Independent autonomy is exalted as a key marker of dignity. On this view, a certain negativity attaches to the passive virtues (meekness, humility, patience). Yet Christ's supreme dignity was manifest in dependence: "Not my will, but thine be done." (Luke 22:42.12.)

For this reason, Drew Christiansen developed a "theology of dependence."[31] For most of our adult lives, we ignore the dependence that ties us to other men and women:

> We keep the realization of our need for others at arm's length by keeping busy. If we can produce enough, if we can win enough, if we can party enough, we don't have to think too long about the meaning of life. Moreover, by manipulating things and managing people, we convince ourselves of our freedom and mastery of the world, and so avoid admitting how much we owe to others and to God.[32]

Christiansen considers this avoidance of dependence mistaken. Dependence is an opportunity—a call to let ourselves go, to open up to God, to cling in trust to a power beyond our control, to see more clearly than ever the source and end of life, much as Christ did in his dying dependence on the Father.

Dependence on others should be a sign of our more radical dependence on God. Because our freedom is intended to lead us to a deeper union with God, it is an interesting paradox that our deep dependence on God establishes our own radical independence: independence in dependence.

Thus, from a theological perspective, dependent old age should represent a flowering, not a wilting. In Christiansen's words,

> Outside of faith, dependence threatens us with subjugation, and our self-assertion may lead to isolation and abandonment. But for those who believe in the Giver of life, the promise hidden in dependence is communion with the Source of life itself.[33]

Similar things could apply to suffering and dying. From the perspective of faith, just as aging is not mere dependence and weakening, so suffering is not mere pain and confusion, dying is not merely an end. Suffering and dying must be viewed, even if mysteriously, in terms of a larger redemptive process: as occasions for a growing self-opening after Christ's example, as various participation in the paschal mystery. Such perspectival nuances may not solve clinical dilemmas—nor are they in any way intended to glorify suffering and dying. They powerfully suggest, however, that in approaching such realities, healing can never be seen as mere fixing; autonomy is not a mere "being left alone" but a condition for life-shaping; care is never merely material provision but a "being with" that reinforces a sense of worth and dignity; and dying can never be seen as "cosmetized passing" whose dignity is measured by the accumulation of minutes.

I have called such influences dispositive because they are rooted in the primacy of charity in a way that one is disposed to view all of life's moments as occasions for a more intense personal assimilation of the shape of the Christ-event.

DIRECTIVE

The biblical materials or stories that pass along the events that are the occasion of faith yield certain perspectives or themes that shape consciousness and therefore constitute the way that faith informs reason. I have attempted elsewhere to identify some of the themes that structure our ethical deliberation in biomedicine: life as a basic, but not absolute value; the extension of this evaluation to nascent life; the potential for human relationships as the aspect of physical life to be valued; the radical sociality of the human person; the inseparability of the unitive and procreative goods in human sexuality; and permanent heterosexual union as normative.[34]

Consider just the first of these themes as an illustration of the "directive" influence of theology on bioethics: life as a basic but not absolute good.

The fact that we are pilgrims, that Christ has overcome death and lives, that we will also live with Him, yields a general value judgment about the meaning and value of life as we now live it. This judgment can be formulated as follows: Life is a basic good but not an absolute one. It is *basic* because, as the Congregation for the Doctrine of the Faith worded it, it is the "necessary source and condition of every human activity and of all society."[35] It is not *absolute* because there are higher goods for which life can be sacrificed (e.g., the glory of

God, the salvation of souls, the service of others). Thus, "There is no greater love than this: to lay down one's life for one's friends."[36] Therefore, laying down one's life for another cannot be contrary to the faith or story or meaning of humankind. After Jesus' example, it is life's greatest fulfillment—even though it is the end of life as we now know it. Negatively, we could word this value judgment as follows: Death is an evil but not an absolute or unconditioned one.

This value judgment has immediate relevance for care for the ill and dying. It issues in a basic attitude or policy: Not all means must be used to preserve life. Why? Pope Pius XII, in a 1952 address to the International Congress of Anesthesiologists, stated, "A more strict obligation would be too burdensome for most people and would render the attainment of the higher, more important good too difficult. Life, health, all temporal activities are in fact subordinated to spiritual ends."[37] In other words, there are higher values than life in the living of it. There are also higher values in the dying of it.

Pius XII was saying, then, that forcing (morally) one to take *all* means is tantamount to forcing attention and energies on a subordinate good in a way that prejudices a higher good—even eventually making it unrecognizable as a good. Excessive concern for the temporal is at some point neglect of the eternal. An obligation to use all means to preserve life would be a devaluation of human life because it would remove life from the context or story that is the source of its ultimate value.

Thus, the Catholic tradition has moved between two extremes: medico-moral optimism—or vitalism (which preserves life with all means, at any cost, no matter what its condition)—and medico-moral pessimism (which actively kills when life become onerous, dysfunctional, or boring). Merely technological judgments could easily fall into either of these two traps. The medically effective could begin to define the humanly beneficial.

Thus far theology. It yields a value judgment and a general policy or attitude. It provides the framework for subsequent moral reasoning. It tells us that life is a gift with a purpose and destiny. Dying constitutes the final or waning moments of this "new creature." At this point, moral reasoning—that is, reason informed by faith—must assume its proper responsibilities to answer questions such as, What means ought to be used, and what need not be? What shall we call such means? Who enjoys the prerogative and/or duty of decision making? What is to be done with now-incompetent or always incompetent patients in critical illness? The sources of faith do not provide direct answers to these questions, in my judgment.

One way to indicate the directive importance of such general themes is by an example. Several years ago, in Louisville, I participated on a panel assessing the artificial heart. The panel included the mandatory Protestant (Robert Nelson), Catholic (myself), and Jew (the late Isaac Franck), along with William Lansing, president of Humana. The question arose about whether the artificial heart works. Dr. Lansing stated, "When Bill DeVries and I decide that it doesn't work, the program will stop." I jumped on that response and asked, "If the artificial heart gives you only an extra ten hours of life, or ten days, does it work?" Somewhat to my surprise at the time—though not as I look back on the incident—my colleague and friend, Dr. Franck, mumbled audibly, "It works." Theology was only thinly disguised in such a reaction. I do not believe the Christian story would support such a response. It views life and death in light of the paschal mystery and has a relativizing influence on both that I found lacking in Dr. Franck's judgment.

I propose, therefore, that theology—and I repeat that I understand theology as a re-flection on Christian faith—can influence bioethics in very important ways. Theology functions not as a *direct* originating influence on concrete moral judgments at the essential level (on this point I agree with autonomists such as Fuchs, Schuuler, Auer, Hughes, and others) but to provide "morally relevant insights," in the words of Franz Bockle.[38] On this view, faith and reason compenetrate to produce a distinct consciousness with identifiable cognitive dimensions or facets. I have identified three such dimensions—overlapping as they are—as *protective* (or corrective), *dispositive,* and *directive.*

Cumulatively, such influences attempt to show how faith informs reason. The out-come of such "informing" is a distinct—though not utterly mysterious—way of viewing the world and ourselves and of hierarchizing values. To claim that such distinct outlooks and onlooks (theology) have nothing to do with bioethics is either to separate faith from one's view of the world (which trivializes faith by reducing it dualistically to an utterly other-worldly) or to separate one's view of the world from bioethics (which trivializes bioethics by isolating it from the very persons it purports to serve).

NOTES

1. This essay previously was published as Richard A. McCormick, "Theology and Bio-ethics," *Corrective Vision: Explorations in Moral Theology* (Kansas City, Mo.: Sheed & Ward, 1994), 133–48; reprinted with permission.
2. Alisdair MacIntyre, "Theology, Ethics and the Ethics of Medicine and Health Care," *Journal of Medicine and Philosophy* 4 (1979): 435–43.
3. Johannes B. Metz, *Followers of Christ* (Ramsey, N.J.: Paulist Press, 1978), 39–40.
4. Joseph Sittler, *The Structure of Christian Ethics* (New Orleans: Louisiana State University Press, 1958).
5. Ibid., 45.
6. John 1: 3.
7. Walter Kasper, *An Introduction to Christian Faith* (Ramsey, N.J.: Paulist Press, 1980), 82.
8. Sittler, *The Structure of Christian Ethics,* 46.
9. Edmund Pincoffs, "Quandary Ethics," *Mind* 80 (1971): 552–71.
10. I take these distinctions from Norbert Rigali, "On Christian Ethics," *Chicago Studies* 10 (1971): 227–47.
11. A good presentation of this discussion is Vincent MacNamara's *Faith and Ethics* (Wash-ington, D.C.: Georgetown University Press, 1985).
12. James M. Gustafson, *Ethics From a Theocentric Perspective, Volume II: Ethics and Theol-ogy* (Chicago: University of Chicago Press, 1984), 98.
13. Congregation for the Doctrine of the Faith, *Declaration on Euthanasia* (Vatican City: Vatican Polyglot Press, 1980) 14; (emphasis added); also in *Origins* 10 (1980): 154–57.
14. Karl Barth, *The Knowledge of God and the Service of God According to the Teaching of the Reformation* (London: Hodder and Stoughton, 1938), 95.
15. Thomas E. Clark, "Public Policy and Christian Discernment," in *Personal Values in Pub-lic Policy,* ed. John Haughey (Ramsey, N.J.: Paulist Press, 1979), 232–42.
16. L. Cerfaux, "La charite fraternelle et le retour du Christ," *Ephemerides Theologicae Lovanienses* 24 (1958): 326.

17. Joseph Fuchs, *Christian Morality: The Word Becomes Flesh* (Washington, D.C.: Georgetown University Press, 1987), 204.
18. *The Documents of Vatican II* (New York: American Press, 1966), 209.
19. MacNamara, *Faith and Ethics,* 120.
20. Ibid., 117.
21. Ibid., 116.
22. Ibid., 119.
23. Ibid., 121.
24. Philip Rieff, *The Triumph of the Therapeutic: Uses of Faith After Freud* (New York: Harper and Row, 1966).
25. Daniel Callahan, "Living with the New Biology," *Center Magazine* 5 (July-August 1972), 4–12.
26. Richard A. McCormick, *Health and Medicine in the Catholic Tradition* (New York: Crossroads, 1984), 37–38.
27. Karl Barth, *Church Dogmatics* (Edinburgh: T. T. Clark, 1958), IV/2, 216.
28. MacNamara, *Faith and Ethics,* 123.
29. Edmund D. Pellegrino, "Agape and Ethics: Some Reflections on Medical Morals from a Catholic Christian Perspective," in *Catholic Perspectives on Medical Morals: Foundational Issues,* ed. Edmund D. Pellegrino, John P. Langan, John Collins Harvey (Boston: Kluwer Academic Publishers, 1989), 277–300.
30. Theodore Minnema, "Human Dignity and Human Dependence," *Calvin Theological Journal* 16 (1981): 5–14.
31. Drew Christiansen, "The Elderly and Their Families: The Problems of Dependence," *New Catholic World* 223 (1980): 100–104.
32. Ibid., 102.
33. Ibid., 104.
34. Richard A. McCormick, "Theology and Bioimedical Ethics," *Logos* 3 (1982): 25–43.
35. Congregation for the Doctrine of the Faith, *Declaration on Euthanasia,* n. 19.
36. John 15: 13.
37. Pius XII, *Acta Apostolicae* Sedis 9 (1957): 1031–32.
38. Franz Bockle, "Glaube und Handelin," *Concilium* 120 (1976): 641–47.

PART IV

Medical Education

Teaching the Humanities in American Medical Schools during the Twentieth Century: A Commentary on the Two Dominant Models

Chester R. Burns

Among today's physician-philosophers, Edmund Pellegrino understands as well as anyone—and better than most—the intimate relationships between medical history and medical ethics.[1] In honor of this understanding, I offer some reflections about the two dominant models that educators have used to teach the humanities in American medical schools during the twentieth century: medical history and medical ethics. After providing some evidence justifying my claims, I offer some explanations and interpretations.

During the 1890s and the early years of the twentieth century, many of the physicians who supported the reform of medical education also supported the teaching of medical history to medical students.[2] Some of these physicians gave lecture courses in medical history, including John Shaw Billings in Baltimore, Nathan Smith Davis in Chicago, Charles Winslow Dulles in Philadelphia, Roswell Park in Buffalo, and Burnside Foster in Minneapolis. These educators were not reactionaries. They were physician-professors who vigorously supported the marriages of medical schools to universities and the biomedical sciences to clinical medicine. At the Johns Hopkins University School of Medicine, William Osler and his colleagues utilized historical knowledge during clinical teaching rounds and during informal sessions with students and house staff, as did Eugene Cordell at the University of Maryland.

In a survey conducted in 1904, Cordell discovered that basic science or clinical teachers at six of fourteen medical schools associated with universities gave medical history lectures or courses.[3] By 1937, forty-six of seventy-seven schools (60 percent) offered regular courses in medical history; these courses were required in twenty-eight of these institutions, elective in the others.[4] In that year, only one teacher was a full-time professor of medical history: Henry E. Sigerist, who had been director of the Johns Hopkins University Institute of the History of Medicine since 1932. The others were experimental scientists and clinical specialists who believed that medical history played an extremely important role in acculturating future physicians.

These individuals—such as William Snow Miller, Harvey Cushing, Henry Handerson, Lewis Pilcher, Charles Dana, C. N. B. Camac, and Chauncey Leake—enthusiastically demonstrated their love of medical history by giving many lectures and seminars, by supporting medical history clubs in schools and medical history societies in major cities, by writing articles for new journals devoted to medical history, and by giving papers during meetings of the American Association for the History of Medicine (which had been founded in 1925).

The teaching of medical history peaked in the 1950s. A survey in 1955 revealed that seventy-one of eighty-one schools (88 percent) offered required or elective courses in medical history, some taught by trained full-time historians of medicine.[5] This situation changed during the 1960s, however. In 1967, only thirty-three of eighty-five schools (39 percent) offered courses in medical history; only eleven of these schools required such courses.[6] The ascendancy of medical history as the dominant way of incorporating the humanities into medical education had ended.

As the teaching of medical history declined, the teaching of medical ethics increased. The first national conference on the teaching of medical ethics was held in Tarrytown, New York, in June 1972. At that meeting, Robert Veatch presented data from a national survey of medical schools. Fifteen of the schools reported no teaching of medical ethics; fifty-six schools reported that ethical issues were addressed in various courses, such as courses on community medicine and legal medicine; and seventeen schools offered special lectures and symposia. Thirty-three schools had electives in medical ethics, and four schools required such courses.[7] In 1980, another survey indicated that 59 of 125 schools offered courses in medical ethics or bioethics.[8]

For another view of these trends, compare the data about the teaching of medical history and medical ethics in the 1978–79 Association of American Medical Colleges' (AAMC) Curriculum Directory with that in AAMC's 1998–99 Directory. In 1978–79, 26 of 124 schools (21 percent) had required courses in medical ethics, whereas only 4 schools had required courses in medical history. Sixty-five percent of the schools offered electives in medical ethics; about 45 percent offered electives in medical history.[9] For the 1998–99 year, every school taught medical ethics, either as a separate required course (50 percent), as part of a required course (81 percent), or as an elective (47 percent). Six of the 127 schools (5 percent) offered required courses in medical history. At 39 percent of the schools, some medical history was provided in required courses such as community medicine or public health. Fifty-one percent of the schools offered medical history as an elective; 28 percent offered no medical history instruction.[10]

I do not claim that medical history and medical ethics were the only disciplinary models used by teachers of the humanities in medical schools. Some of the most engaging courses in recent years have involved literature and medicine, death and dying, and spirituality in medicine. Nor do I claim that medical ethics was ignored during the first half of the century or that medical history was ignored during the second half.[11] I do claim that medical history was the dominant pedagogical model during the first half of the century, whereas medical ethics has become the dominant model during the second half. Even courses in literature and medicine are often considered inadequate if they do not focus on ethical problems in contemporary medicine.

Why did teachers in American medical schools give so much allegiance to medical history before the 1960s, and why have teachers in these schools given so much allegiance to medical ethics since the 1960s? As someone who straddles both movements, I offer my reflections only as prologue to more thorough inquiries.

Physician-professors at the turn of the twentieth century experienced profound changes in medical science and medical practice—changes they deemed progressive and salutary. William Osler's *Principles and Practice of Medicine* (published in 1892) symbolized the scientific dimension of the moral ideals animating the new group of clinical specialists emerging at the turn of the century. Their brand of medical ethics was enshrined on every page of Osler's textbook. Physicians who ignored the knowledge in that text were immoral. Loyalties to particular religious groups, philosophical systems, or codes of professional societies could never be acceptable substitutes for learning and applying the contents of Osler's text in caring for individual patients with specific diseases.

The values associated with experimental science and clinical specialization created new perplexities, however. Was allegiance to experimental science and clinical specialization sufficient to determine the morality of the medical profession? Was the philosophy of medical science in Osler's text sufficient for the ethics of medical practitioners? Osler did not think it was. He did not turn to religion, philosophy, or law for humanistic values, however; he turned to biography and history.

Persons, not abstractions or codes, were Osler's foci for humanistic values. Osler wrote numerous biographical essays about British and American physicians, including William Harvey, Sir Thomas Browne, Elisha Bartlett, and Oliver Wendell Holmes.[12] For Osler, these essays were case studies in professional values. For example, in an essay about John Bassett, Osler wrote, "We honor those who respond to the call; we love to tell the story of their lives; and while feeling, perhaps, that we could not have been, with them, faithful unto death, yet we recognize in the power of their example the leaven which leavens the mass of selfishness about us." Later in this essay, Osler added, "To have striven, to have made an effort, to have been true to certain ideals—this alone is worth the struggle."[13] Osler used biographical studies of physicians as a vehicle for conveying professional ideals to fellow practitioners and students.

Osler's approach to human values was liberal and pluralistic. As *Evolution of Modern Medicine* revealed, Osler's approach to historical knowledge was as open as his approach to scientific knowledge.[14] An open mind, a willingness to investigate in the laboratory and at the bedside, and an enduring commitment to revising one's understanding of disease and therapy were the hallmarks of such values for Osler and the new specialists who valued science as a foundation for morally acceptable medical practice. An open mind about human greatness and human foible, a willingness to investigate the stories of past doctors and past medical institutions, and an enduring commitment to historical narrative as a method for recognizing and honoring those who sustained the most worthwhile values of the medical profession were the hallmarks for Osler and others who chose history as the principal source of humanistic values in medicine.

Medical science would provide the knowledge needed to deal with the diseases of sick persons. Medical history would provide the knowledge needed to manage relationships within the medical profession and those of the profession with the larger society. These and related beliefs satisfied the cultural needs of hundreds of students, teachers, and doctors during the first half of the twentieth century—as well as many during the last half of the century.[15] Osler's legacy was institutionalized in the establishment of the American Osler Society in 1970—a society that still vibrates with much energy today.[16]

Especially after 1960, this paradigm of medical history and humanistic values became less influential as some medical leaders and many savants outside medicine recast the meaning of humanistic values in terms of bioethics and medical ethics. Critics assailed the Oslerian approach as too paternalistic and naive. Learning about the lives of individual doctors or about the progressive accomplishments of the medical profession did not automatically transform students into caring physicians, nor did it transform medicine into a socially judicious profession. An approach based on custom and tradition was insufficient, these critics argued, as a method for adaptation to the profound technological and social changes of contemporary society. Religious professionals, philosophers, and legal scholars were among the commentators who expected physicians to reexamine their professional values and renegotiate their covenants and contracts with multiple American publics. For these observers, history was not sufficient for determining how to behave during the new evangelical era of rights for women, children, blacks, and patients.

Bioethics and medical ethics became the new models for teaching the humanities in medical education. Spurred especially by the Institute on Human Values in Medicine project of the Society for Health and Human Values (1971–1981), the Hastings Center project on the Teaching of Ethics in Higher Education (1977–1982), and Georgetown University's support of the first edition of the *Encyclopedia of Bioethics* (1975), administrators of medical schools employed new faculty members (mostly trained in philosophy or theology) who introduced students and faculty to various patterns of ethical discourse and argumentation.

At Pennsylvania State University's College of Medicine, for example, Dan Clouser has taught ethics in ways that nurture the development of certain skills in medical students: moral discernment, critical thinking, imaginative empathy, and nondogmatic appraisal of varying perspectives.[17] Often using patient-centered cases brimming with ethical conflicts, Clouser and other teachers have engaged students and faculty members with action-oriented, problem-solving, life-or-death issues in contemporary medical practice. As a strategy for addressing humanistic values in medical education, medical ethics (especially bioethics) appears to be more popular than medical history. Every medical school has one or more persons specifically designated to teach ethics—a practice that never occurred with medical history.[18]

Several factors may explain the fall of medical history as the dominant humanistic model in medical schools. The first is an irony of professionalization. As the number of professional historians of medicine teaching in medical schools increased, there was a substantial decline in the numbers of basic science and clinical professors who displayed an interest in history. A cultural segregation occurred between the "amateurs" and the "professionals" because the professional historians assigned more value to their research endeavors than they did to transforming their knowledge into patterns of understanding that would meet the cultural needs of graduate students in the biomedical sciences and medical students. This segregation produced a loss of engagement with many students and faculty members.[19]

A second reason involves our submergence in a popular culture that judges the events of yesterday as instant history. Curiosity about a more remote past is stifled by the compelling, even oppressive, emotional dramas of the present, which are displayed in countless media images every moment of every day. Not a few of these dramas involve ethical conflicts in the practice of medicine—as anyone who watches *Chicago Hope* or *ER* can attest. The behaviors and beliefs of ancient Greeks, medieval scholastics, and colonial North American clergy seem more disconnected than ever from today's technology-driven global cosmopolitanism.

Likewise, a variety of factors may explain the rise of interest in the teaching of medical ethics and bioethics. The basic science and clinical teachers who previously attended to medical history now must deal with the ethical challenges associated with the many technological, social, and cultural changes of the past forty years. Every academic medical center that accepts federal dollars for research must now offer a required course in ethics to its graduate students in the biomedical sciences—who later become teachers in medical schools.[20] Most clinical professors acknowledge the ever-present ethical conflicts that arise daily in the care of sick persons. Full-time professionals who teach bioethics or medical ethics in today's medical schools have little difficulty engaging the minds of students who usually acknowledge the relevance of ethics to their roles as future scientists or physicians.[21] The allure of timeless ideals and ethical critiques appears more powerful than any fascination with stories about dead persons and dead cultures.

There are other interpretations of the vicissitudes of teaching medical history and medical ethics in twentieth-century American medical schools. The social environment of these schools exerts a peculiarly compressive force. Throughout this century, these schools have employed mostly clinical specialists and biomedical scientists as teachers. Administrators and faculties have expended their financial resources in support of the scientific and specialty ideals espoused by Osler and others at the turn of the century.

Compared to the number of biomedical scientists and clinicians constituting medical school faculties, only a small number of professors in the behavioral sciences, the social sciences, and the humanities have been employed to teach in these schools. Moreover, these nonclinical professors have been allowed to offer their knowledge only in tightly controlled and relatively tiny parts of the medical school curricula. In these circumstances, teachers of medical history and teachers of medical ethics are happy just to have their feet inside the doors. Because only a few professors are designated or employed to teach these subjects, their approaches seem to be dominant because in many cases colleagues from other humanities disciplines are not allowed or encouraged to present their perspectives.

Another interpretation involves the intellectual sensibilities of the professors who teach medical history and medical ethics. These teachers may be less liberal and less open than they might appear at first glance. Exclusivist—perhaps ethnocentric—salvation themes tend to appear. Some of the professors who taught medical history in the first half of the century believed that medical history embraced all of the humanities and offered eclectic views that they considered sufficient for transmitting the everlastingly "best" cultural values. Some of the teachers of medical ethics and bioethics also appear to move into reductionist or fundamentalist modes of thinking—as Tristram Engelhardt argued in his keynote address during the first annual meeting of the American Society of Bioethics and Humanities in November 1998.[22]

The changing patterns of dominance between medical history and medical ethics may be a manifestation of the tendencies for teachers of the humanities in medical schools to narrow their intellectual approaches as ways of coping with the scope and complexity of cultural values and pluralistic behaviors in today's world. Specific paradigms of historical knowledge and philosophical arguments provide some illusions of certainty in an ever-changing world.

Surely both medical history and medical ethics have a place in the education of physicians. Neither, however, provides exclusive paths to value-salvation in medicine, and neither has earned exclusive rights to pedagogical dominance in the teaching of the humanities in medical schools. The future of these teaching endeavors depends on the educators who administer medical schools and those who are invited to teach in these schools.

As the twentieth century ends and the twenty-first century dawns, administrators in medical schools have opportunities to foster more constructive dialogues between the humanities and medicine than ever before. They can choose to support small cadres of humanities professionals with a variety of disciplinary perspectives, including—but not limited to—history and ethics. They can employ teachers who are willing to offer their perspectives in ways that genuinely respond to the cultural needs of today's students, professors, and practitioners.

Eschewing exclusivist postures, these teachers can display suitable respect for the relevance of multiple disciplines in today's pluralistic cultures. Humanistic values are cultivated for one student by history, for another by ethics, for another by literature, for another by religion. With a willingness to explore interdisciplinary approaches, these teachers can provide perspectives that nurture the cultural integrity of students as individuals and as young professionals.

For three decades, Edmund Pellegrino has pleaded with humanities teachers in medical schools to pursue more effective styles of teaching.[23] Inspired by his visions and energies, numerous teachers have improved the teaching of medical humanities in medical schools during the twentieth century.[24] Many more interdisciplinary opportunities await those who will sustain and enrich these legacies in the new century.

NOTES

1. For samples of this understanding, see Edmund D. Pellegrino, "Medicine, History, and the Idea of Man," *Annals of the American Academy of Political and Social Science* 346 (March 1963): 9–20; Edmund D. Pellegrino, "Percival's Medical Ethics: The Moral Philosophy of an 18th-Century English Gentleman," *Archives of Internal Medicine* 146 (November 1986): 43–47.

2. Genevieve Miller, "Medical History," in *The Education of American Physicians Historical Essays*, ed. Ronald L. Numbers (Berkeley: University of California Press, 1980), 290–308.

3. Eugene F. Cordell, "The Importance of the Study of the History of Medicine," *Medical Library & Historical Journal* 2, no. 4 (1904): 268–82.

4. Henry E. Sigerist, "Medical History in the Medical Schools of the United States," *Bulletin of the History of Medicine* 7, no. 6 (1939): 627–62.

5. Edward L. Turner, Walter S. Wiggins, and Anne Tipner, "Medical Education in the United States and Canada," *Journal of the American Medical Association* 159, no. 6 (1955): 579.

6. Genevieve Miller, "The Teaching of Medical History in the United States and Canada: Report of a Field Survey," parts 1–4, *Bulletin of the History of Medicine* 43, no. 3 (1969): 259–67, no. 4 (1969): 344–75, no. 5 (1969): 444–72, no. 6 (1969): 553–86.

7. Robert M. Veatch, "National Survey of the Teaching of Medical Ethics in Medical Schools," in *The Teaching of Medical Ethics,* vol. 14, ed. Robert M. Veatch, Willard Gaylin, and Councilman Morgan (Hastings-on-Hudson, N.Y.: Institute of Society, Ethics and the Life Sciences, 1973), 97–102.

8. Edmund D. Pellegrino and Thomas K. McElhinney, *Teaching Ethics, the Humanities, and Human Values in Medical Schools: A Ten-Year Overview* (Washington, D.C.: Institute on Human Values in Medicine, Society for Health and Human Values, 1980), 15.

9. Association of American Medical Colleges, *1978–79 AAMC Curriculum Directory* (Washington, D.C.: Association of American Medical Colleges, 1978), 300–301. I counted required courses by analyzing the entries for each school.

10. Association of American Medical Colleges, *Curriculum Directory 1998–1999* (Washington, D.C.: Association of American Medical Colleges, 1998), 12.

11. For details about the historical evolution of medical ethics teaching in medical schools, see Chester R. Burns, "Medical Ethics and Jurisprudence," in *The Education of American Physicians: Historical Essays,* ed. Ronald L. Numbers, 273–89.

12. For a list of Osler's historical and biographical writings, see Richard L. Golden and Charles G. Roland, eds., *Sir William Osler: An Annotated Bibliography with Illustrations* (San Francisco: Norman Publishing, 1988), 75–96.

13. William Osler, *An Alabama Student and Other Biographical Essays* (New York: Oxford University Press, 1908), 1–2, 18.

14. William Osler, *Evolution of Modern Medicine* (New Haven, Conn.: Yale University Press, 1921).

15. To appreciate the extent of Osler's influence, one need only know that physicians and others had written 1,367 publications about Osler and his legacy by 1976; see Earl F. Nation, Charles G. Roland, and John P. McGovern, eds., *An Annotated Checklist of Osleriana* (Kent, Ohio: Kent State University Press, 1976). Readers unfamiliar with Osler can find a good sampling of Osleriana in a commemorative issue of the *Journal of the American Medical Association* 210 (Dec. 22, 1969): 2213–71.

16. To sample this energy, see two collections of papers presented during meetings of this society: Jeremiah Barondess, John P. McGovern, and Charles G. Roland, eds., *The Persisting Osler: Selected Transactions of the First Ten Years of the American Osler Society* (Baltimore, Md.: University Park Press, 1985), and Jeremiah A. Barondess and Charles G. Roland, eds., *The Persisting Osler II: Selected Transactions of the American Osler Society 1981–1990* (Malabar, Fla.: Krieger Publishing Company, 1994). Two essays by Edmund Pellegrino appear in the 1994 volume.

17. K. Danner Clouser, "Humanities in Medical Education: Some Contributions," *Journal of Medicine and Philosophy* 15, no. 3 (1990): 289–301; K. Danner Clouser, "Humanities in the Service of Medicine: Three Models," in *Philosophy of Medicine and Bioethics: A Twenty-Year Retrospective and Critical Appraisal,* eds. Ronald A. Carson and Chester R. Burns (Dordrecht, The Netherlands: Kluwer Academic Press, 1997), 25–39. For Clouser's earlier and more extensive analysis of ethics teaching, see K. Danner Clouser, *Teaching Bioethics: Strategies, Problems, and Resources* (Hastings-on-Hudson, N.Y.: Institute of Society, Ethics and the Life Sciences, 1980).

18. To sample the voluminous literature on the teaching of medical ethics, consult the annual volumes of the *Bibliography of Bioethics,* which began in 1975; search under the heading "Teaching Medical Ethics" in earlier volumes, "Bioethics/Education" in more recent volumes.

19. Chester R. Burns, "History in Medical Education: The Development of Current Trends in the United States," *Bulletin of the New York Academy of Medicine* 51, no. 7 (1975):

851–69; Chester R. Burns, "Liberating Medical Minds: Can Historians Help?" in *The Role of the Humanities in Medical Education*, ed. Donnie J. Self (Norfolk, Va.: Bio-Medical Ethics Program, Eastern Virginia Medical School, 1978), 8–20; Chester R. Burns, "Medical History and Medical Humanities: Some New Styles of Learning and Teaching," in *Teaching the History of Medicine at a Medical Center*, ed. Jerome J. Bylebel (Baltimore, Md.: Johns Hopkins University Press, 1982), 31–40.

20. I do not know of any graduate school in the biomedical sciences that offers a required or elective course in the history of medicine or history of science.

21. The rise of interest in teaching is concurrent with the rise of interest in scholarship. For a substantial analysis of the scholarly origins of bioethics, see Albert R. Jonsen, *The Birth of Bioethics* (New York: Oxford University Press, 1998), 3–89.

22. H. Tristram Engelhardt, Jr., "Bioethics in the Third Millennium: Some Critical Antici-pations" (paper presented at the annual meeting of the American Society for Bioethics and Humanities, Houston, Texas, November 1998). Engelhardt claimed that quests for single, universal, unified, correct moral visions among bioethicists denied or discounted today's moral pluralism.

23. Edmund D. Pellegrino, "Reform and Innovation in Medical Education: The Role of Ethics," in *The Teaching of Medical Ethics,* eds. Robert M. Veatch, Willard Gaylin, and Councilman Morgan (Hastings-on-Hudson, N.Y.: Institute of Society, Ethics and the Life Sciences, 1973), 150–65; Edmund D. Pellegrino, "Medical History and Medical Education," *Clio Medica* 10, no.4 (1975): 295–303; Edmund D. Pellegrino, *Humanism and the Physician* (Knoxville: University of Tennessee Press, 1979), 153–230; Pellegrino and McElhinney, *Teaching Ethics, the Humanities, and Human Values in Medical Schools,* 41–55.

24. For a splendid introduction to innovative teaching, see the special issue of *Academic Medicine* vol. 70, no. 9, (September 1995): 755–813, which was devoted to the human-ities and medical education.

Reflections on the Humanities and Medical Education: Balancing History, Theory, and Practice

Thomas K. McElhinney

Physician education is an interweaving of the three common themes of all professional education: theory, practice, and history.[1] In medicine, the role of history has been the least understood of this triad. For musicians, history is the story of the music that helps in the understanding of theory and the interpretation that guides performance. For a lawyer, history primarily means precedents: prior rulings upon which a new case can be constructed. Neither law nor music, however, shares with medicine the constant pressure of a rapidly developing scientific knowledge base that requires doctors to maintain an awareness of the most current findings and the most recent diagnostic and therapeutic methodologies. If *history* means anything to a doctor, it relates to the individual patient's record of health and illness—a recounting of personal and family illnesses. Less recognized in medicine is the role that prior experiences and controlled trials have as a history of what does and does not work effectively.

In these three professions—as in engineering, ministry, and other fields—the theme of history in professional education must be reconceptualized. It must be perceived in very broad terms as not only the story of a profession but also its context within its society.

Beginning in the 1960s, this broader sense of history was captured in physician education through the development of human values and humanities programs. Yet finding agreement about a word or phrase to describe the new emphasis on humanities and human values in the professions has been difficult.[2] The choices include humanities, humanistic studies, humanistic social sciences, behavioral sciences, liberal arts, general studies, bioethics, and medical humanities. One or more of these terms may appear in a particular medical school's program, and many are used interchangeably. I have argued that the phrase "humanities perspective" indicates the importance of the academic humanities without excluding efforts in the social sciences, law, and other fields.[3] A humanities perspective in this sense is the historical overview that complements and completes theory and practice.

During the four years of undergraduate medical education, the areas of theory and practice—presented as basic medical sciences and clinical training—cause the greatest tensions and the most powerful conflicts as they compete for curriculum time and recognition. Consequently, little time is provided for a humanities perspective—a matter that is assumed to have been completed during the undergraduate college years. The residency years extend

267

the clinical training, with some attention to basic science as well as ethical problems. Continuing education emphasizes what a physician needs to know to be up-to-date, thereby mingling theory and practice. Continuing education conferences sometimes focus on ethical problems, and other aspects of practice that incorporate a humanities perspective that some practitioners may not have experienced in their previous medical training.

In this essay, I review the events that brought a humanities perspective and human values teaching into more prominence in undergraduate medical education as well as throughout a physician's education. This movement helped to restore in health education a critical balance among the themes of history, theory, and practice.

BACKGROUND: RECOGNIZING THE NEED

About fifty years ago, developments in the science of medicine and in new technologies experienced an acceleration that had profound effects on the practice of medicine and in the traditional methods of delivering health care. Building on the dramatic political, social, and technical changes that resulted from World War II and the threat of the developing Cold War, the United States committed significant resources to research in all areas, including medicine. During World War II and the decades that followed, new drugs began to increase survival from infectious diseases. Meanwhile, new technology required that patients receive more and more of their treatments at doctors' offices and in hospitals. A "cottage industry" became a "techno-industry," and physician practices became businesses as private payers increasingly gave way to insurance, government, or other third-party providers.

By the end of the 1950s, the changes that technology was introducing called for critical reviews of the issues that the new science had raised. C. P. Snow's controversial thesis on *The Two Cultures and the Scientific Revolution* was released in 1959. That year was also significant because it marked the 100th anniversary of the publication of Charles Darwin's *On the Origin of Species*—a scientific revolution whose centennial celebration occasioned several conferences and studies. These reports that were generated demonstrated not only an appreciation of Darwin's impact but also an awareness of the major advances in genetics that had occurred in the 100 years that followed. These advances included the then-recent proposal by Watson and Crick regarding the double helix structure of the DNA molecule. The Darwin centennial articles and conferences called attention to problems and ethical dilemmas that an increasing knowledge of the basic genetic mechanisms of life, coupled with the development of more invasive technology, would produce.

The manner in which the increased complexity of the science of medicine was affecting what needed to be taught in the four years of medical school was critical. The more technically oriented medicine had two effects in undergraduate medical education: the creation of new specialties—with their demands for curricular time in clinical training—and increased pressure for clinical preparation in the first two years of undergraduate medical education. These first years of undergraduate medical education, which were reserved primarily for the basic medical sciences, were also becoming more crowded as the knowledge base for medicine not only expanded but also underwent continued revision. New discoveries were being announced in each new edition of the major journals, and physicians increasingly were relying on technology in diagnosis and treatment, so ensuring that basic science concepts were reviewed and taught in the last two years of undergraduate medical education, as well as in the residency years, became increasingly important.

The pressure from the growing body of medical knowledge also required that students entering medical school have substantial preparation in the sciences, particularly the biological sciences. Premedical preparation increasingly emphasized science—at the cost of other studies, including the arts and humanities. The broad general education offered by universities was also crowded from the curricula of undergraduate professional education in allied health and nursing, which also felt a need to increase basic science requirements.[4]

The same post–World War II period that saw so many changes in the science of medicine also produced social and political revolution. Throughout the world, nations freed themselves from colonial rule that had been established in earlier centuries through the expansion of Western culture. In the United States, a civil rights movement carried on work begun by free and enslaved blacks and white abolitionists from the beginning of the country's history. An almost 100-year pattern of segregation that developed in the southern states following the Civil War was challenged and then broken in the mid-1950s with the integration of the public schools. In the following years, these efforts to achieve civil rights for racial minorities were expanded to include women's rights, gay rights, and the recognition of other rights—including the rights of patients to be involved in decisions related to their medical care and the rights of experimental subjects to know the risks occurred through their participation in research.

The social setting for the practice of medicine also changed because of technological developments. Physicians visited the home less commonly, and patients more regularly found it necessary to undergo invasive diagnostic procedures that could only be conducted in a doctor's office—or, with increasing frequency, in a hospital setting. The technology itself shrouded doctors in more mystery because of the complexity of the interventions. Through this technology, the physician also gained more power and authority to control the progress of the patient's treatment. Research subjects were even more likely to be kept unaware of the protocol being followed or the procedure being done. In the mid-1960s, the efforts of Beecher, Pappworth, and others called attention to research abuses and engendered the movement toward civil rights for patients. Ultimately, physicians and researchers were forced to recognize the ethical problems of authority in medical research.

The twin challenges of an expanding recognition of individual rights and the increased complexity and invasive nature of health care led to a review of the education and training of health professionals. Medical educators and physicians in practice, inspired by their own social involvement and by discontent with their own medical education, were joined by the demands of a newly energized public and the protests of activist students. Questions were raised about the absence of women and minorities in medical school, and admissions committees responded. As women and minority students increased in number among medical students, there was pressure for recognition of patients' rights, for community involvement by the medical schools, and for a restructuring of authority. With increasing frequency, humanities-trained professionals began to appear on the faculty rosters of the nation's medical schools.

The changes in medicine caused by scientific discovery and technological developments, on the one hand, and social and political transformations, on the other, increasingly highlighted the impossibility of a complete medical education structured only on theory and practice (i.e., basic science and clinical training). The study of basic sciences raises questions about what science does and the direction science should take. Science, once viewed as the great liberator, had a darker side that appeared too frequently for public confidence to be sustained. Clearly, basic science studies in medical school needed to involve discussions of values and priorities. Similarly, clinical practice often furnishes multiple pathways for a physician to pursue in diagnosis and treatment. When choices can be made, medical students must think about the values of the profession, about their own values, and—with the impact of patient rights—about the wishes of their patients. Furthermore, medical practice was beginning to be sharply limited by a demand for services that outstripped the resources that were available. Economic pressures raised the question of who would get treatment and who would pay the cost of treating the uninsured.

The introduction (or reintroduction) of the humanities and human values—including value questions raised in law, in the politics of medicine, and in questions of rights to health care—into medical education came about as a response to questions that could not be answered in a basic science class or in the clinic. The balance among history, theory, and practice was restored.

EXPLORING THE HUMANITIES PERSPECTIVE

Two major vectors must be considered in the introduction of the humanities into medical education. One vector addresses the question, What can the humanities be used for? The other addresses a less-explored question: How do differences among students affect humanities methodologies?

The Uses of the Humanities

Students learn the skills of critical analysis, reasoning, decision making, and judgment through the humanities. Commentators have often noted that these skills are a necessary part of medical education.[5] Edmund Pellegrino has frequently and persuasively argued for the role of the humanities in medical education. Pellegrino regards the humanities as vehicles for the liberal arts. Why are the liberal arts important for the medical student? Pellegrino says that the liberal arts are "a set of skills which truly set us free, and without which we cannot consciously be free men in any other domain. The freedom to which I refer is freedom from the tyranny of the opinions, ideas, words and productions of other men."[6] Pellegrino outlines the necessary components as "capacities":[7]

- The capacity for critical thinking
- The capacity to listen and read intelligently
- The capacity to make judgments about the beautiful
- The capacity to make judgments about morals
- The capacity to comprehend the notion of continuity—that is, history

The humanities are the cognitive instruments that are the working tools of the educated person, and Pellegrino hopes that the physician will be an educated person. He also acknowledges the importance of the affective domain—especially the role of the physician as a compassionate individual. He also notes that these areas of human understanding are sources for the "delectation of the human spirit," a theme he develops in writings on the "post-Evangelical era" of medical humanities.[8]

In medical education, the humanities have been dominated by the development of skills needed to cope with moral issues (bioethics and medical ethics). The frequency of ethical dilemmas in the changing environment of medicine and the great interest within medicine and among the general public reinforce the need for ethical instruction throughout the formal years of medical training and into continuing education. Additionally, all professional education is value-laden. In the first days of medical school, in a "white coat ceremony," medical students receive a jacket traditionally worn by undergraduate medical students and take the Hippocratic Oath. This increasingly popular ritual demonstrates that medicine expects that its students know and practice the values of their profession early in their training.

Many areas of medicine can be informed by any of several disciplines. For example, many medical students have awakened to value conflicts in certain situations by reading a short story by Richard Seltzer or poetry by John Stone or Jack Coulehan. Practitioners of individual disciplines have developed their own journals, hold their own conferences, and have interest groups in other professional organizations. Although bioethicists are the most numerous group in the humanities in medicine activities, other disciplines—such as law, religion, the social sciences, history, and literature—are usually well represented at any meeting. In Charon and Williams' overview of the humanities in medicine,[9] discipline-specific articles follow brief introductory material. These studies of individual disciplines help to deepen the foundation for the study of humanities in medical education. One need not demonstrate that one discipline—even ethics—has priority. A comprehensive approach to the triad of history, theory, and practice will draw profitably not only from the traditional humanities but also from law, economics, psychology, and other nonmedical fields.

Individual Responses to the Humanities

Admission to medical school is a formal process that ordinarily includes a standardized examination and requires outstanding academic achievement in college. Nevertheless, medical students differ greatly; the variances among students are reflected in their readiness for and reception of the many elements of a medical education. The humanities will be a distraction to some but an oasis in an otherwise arid environment for others. For example, for a medical student with an undergraduate degree in literature, Tolstoy's *Death of Ivan Illich* might provide welcome insight that combines information gained in the college experience with the realities of a dying patient in a clinical setting. The use of this reading might have negative effects, however, if the material is presented in a manner that the student perceives as simplistic or inaccurate.

The differences among medical students include the amount of prior education in the humanities, the maturity of the individual student, the correlation between the approach used and the learning style of each individual, and the goals and values that each student possesses. Because of these contrasts, no specific method can alone provide a humanities perspective that will reach all students. Individuals come into medicine with different educational backgrounds and life experiences; they must be given multiple opportunities to explore the humanities perspective, just as they find theory and practice interwoven throughout their educational experiences.

Thus, the humanities perspective draws together many traditional academic disciplines to provide the theme of history in addition to the dominant interaction of theory and practice in physician education. Where medical educators recognize the need for the humanities perspective, medical school admission committees will indicate to college and university premedical advisors that a science background is a necessary but not a sufficient preparation—that a prospective medical student must have a more comprehensive education. Just as experiences in research laboratories and volunteer clinical services are desirable achievements to list on an application form, so other more general coursework will receive weight in candidate selection when admissions committees indicate the importance of such achievements.

In undergraduate medical education itself, formal and informal time is devoted to humanities education. At times these activities will focus on a discipline in the humanities, such as a reading club or a history club; at other times, humanities education will entail team teaching, as part of rounds or at case conferences. Because several residency programs (e.g., ophthalmology) require ethics conferences, many medical students find ethics taught for house staff and attending physicians. The variety of approaches helps to meet the diverse needs of students and the house staff.

How much of the humanities is enough? A humanities perspective that begins in college as the student is preparing for medical school, is integrated into classroom and clinical experiences throughout medical school and residency training, is prominent in continuing education, and is reinforced in professional journal articles as well as by the national media is necessary to provide a balance of history, theory, and practice to all physicians throughout their training and careers.

Medicine without the proper blending of science and technology, on the one hand, and caring and reasoning in human values, on the other hand, is incomplete and its practitioners incompetent. Happily, for at least the past thirty-five years many physicians, humanists, and other interested persons have advocated the development of humanities programs. I turn now to their efforts.

METHODS OF PROMOTING HUMANITIES TEACHING IN MEDICAL EDUCATION

By the early 1970s, several organizations devoted to human values and ethics had been created in response to concerns about medicine—prompted by social changes and technological developments—that were raised in the late 1950s and throughout the 1960s. These groups promoted and developed human values programs in individual medical and health professions schools, developed faculties, responded to societal concerns about specific ethical issues, and provided guidance for governmental agencies. The Hastings Center and the Kennedy Institute for Ethics were two of the important early leaders of this movement; both remain active today. The Society for Health and Human Values, which began preliminary meetings in 1963, recently merged with the Society for Bioethics Consultations and the American Association of Bioethics to become the American Society for

Bioethics and Humanities. This new organization is now the major professional organization for persons working in the humanities in medical education. Many other fine programs exist in individual medical schools or on a regional basis.

Each group has its own specific interests and particular methods of resolving issues; nevertheless, a considerable amount of overlap exists. Especially in the formative years of the development of programs in ethics and humanities, many individuals actively participated in two or more of these organizations. The needs first identified by these pioneers remain important for continued retention of the humanities perspective in medical education.

Program Development within Individual Schools

A presentation at the second meeting of the Institute on Human Values in Medicine of the Society for Health and Human Values, in 1972, reported that there were twelve programs in human values in medical schools. Defining these efforts as "programs" was generous; some were in the planning stage rather than actively funded and staffed efforts. Nevertheless, these activities were the forerunners of a movement that is now an accepted part of medicine. Several individual programs today probably have as many persons engaged in human values teaching as the total faculty of the twelve schools that reported doing so in 1972.

Because the accreditation of humanities programs in medical schools is controversial, it has not yet been effected. In the environment of medical education, there is merit to the case for establishing and enforcing national standards and for receiving recognition within organizations such as the Association of American Medical Colleges. Yet the vast differences among programs, centers, and institutes among individual schools; the breadth of interests that can legitimately claim to be humanities programs; and the scarcities of resources temper the need to create the fixed measures that accreditation would impose.

Even in the absence of accreditation, evaluation is possible. Such assessment should be a goal of all humanities programs. Internal reviews of all programs are a matter of course in the medical school setting. External visits by teams of humanities-trained professionals largely drawn from other medical schools could suggest new ideas, provide impartial review, and give stature to a local humanities program.

The building of humanities programs in medical schools began more than thirty-five years ago. Although the need for a humanities presence as an integral part of medical education probably is firmly rooted, the presence of distinct programs is not guaranteed; therefore, continued effort must be devoted to developing and refining individual humanities programs in medical schools to sustain a balance among history, theory, and practice.

Faculty

When the new interest in humanities teaching for medical students began, few faculty members were prepared to engage in such efforts. Some medical doctors had the expertise to understand a specific humanities discipline and how it might affect students. Some physicians had found individual methods with which they had success, but there was little discussion among colleagues—many of whom regarded such interests as irrelevant at best or, at worst, a sign that the physician did not understand the priorities of basic science and clinical practice.

A few humanities scholars had given occasional lectures to medical students, and a few had regular courses, often taught as they would be taught to non-medical students. Because of differing academic calendars, medical students rarely took courses with other students in the university. The major problems for humanists were lack of contact with the clinical setting and failure to grasp the technological inroads that new scientific discoveries had produced. One early source of humanist-trained faculties were chaplains, directors of pastoral counseling, and other religiously trained persons who had patient contact as well as liberal arts backgrounds. The new generation of faculty members and practitioners who have come to the medical humanities from more academically oriented backgrounds owes more to these early religious leaders than they commonly understand.

Thus, chaplains, some physicians, and a few humanities teachers were the only available faculty members for the first programs that were created. Unfortunately, there were also negative models: clergy who saw teaching as proselytizing; humanists whose rigidity about presentation of their disciplines kept them from real dialogue with medicine; physicians who had simple but largely ineffective solutions, such as "require all medical students to read the works of Shakespeare."

One means of developing a cadre of faculty members with the skills to teach the humanities in medical education was to provide short-term training with the few experienced humanities teachers that were available or to have faculty members spend time in the individual schools where the first programs had developed. As the stream of persons seeking such experience increased, the Hershey (Pennsylvania) program finally had to set designated days for visitors so that the Hershey faculty members could pursue their other efforts. The Institute for Human Values in Medicine offered individual fellowships for persons in a wide range of settings; the Kennedy Institute for Ethics ran its successful summer institutes, and the Hastings Center and several local bioethics centers had fellowship and intern programs. Growth in the number of faculty members available for medical humanities programs was stimulated by the expansion of M.D./Ph.D. programs—which traditionally specialized in the sciences and medicine—to include the humanities and medicine, by the creation of doctoral programs in medical humanities, and by allowing students in individual disciplines to specialize in topics related to medicine.

Most of the first generation and many of the second generation of physicians and humanists who developed the initial programs in medical schools are no longer active in medical education. One successful aspect of their efforts has been that many younger faculty members have now entered into positions of leadership and are energetically creating yet a new generation of students trained in the study of medical humanities. Although the number of active bioethicists and other medical humanities professionals continued to grow, the field does not yet seem to be saturated, and the issues these professionals address require continued exploration. Continued study of where the needs for future faculty members will be and what positions are held by those who have degrees related to medical humanities will be useful.

Conferences and Professional Meetings

Every year, members of professional organizations or subscribers to journals in the field of medical humanities receive many notices about upcoming international, national, and regional conferences. Although the casts of speakers contain duplications among various conferences, they reveal broad diversity that bodes well for the continued growth of the intellectual component of the medical humanities. Most of these conferences focus on ethical problems, which have long been the central attraction of the humanities in medicine. The issues raised in these conferences—such as abortion, terminating life, and assisted suicide—represent continuing conflicts occurring in national and international contexts; it is not surprising that ethics claims such attention.

With rare exceptions, issues in the field of medical humanities are most likely to be considered at these professional meetings (where ethical concerns maintain a certain primacy). Discipline-specific groups have opportunities to continue their discussions of special interests, administrators consider strategies for developing and continuing the individual school programs, and other interest groups are formed to address their issues.

The humanities movement was first defined and developed as a discipline at early conferences. Such conferences continue to be an important resource in bringing together members in the field to consider new issues and to test their concepts against the opinions of others. Because medical humanities faculty members often work in very small departments and lack the stimulation of a large academic department with persons of similar educational specialization, the interpersonal dimension of conferences and professional meetings is a significant contribution to the field.

Publications

The most comprehensive index in medicine—Medline—began indexing electronically in 1963—coincidentally, just as the medical humanities were being established. The following table shows the growth of articles related to the topic of "humanities" in a recent search of Medline.

In the first five years of this period, only nineteen humanities articles appeared in Medline. The number of articles in the next five years almost doubled. Overall, in the first ten years of electronic indexing (1963 to 1972—about 30 percent of the time period), about 14 percent of the articles indexed were humanities articles. The difference between the earlier period and more recent years is further reflected in the ratio of English articles to the non-English articles, which has almost doubled as humanities programs have grown in the United States.

In addition to the significant increase in articles on humanities published in major journals, there have been special theme issues (such as the 1995 report by *Academic Medi-*

TABLE 1. *Humanities Articles*

Date	Total	% of all Articles	Number in English	% in English
1963–1967	19	5	8	42
1968–1972	36	9	28	78
1973–1998	350	86	301	86
All Articles	405	100	337	83

cine). The Hastings Center *Report*; the Kennedy Center's *Encyclopedia, Notes,* and *Bioethicsline;* and several journals have been created for the specific purpose of exploring medical humanities, bioethics, and specific disciplines. All of these efforts have helped to develop the field and capture public interest in key humanities issues. The Society for Health and Human Values and its Institute for Human Values in Medicine have published several books, monographs, and reports. Other institutes and centers provide an important service through newsletters, as well as other means of publication. Many conferences result in the publication of the proceedings, and several government task forces and commissions on medical ethics have released important reports. Finally, the medical specialties and other health profession journals have devoted space to articles on the impact of the humanities on their disciplines; many have regular commentaries on ethical issues.

Government

The federal government has become actively involved in addressing ethical concerns raised by changing technology, the civil rights movement, and unethical research procedures revealed by Beecher, Pappworth, and others. Committees and commissions were created, regulations were developed that became legally binding, and a climate of responsibility in science and the practice of medicine was created. Although some researchers resisted these inroads on their autonomy, others were leaders in the setting of standards. The Department of Energy, through its major project for the mapping of the human genome, required that 3 percent of its funding be set aside for an ethical, legal, and social implications (ELSI) program to maintain continuing review of the work.

The government's actions in passing informed consent regulations for patients and in developing institutional review boards for the approval of research signaled a commitment to respond to ethical concerns. More recently, the need for decisions about cloning has posed formidable questions of governmental action for ethical advisors. Regardless of the rightness or wrongness of the decisions that have been made, and regardless of whether regulations are followed or abused, ethical and human values considerations have led to government intervention that has had a powerful effect on science and medicine.

CONCLUSION

Medicine is neither as distinct from the humanities nor as rigorously scientific as many observers believe. Developing means whereby history, theory, and practice continually interact can thereby provide the basis for medical education—as well as standards and guidelines for clinical practitioners and biomedical researchers—to avoid the imbalance that developed during the 1950s and1960s. The humanities perspective is the arena in which humans pose questions about the meaning of change in their society, the moral uses of their discoveries, and the rights of individuals and groups. No profession—especially a profession as closely involved with persons in their most vulnerable and personal needs as medicine—can avoid conversation with the society in which it performs its duties and that provides it authenticity to carry out its tasks.

The development of new humanities programs in medical education and the continuing presence of a humanities perspective in medicine are the legacy of physicians, medical students, medical administrators, clergy, scholars in humanist disciplines, government leaders, and others who took risks with their careers, subjected themselves to the scorn of their more traditional colleagues, and pursued the task of redressing an imbalance that had arisen through the post–World War II influx of science and technology into the practice of medicine. The work that remains is to continue to develop humanities programs, to increase the effectiveness of humanist faculty members, and to refine the base of scholarship that has been produced. Most important, we must sustain the interaction of physicians and humanists—for it is in the conversation between disciplines that history, theory, and practice are most closely kept in creative tension.

NOTES

1. D. Hughes, "Introduction," in *Education for the Professions of Medicine, Law, Theology, and Social Welfare* (report prepared for the Carnegie Commission on Higher Education), ed. E. C. Hughes et al. (New York: McGraw-Hill, 1973).
2. E. D. Pellegrino, "Medical Humanism: The Liberal Arts and the Humanities," *Review of Allied Health Education* 4 (1981): 1–15.
3. T. K. McElhinney, "Placing the Humanities Perspective in the Health Professional Curriculum," *Journal of Allied Health* 12, no. 3 (August 1983): 221–28.
4. The arts and humanities were themselves experiencing a time of narrowing of focus: The training of specialists in each discipline often was regarded as the primary if not exclusive goal. See E. D. Pellegrino, "The Most Humane of the Sciences; the Most Scientific of the Humanities," chap. 2 in *Humanism and the Physician* (Knoxville: University of Tennessee Press, 1979).
5. See, e.g., R. Charon and P. Williams, "Introduction: The Humanities and Medical Education," *Academic Medicine* 70, no. 9 (September 1995): 758–60; E. D. Hook, "Humanities in Medicine: Treatment of a Deficiency Disorder," *Transactions of the American Clinical and Climatological Association* 108 (1997): 203–21.
6. Pellegrino, "Medical Humanism," 9.
7. Ibid., 9–12.
8. E. D. Pellegrino, "The Humanities in Medical Education: Entering the Post-Evangelical Era," *Theoretical Medicine* 5 (1984): 253–66.
9. Charon and Williams, "The Humanities and Medical Education."

Religious Elements in Healing

Glenn C. Graber and Bradford R. Smith

Morris Payne is a forty-three-year-old truck driver who is hospitalized with a back injury. The injury occurred when Morris fell from a ladder while he was painting a classroom in the education building of the church his family regularly attends. Morris himself is not a regular churchgoer. He typically visits only a few Sundays a year, and he does not take much interest in the activities or needs of the church. He was helping with the painting project only at his wife's insistence. The fall occurred when another painter bumped into the ladder on which Morris was standing.

Reverend Concern, the minister of the church, is on the way to Morris's hospital room to pay a call. Rev. Concern seeks out Morris's physician, Dr. Care, to inquire about Morris's condition. In particular, Mrs. Payne has requested him to ask about Morris's ability to return to active work.

Dr. Care greets Rev. Concern by saying, "I'm glad you came to see Mr. Payne. I was preparing to call you to tell you that he has asked to talk with you. He has authorized me to discuss his case with you, and I would like to do so." At this point, Dr. Care leads Rev. Concern into a nearby staff room and closes the door.

"I want to enlist your help in dealing with Mr. Payne," Dr. Care explains when they are alone. "My clinical evaluation is that Morris's injury was relatively minor, and his medical condition is stable. The organic pathology is not severe enough to interfere with his returning to work immediately. Nor is it sufficient to account for the level of pain he reports. However, he appears to have a lot of pent-up hostility and resentment—not so much about the conditions of his accident but relating more to the frustrating nature of his job and certain elements in his home life; that frustration is probably sustaining his symptoms.

"Morris is demanding narcotic medication to relieve the pain, but I am very reluctant to give it to him. He fits the classic pattern of a potential addict; I'm afraid that once we introduce him to narcotics, a lifelong relationship may be established.

"I've brought in a physical therapist to teach him some exercises that might help to control the pain, but Morris has been uncooperative. And he adamantly refuses to talk with a psychotherapist."

"One component of Morris's mental state might be classified as theological in nature. Because the accident took place in a church building, he harbors the belief that God

278

was 'striking him down.' His reaction to this belief vacillates between anger toward God and fear of further divine wrath.

"What I propose to do is to prescribe a placebo but tell Morris that it is a narcotic. You can help in two ways: first, by reinforcing my assurances that the medicine can be expected to be effective in controlling the pain; your endorsement added to mine should strengthen the placebo effect. The second thing you can do is to counsel Morris, focusing especially on the theological questions with which he is wrestling but also helping him begin to resolve some of his hostility and resentment. I really think it would be best in the long run if you could persuade him to cooperate with the physical therapist and begin long-term psychotherapy."

Dr. Care concludes by asking Rev. Concern, "Will you assist me in helping Morris?"

INTRODUCTION

The greatest experience open to man, then, is the recovery of the commonplace.[1]

Author Peter DeVries insightfully expressed a truth that patients who have been uprooted from the familiar and thrown into the foreign because of illness recognize all too well. Part of the health care experience involves the replacement of the intimate comfort and warmth of home, and all that symbolizes, with the sterile, detached, and unknown environment of a hospital. Even more significant, however, the total experience of illness has at least as much, if not more, to do with the patient's confrontation with a condition that affects her or him at a deeply existential and spiritual level, as with the alien surroundings of the hospital. In other words, the experience of patienthood is best understood not merely in terms of a struggle with data external to the self but more significantly as the patient's struggle with *internal* data. This tension can be spurred by questions of self-identity, which often include religious issues. In this essay, we focus on this religious dimension—specifically, the religious dimension of healing.

ILLNESS AND RELIGION

All questions of ultimate meaning are spiritual in nature, even if they do not take an explicitly religious form. Often, however, such personal elements of the patient's experience are discovered within an intricate web or context shaped by religious values and beliefs. Morris is an obvious example of a patient who views his plight from within an explicitly religious framework. He reveals to his physician the belief that "God is striking me down." The cancer patient who asks, "Why me?" or "What does this all mean?" is asking a no less spiritual question, even though these questions make no explicit reference to religious concepts or a religious vernacular per se.

Illness and healing are very significant circumstances in anyone's life. For a believer, these experiences are especially significant because the patient's life is profoundly shaped by faith in God. Illness and healing challenge faith in important ways that affect the believer's ethical deliberation and understanding not only of her or his surroundings but also of the motivations of her or his family, physician, and others. A negative interpretation, for example, could lead to conflict in the patient-physician relationship—as in our case study—and a difficult experience for everyone involved. A patient who feels that her or his illness is a punishment inflicted by God may be less willing to cooperate in efforts to overcome the condition by medical means than a patient who regards the physician as an instrument of God. Such dynamics are reciprocal, of course; they affect not only the patient's understanding of the physician but the physician's understanding of the patient and the patient's own role in her or his healing.

A believer's understanding of illness and healing involves not merely an awareness of the physical by itself but an awareness of the spiritual aspects of life as well. Because illness affects both the physical and the spiritual aspects of life, the physician's healing efforts affect the physical and the spiritual, as well. This conclusion does not imply that the physician must also serve as a priest or rabbi, but it does indicate a need for the physician to be sensitive to how the patient interprets her or his treatment efforts and decisions. It may also suggest calling in a priest or other spiritual counselor to assist in the healing effort (as the physician in our case does).

Considering illness in a Christian context, Swiss psychiatrist Paul Tournier explains that all diseases and illness present some threat of death.[2] Sometimes the threat is negligible; at other times it is so close that the threat alone might seem worse than death itself. Illness reminds us of our human condition: our susceptibility and ultimately our vulnerability to death. It reminds us of our mortality and evokes questions about the great unknown. This point is nicely illustrated by a cartoon that appeared years ago in *The New Yorker* magazine. A man answering the door of his apartment encounters a waist-high, miniature "grim reaper." The figure looks up at the scared man and says, "Relax, I'm only a sore throat." The point, of course, is that even a sore throat reminds us of our mortality.

For believers, illness can instigate reflection on their relation to God. This reflection can be a source of anxiety and a source of hope. Interpreted hopefully, illness is an invitation to reflect positively on one's relation with God; on the other hand, it may serve as a definitive mark of (or punishment for) sin and spiritual weakness. Illness might therefore be interpreted as much more than an unfortunate condition that is explainable merely in physiological terms.

Although parts of the Bible imply that illness and sin are related, theological interpretations vary dramatically. Tournier, for example, argues that the association is not a direct association—that is, a particular illness resulting from a particular sin—but that the connection is general and is intelligible by virtue of a recognition of human interdependence and freedom. Accordingly, disease reflects and results from an overall disorder in the world caused by sin.

Evidence that reflects a patient's belief in the association between sin and illness can be found in the feeling of guilt that often is present. In such situations (as in our case study), a patient may feel guilty because of past misdeeds. The patient therefore views her or his condition as punishment by God for her or his sins. Serving as a hospital chaplain, one of the authors of this essay (Smith) has encountered numerous Christian patients, for example, who conclude that God is punishing them for their sins or lack of faith. Sometimes, a patient's family members take this association of sin and illness a step further by attributing a causal connection between their own wrongdoing and the patient's illness. Furthermore, when the illness is fatal, Smith has also encountered numerous families who believe that their own spiritual weakness and/or failure to pray enough led to their loved one's failure to recover.

One can find specific references to sin's causal role in illness throughout the Bible. For example, Matthew, Mark, and Luke contain references to evil or sin causing particular maladies: In Matthew 8:26–36, sin causes insanity; in Matthew 12:22, it causes blindness; in Mark 9:22, it causes suicidal mania. Similarly, in the Hebrew testament, Micah 6:13 speaks of sickness caused by sin; Genesis 3:16–19 describes mankind's original sin and its consequences; and 2 Kings 5:25–27 describes a case of sickness caused by actual sin.

Indeed, one need only consider some of the more fundamentalist views on AIDS and homosexuality to find stark examples of belief in the direct association between sin and illness. Some people believe that AIDS is the manifestation and direct expression of God's anger toward homosexuals for their disregard of God and His moral laws.[3] In other words, if one disobeys God, God punishes; illness and disease are forms of that punishment. Presumably, if this is the way of God, all persons are subject to the consequences of blatantly disregarding God's laws.

A few things must immediately be noted about the aforementioned Biblical references to sin and illness. First, one might take a theologically literal stance and argue that the Bible supplies evidence of sin as a direct cause of particular illnesses. One might also believe that sin has a causal role in illness without assuming a direct relationship as in the literal perspective. One might interpret sin as a condition of being separated from God. Second, two of the foregoing references cite mental conditions as being affected by sin. Needless to say, much has been learned about mental health since the days when sin was claimed to be a direct cause of insanity and suicidal mania. Again, one might view separation from God as the foundation for psychological depression (in at least some cases), feelings of meaninglessness, or the perpetuation of a fatalistic world view. Third, whether we advocate the literal or the liberal interpretation of these references is irrelevant; the point is that anticipating these or other similar interpretations can help the medical staff communicate more effectively with the patient at the patient's point of experience.

In contrast, consider how a believing patient might view illness as a positive experience:

> [C]ourage . . . is that which listens to what God is saying to us through disease and the threat of death. If this is our attitude, sickness . . . will take on meaning for us, [it] will have something to teach us, something to bring us, and . . . will also help to make us revise our scale of values.[4]

In this way, one's experience can be viewed positively as an opportunity to assess her or his relationship with God. Any parent whose child develops a serious disease will ask, "Why me?" A believing parent may have at least a partial answer to this question, which might be, "God is trying to tell me something." (Of course, this answer may vary depending on the religious persuasion of the believer.)

Furthermore, the believing patient, through her or his experience of illness, could positively affect her or his relationships with members of her or his faith community. The patient's own experience can actively reinforce religious values. Thus, the patient is not simply a passive recipient of others' support but a profound example of faith in action.

Some Christian scholars (e.g., Stanley Hauerwas and Charles Pinches) have raised important considerations about euthanasia and the role of the person who exemplifies courage and faith in the face of suffering and adversity; this role, they argue, reflects the Christian's obligation to strive to be Christ-like at all times—a role that would be nullified by euthanasia.[5] Admittedly, this view is a strict interpretation of religious obligations, but it may indeed be part of some Christians' value systems. This pattern of values is not foreign to other religious traditions or even to secular thought. Most people admire courage in the face of suffering; many would experience at least some lack of admiration for a person who insisted vigorously that she or he was unwilling to endure even a moment of discomfort.

A believing patient can also approach a time of illness as a time for reconciliation with other members of the community of which she or he is a part, whether they are immediate family or friends within that community. Believers value reconciliation because of the opportunity to make amends with "brothers" and "sisters"—which is essentially to make amends with God through them. One can also make this point with regard to a view of healing. Regret for things said and done can be a source of great emotional pain and guilt. For a believer, a time of illness is not just a chance to apologize or accept apologies because the patient may be on the brink of death ("speak now or forever hold your peace"). It is a chance to reevaluate one's order of priorities, one's relationship with others, one's system of values, and one's basis of faith. The focus is on the particularities of the spiritual context as they distinctly impact the patient's response to his situation.

Many ancient Christian mystics—including Hildegard of Bingen, Mechtild of Magdeburg, Julian of Norwich, and the Beguines (an order of mystic nuns)—have proclaimed that times of illness are beneficial. Some have described illness itself as a purging or an opportunity for revelation.

Edmund Pellegrino and David Thomasma echo this view of positive opportunities in illness.[6] They describe three different ways that illness can be valued in a Christian context. First, "Illness can be seen as an enablement; it may enable one to grow spiritually and emotionally. It teaches finitude and appreciation for the smallest thing."[7] Second, "As empowerment, illness can be an invitation to selflessness, calling individuals to imitate Christ . . . in their devotion to the building up of the community."[8] Third, they argue that illness offers the believing patient the chance to atone:

> Atonement in the religious sense has little to do with "making up for." Rather atonement should be taken as "at-one-ment," in an effort to unite with all persons through being.[9]

This analysis would appear to correlate with the patient's consideration of the treatment options that are acceptable and how the patient understands healing. Some patients may prefer to be very aggressive in fighting illness; others might not. For example, Hauerwas and Pinches discuss the meaning of patience in a Christian context and how such a patient should be sick—in other words, how a Christian patient can exemplify faith-in-action in the midst of sickness and suffering. Indeed, they argue that illness is a chance for the patient to minister to others by enduring sickness.[10]

A similar viewpoint is expressed in the National Conference of Catholic Bishops' *Ethical and Religious Directives for Catholic Health Care Services*, which describe suffering as "a participation in the redemptive power of Christ's passion, death, and resurrection."[11]

Christian responses to illness indeed vary, but as Hauerwas explains in *Suffering Presence*, perceiving illness as an opportunity for growth and wisdom has always presented Christians with the challenge of reconciling medicine for the soul with medicine for the body.[12]

HEALING AND RELIGION

The association of sin with illness can play a direct role in deliberations about healing and treatment goals. Patients can understand healing, like illness, not just in a physical sense but also in spiritual and emotional terms as well. Whereas a religious/sacred world view finds significance in daily affairs, healing is more than just a physical event; it is an example of seeing sacredness in the mundane. This perspective again illustrates how different meanings can be attributed to the same data because of different contexts: "Healing of physical infirmity is a spiritual affair. It has to do with a person's spirit."[13] This perspective also is evident in the Jewish context:

> [A]ttending to the needs of the sick has been seen in Jewish tradition as being more than general benevolence, it is an act having even mystical connections. This appears in the many biblical texts that see illness and healing as specifically supernatural interventions (e.g., Gen. 18:14, 25:21–22; Exod. 15:26; Lev. 26:16; Num. 5:21; Deut. 28:20–22, 32:39; 2 Kings 5:7–8, 20:1–5; Jer. 17:14; Ps. 103:1–3; 2 Chron. 16:12).[14]

Believers often view healing in terms of reconciliation, although different religions may have different interpretations of reconciliation. Closely tied to reconciliation is forgiveness, which can be associated with healing. The connection between reconciliation and forgiveness might be tied to specific actions of repentance and absolution, or they might be interpreted as enduring aspects of the human condition that underlie any and all specific actions.

To explore the religious meanings of healing further, consider the following case:[15] Suppose that a certain man is afflicted with a serious physical illness. Let us say that he has been diagnosed as having cancer of the lung and has been told that he has only a few weeks to live. He is too weak to get out of bed. He has difficulty breathing and requires oxygen frequently. He is in constant, severe pain. Fellow members of his religious community visit to talk with him and to pray with and for him.

Here are some logically possible outcomes in this case:

> Outcome 1: The man is completely cured. He becomes free of the pain and the breathing difficulty. He regains his strength, gets out of bed, and goes back to his job. All diagnostic signs of cancer disappear, including X-ray indications and tissue features. He lives a life of prime health for twenty years—until he dies in an automobile accident.

> Outcome 2: The man's cancer goes into remission. He feels stronger and finds breathing easier, and the pain is no longer constant and is less severe. He is able to

get out of bed—and even out of the house from time to time—but he does not re-gain the energy he needs to return to his job or to fulfill his life-long dream of a trip around the world. After two years, his condition again worsens, and he dies after three weeks of intense suffering.

Outcome 3: The end comes much more slowly than the doctors predicted. The man remains in his present condition for more than a year before he dies.

Outcome 4: The man suddenly slips into a coma and dies within twenty-four hours of the prayer session conducted by his religious community.

Outcome 5: The man's physical condition does not improve at all, and he dies six weeks later. His attitude changes dramatically, however. Whereas he had been bitter about his fate and hostile toward everybody who did not share it—including his wife and family—now he accepts his impending death with equanimity, and he is a great help in getting his wife and family to come to grips with it, too. He writes a will and plans his own funeral service.

Outcome 6: Neither his physical nor his mental condition changes at all. The man dies in six weeks, still bitter and hostile.

Which of these outcomes counts as a healing? Clearly Outcome 1 does; equally clearly, Outcome 6 does not. Each of the other outcomes is likely to be disputed.

Outcome 2 certainly does not involve a cure of the disease, but it does involve some relief from some of the more agonizing aspects of the disease. Although this outcome is a welcome departure from what was expected to occur, one might have hoped for still more (in particular, the complete cure of Outcome 1). The patient's reaction to this outcome depends largely on the kind of person he is. If he is strongly oriented toward an active life, if his job is all-important to him, or if he has little tolerance for uncertainty, he may not find the extra years of life especially worthwhile. Many people who find themselves in this situation react thusly. They do not find much reason for gratitude in such circumstances. They are more likely to describe the situation in Outcome 2 as "prolonging the agony" than to call it a healing or a benefit. Others, however, manage to adapt to the uncertainty and the diminished activity; they would describe this two-year period as meaningful and be grateful for it. Some even go so far as to say that life is more meaningful in this situation than it was before death was near. These people might well describe this extension of life as a healing or a gift.

Calling Outcome 3 a case of healing would strain that concept beyond the natural limits of its use. Yet some persons would consider this extension of a pain-racked existence valuable. After all, the key elements that give meaning to human life would still be present—in particular, conscious awareness and interpersonal relationships. Understandably, however, the number of people who respond to Outcome 3 with gratitude would be much smaller than those who respond that way to Outcome 2. Many people would regard an extension of this kind of life as a burden rather than a benefit.

This same attitude may apply with regard to Outcome 4: "It was a blessing that he died quickly. At least he did not have to suffer weeks and months of agony." Although many people would describe this outcome as a benefit or a blessing, calling it a case of healing would be bizarre indeed. (On the other hand, Socrates described his own death in precisely this way by implication when, with his last breath, he asked that a sacrifice be made on his behalf to the god of healing.) Yet many people would describe this outcome as a benefit or a blessing.

Outcomes 3 and 4 illustrate some interesting features of our attitude toward life and death. Life is a value, yet it is not absolute or unconditional. All of us have a "will to live," but none of us wants to live *no matter what.* Each of us could describe situations too horrible to endure. The limits to the value of life are different for different people. Some people commit suicide because of situations that most of us could take in stride. What is important, however, is that the value of life has a limit; beyond that point, death is welcomed as a benefit.

There is little indication that doctrines of immortality have a major effect on our thinking on this point. This is partly because the positive aspects of the afterlife, which might incline us to welcome death, are balanced by the affirmation of the value of this life that is also contained in doctrine and by the conviction that we have a responsibility to God to make the most of the gift of earthly life.

We might naturally and usefully describe Outcome 5 as a case of "healing of attitude." Many patients have experienced moments of reconciliation and healing, regardless of their religious affiliation (or lack thereof). For many believers, however, the notion of reconciliation is typically defined in terms of love for God and God as love. If God is love, then not loving is not Godly. Believers strive to be Godly. Therefore, reconciling differences by which the love relationship is threatened carries a great deal of weight in a religious community. Believers do not necessarily regard such reconciliation in terms of its being psychiatrically healthy; instead, they regard it as the God-like thing to do.

Along these same lines, a second dimension—forgiveness—is often implicated with reconciliation and thus healing. For example,

> Jesus' contemporaries thought that sickness was the result of sin. The common understanding was that God sent sickness to punish and rehabilitate the sinner. Consequently, physical healing required and was accomplished only by forgiveness of sins.[16]

Forgiveness closely parallels, and is symbolized by, healing in the physical sense. Healing is also a spiritual experience, however. Thus, we speak of healing in an "attitudinal" sense, which is no less significant for the believing patient than the healing of physical infirmities. "Sickness is cured by forgiving sins and renewing the spirit."[17] This additional dimension of healing was recognized even in Jesus' time. Indeed, the New Testament accounts of Jesus' healings exemplified overcoming not just physical infirmities but, more important, spiritual infirmities. Thus, some Christians might interpret accounts of healing of blindness not merely as actual renewal of physical sight but as bestowal of spiritual sight and wisdom. In Matthew 13:13, Jesus explains to His disciples why He speaks to the crowds in parables: "Therefore I speak to them in parables, because seeing they do not see, and hearing they do not hear, nor do they understand." This passage illustrates an awareness by Jesus that people are spiritually blind and deaf and thus lack true spiritual wisdom.

Such spiritual infirmity requires healing no less than physical infirmities do. In the Hebrew testament, the story of King David suffering over his sin in sending the husband of his paramour to the front lines of battle is an account of physical illness resulting from a spiritual ailment; David addresses his suffering through the spiritual means of repentance.

Although believers of different faiths might define forgiveness differently, all definitions are shaped by a relationship to God and/or to one another. Ultimately, to forgive is to love, even amid differences. Forgiveness often requires compromise (where compromise is based on trust not only in God but in one another) because compromise requires letting go of pride. "Jesus proclaimed God's offer of salvation. Through forgiveness of sins, man could become reconciled to God."[18]

Thus, healing in a religious sense means more than just reestablishing physical functionality. It means reconnecting wounded relationships and attitudes. These relationships might involve reconnecting with oneself, with others in the community, and even with God. Sometimes this reconnection takes place in suffering—a suffering that occurs within God's presence. An awareness of God's presence profoundly affects how one responds to the world and those in it, especially considering that reconnection often entails granting and/or asking for and receiving forgiveness. Where a relationship has suffered because of separation from God—an earlier definition of sin—one can see how the association of sin with illness affects the view one might have of how to be healed.

Tournier describes how healing can also be viewed as indicative of God's patience.[19] God has compassion on man. In Exodus 23:25, we find that God wishes to protect humans against disease. In Jeremiah 30:17, God wishes to heal human wounds. In Proverbs 3:2, God wishes to prolong our days. This latter reference can be abused, just as the notion of accepting all healing as God's gift can be abused.

To what extent does God want to prolong life? Obviously, there is room for critical ethical consideration. The belief that God wants to prolong life can motivate a vitalist approach as well as a more liberal approach based on compassion. The idea of patience, however, is important. The presence and function of religion in the world is often regarded as an extension of God's desire to heal the world of its illness.

In sum, there are several religious understandings of healing, all of which can implicate the idea that sin has shaped the patient's circumstances. Healing implicates both the physical and the spiritual. To approach healing without regard for this dualism is to risk overlooking certain important values and beliefs that profoundly affect a patient's response to the care being delivered. For a believing patient, "care" that focuses exclusively on the physical conditions of healing might not be regarded as "caring" at all. (Families often experience this reaction to the visitor limitation in intensive care units, although administration may have sound justifications that are based on clinical efficiency and effectiveness.)

As such, healing implicates reconciliation and forgiveness. These two aspects presuppose some type of wounded relationship either within oneself, with others, or with God. This notion of healing can further entail a sense of community—an important element within a religious perspective.

Healing can also indicate belief in God's presence, grace, and patience. These aspects of healing affect the patient's experience in significant ways that can spark conflict between the patient and physician if the physician and the patient do not try to understand the values at stake and how they might relate differently to each other.

PHYSICIAN AND PATIENT

Because of the patient's vulnerabilities and the power imbalance (which favors physicians), the onus of communication lies with the physician. The patient is entering unfamiliar territory. The patient may not fully understand the medical vernacular. The patient's mere visit to the physician is an implied act of trust. Consequently, as Pellegrino and Thomasma argue, the physician has an especially compelling ethical obligation to avoid abusing the patient and to nurture the patient out of respect for the patient as a person in such a vulnerable state.[20] The physician can fulfill this obligation only by engaging and getting to know the patient—by meeting the patient at the patient's point of experience, by striving to understand the patient as a person, and by recognizing the patient's motivations, fears, hopes, values, and beliefs.

Key to the physician's efforts to learn about the patient is asking probing questions as part of active listening. This process is very different from simply not talking to allow participatory space for the patient's input. Active listening is more than merely hearing. Beyond simply giving the speaker "air time," active listening involves an interpretive effort to comprehend not only the speaker's message *qua* words but the message being conveyed without words or between words (e.g., through facial expressions, pauses between sentences, body posture, and voice inflection). Indeed, many distinct, nonverbal messages are transmitted simultaneously with verbal ones. Therefore, words alone do not constitute all of what a speaker is communicating. Words must be taken as only one element among many within a communicative context.

The physician should listen to how the person's beliefs inform his or her perspective about himself, his or her reaction to the medical environment, and the treatment choice(s) with which he or she is presented. This information is particularly important for patients of religious faiths. When the patient's perspective is informed by an institutionalized religious context, there is a systematic body of knowledge and data to which a physician can refer in relating what he or she learns about the particular patient. This body of information frequently includes formal doctrines, outlined value systems, traditions, rituals, and a community of believers that informs and reinforces the patient's own beliefs.

Daniel Sulmasy discusses the role of "God-Talk at the Bedside" instructively in his essay by that title:

> I have begun to include questions about religion in the social history as part of my routine new patient history. . . . I have begun to ask the fairly open-ended and, I think, nonjudgmental question: "What role does religion play in your life?"[21]

Gathering this information does not mean that the physician can assume that the patient rigidly adheres to these religious beliefs. However, it does offer an opportunity for the physician to anticipate how the patient's religious background might factor into the patient's medical experience, which will certainly affect the patient's relationship with the physician. The power imbalance created by patient vulnerabilities thus obligates the physician to take the first step by getting to know the person behind the patient through active listening. This process leads to a mutual respect—the groundwork for a productive working relationship.

CONCLUSION

With regard to the case with which we began this essay, we would contend that the physician was correct in enlisting the help of the minister. The patient's religious conceptualization of his illness calls for spiritual counseling (by both minister and physician) as well as physical healing measures. We would maintain, however, that the proposal to employ a placebo and enlist the minister in the deception is the wrong direction to take. Open and honest communication—not trickery and deception—should be initiated. The personal and spiritual issues at work in this situation need to be dealt with directly, not swept under the rug. Ideally, the minister and the physician could work together (enlisting as well the patient's family and the members of his wider support circle—including, perhaps, the religious community in which his wife is active) to bring about reconciliation, a sense of forgiveness, and thus a more complete healing for the patient.

NOTES

1. Peter DeVries, *The Blood of the Lamb* (Boston: Little, Brown, 1961), 166.
2. Paul Tournier, *A Doctor's Casebook: In Light of the Bible* (New York: Harper & Row, 1960).
3. If AIDS is a punishment for homosexuality, why do we not find a proliferation of this disease among female homosexuals as we do among male homosexuals?
4. Tournier, *A Doctor's Casebook,* 174.
5. Stanley Hauerwas and Charles Pinches, "Practicing Patience: How Christians Should Be Sick," *Christian Bioethics* 2, no. 2 (1996): 202–21.
6. Edmund D. Pellegrino and David C. Thomasma, *Helping and Healing: Religious Commitment in Health Care* (Washington, D.C.: Georgetown University Press, 1997).
7. Ibid., 14.
8. Ibid.
9. Ibid., 15.
10. Hauerwas and Pinches, "Practicing Patience." Hauerwas and Pinches challenge Christian patients in particular to fully exploit the opportunity they have to minister to others. All too often, society perceives patients as weak and incapable. Hauerwas and Pinches raise the possibility that we might understand patients, especially in their suffering, as possessing great strength through opportunities to teach others by their responses to their condition. They readily acknowledge personal limits to this challenge, however, and do not neglect the patient's freedom to choose when enough is enough, should such a choice arise.
11. National Conference of Catholic Bishops, *Ethical and Religious Directives for Catholic Health Care Services* (Washington, D.C.: United States Catholic Conference, 1995), 2.
12. Stanley Hauerwas, *Suffering Presence: Theological Reflections on Medicine, the Mentally Handicapped, and the Church* (Notre Dame, Ind.: Notre Dame University Press, 1986).
13. Laurence A. Gipson and Glenn C. Graber, "Spiritual Healing: A Theological and Philosophical Study," unpublished manuscript, 24.
14. David Novak, "Judaism," in *The Encyclopedia of Bioethics,* revised ed. (New York: Macmillan Library Reference USA), 1304.
15. This case and the discussion of it are drawn from Gipson and Graber, "Spiritual Healing."
16. Gipson and Graber, "Spiritual Healing," 23.

17. Ibid., 24.
18. Ibid., 21.
19. Tournier, *A Doctor's Casebook.*
20. Pellegrino and Thomasma, *Helping and Healing.*
21. Daniel P. Sulmasy, "God-Talk at the Bedside," in *The Healer's Calling* (New York: Paulist Press, 1997), 65.

Index

Medical education, 32, 89, 129. *See also*
  Education
  for basic sciences, 267–69, 270
  ethics in, 259–66
  Flexner Report and, 124–26
  history of, 114–15, 120, 124–26, 268–70
  humanities in, 259–66, 267–77
  managed care and, 128–30
  M.D./Ph.D. programs in, 274
  research in, 117–20, 126
  standards for, 116
  values and, 261–62, 264
Medical errors
  disclosure of, 21, 90, 102–03
  self-forgiveness and, 92–93, 101–03
Medical humanism, 150–53
Medical knowledge. *See* Scientific knowledge
Medical procedures, 21, 109, 155–56, 157
Medical students
  humanities and, 271–72
  moral agency and, 30–31
Medically indicated services, 155–56, 157
Medicine, 81, 83
  American, 113–32
  art of, 151
  belief systems in, 82–83
  as a commodity, 153
  communal, 153–60
  cultural differences in, 68, 81
  defensive, 128
  ends of, 77–80, 82–84, 88–89
  evidence-based, 14, 60
  goals of, 77–78
  history of, 113–32, 268–70, 276
  institutional focus of, 153–60
  internal morality of, 75–86, 203–04
  limits of, 109
  vs. medical knowledge, 77–80
  social constructs of, 81
  traditional, 68, 149–53, 157
Mental illness, 141
Mental retardation, 140, 141
Mercy killing, 141, 142
Messianic complex, 22
Metz, Johannes, 245
Midwifery, 115
Mission, institutional, 5–6
Mistakes, medical. *See* Medical errors
Mistrust, 4–7, 71

Moes, Josephine, 121–23
Moral agency, 30–31, 51, 52–55, 58
Moral courage, 106–12
Moralism, 59
Morality, 18, 26, 32
  external, 75–86
  internal, 32, 75–86, 203–04
  public policy and, 7, 173
  society and, 2
  of therapeutic relationships, 200–201
Mothers, surrogate, 171
Mutuality, 29, 41, 42

N
Narratives, 58–59, 230, 248
National health care, 127, 140, 241
Native Americans, 185
Natural law, 166–67
Nature, control of, 133–34, 250
Nazi Germany, 139–43, 145, 220–21
  euthanasia in, 139–40, 141–42
  genetics in, 140–41
Needs, 44, 45–46
Negligence, 102–03
New York Pathological Society, 119
Nightingale, Florence, 49
Nonmaleficence, 235
Nuland, Sherwin, 100, 101
Nurse-patient relationships
  emotional engagement in, 53–58
  experiential learning in, 51, 59
  trust in, 65–66
Nursing education, 58–59, 62
Nursing practice, 49–64
  caring in, 50, 52
  experiential learning in, 51, 55–59, 61–62
  goal of, 50–51
  history of, 121–22
  knowledge development in, 58

O
Oaths, 15
Obitiarists, 140
Objectification, 137
Obligations, 213, 241. *See also* Responsibility
O'Donovan, Leo J., 1–9
Omnipotence, 89
Optimal care, 108
Oregon Death with Dignity Act, 202–07